Intramedullary Nailing

Intramedullary Nailing

Dietrich Hempel &
Siegfried Fischer

Translated by
Hans Koening, M.D. and
Thomas Koening

English edition edited by
Benno Lotz
President, OEC. International, Inc.

1982
Georg Thieme Verlag Stuttgart · New York
Thieme-Stratton Inc., New York

Publisher: Thieme-Stratton Inc.
381 Park Avenue South
New York, New York 10016

Intramedullary Nailing

GTV ISBN 3–13–623101–5
TSI ISBN 0–86577–045–X

 Library of Congress catalog card number 81–52634.

Last digit is print number 4 3 2 1

Contents

General Considerations

Detailed Section

Foreword

In December 1980, Gerhard Küntscher would have celebrated his 80th birthday. After his death, two of his outstanding students, Dietrich Hempel and Siegfried Fischer, wrote this book as a special gift to the late master of intramedullary nailing.

The same year this book was written marked the 40th return of the historical presentation of Küntscher's revolutionary first paper on intramedullary nailing in Berlin in 1940. Therefore it is significant to learn from this book that 40 years after the first presentation, and eight years after his death, Küntscher's idea is not only alive and well but continues to inspire his former students toward further improvements and modifications that widen the range of indications and lead to higher perfection.

For many years, I enjoyed the pleasure of working with Gerhard Küntscher on the development of implants and instruments for his procedures, which received worldwide acknowledgement and respect. In the countless hours I spent with him, I gained a close insight to his genius. When he died, far too soon in December 1972, I felt a great void would be left unfilled.

In memory of his accomplishments, I met with some of his closest friends and students to form the "Küntscher Kreis," an association to spread the inspiration that Gerhard Küntscher had implanted in us. This book has the same purpose. The authors have succeeded in describing the fundamentals, details, and benefits of the Küntscher idea, which became a significant contribution to orthopedic surgery.

The English edition is amended by a chapter written by Robert Winquist of Seattle, Washington. This represents the realization of one of Küntscher's longtime dreams to inspire the "new world" with his ideas, which he did not live long enough to see.

A special note of thanks is owed to another student of Küntscher, Hans Koenig, M.D. of Pittsburgh, Pennsylvania, and his son Thomas, who translated the original German work in their spare time into English, which made this publication possible.

It is my sincere hope that many English speaking surgeons, and ultimately their patients, will benefit from the contents of this work.

Benno Lotz, President
OEC International
Bourbon, Indiana

Introduction

It has been nearly twenty years since the last German edition of Gerhard Küntscher's *The Practice of Intramedullary Nailing* was published. Küntscher died in 1972 while writing a new edition of this book. Because his intramedullary nailing methods are being more widely accepted, there is a marked increase in the number of inquiries concerning the detailed procedures of Küntscher nailing and closed osteotomies. As long-term students of Küntscher, we felt called upon to publish an operational guide for closed intramedullary nailing and closed osteotomy. We will limit ourselves to only the most common Küntscher methods. The more recent further developments, for example, the standardized interlocking and the compression nailing as well as the closed osteotomy, are described in detail. Other procedures of Gerhard Küntscher, which have been replaced by more successful methods, such as the nail-arthroplasty of the elbow joint by more appropriate joint replacement implants or the nailing of joint-fractures with split nails by AO-osteosynthesis, and other procedures no longer practiced, will not be discussed. The reader should draw primarily from the informative operating illustrations. The text is designed only to give the necessary explanations of the accompanying illustrations and roentgenograms. For this reason, illustrations and discussions concerning the known scientific basics of fracture healing have been omitted. For an easy transition from the theoretical illustrations to the practical operational situation, the illustrations are drawn with the bones in the same position as they would be seen on roentgenograms or image intensifier monitors. All the illustrations were drawn directly from original roentgenograms. This type of illustration demands large amounts of intuitive thinking and technical capability. We would like to thank our artist, Mrs. Ingrid von Marchtaler, for the successful application of this idea. The roentgenograms prove the success attainable by the nailing procedures discussed in their respective chapters.

In the preface of this book, *The Practice of Intramedullary Nailing,* Gerhard Küntscher wrote in 1962 that the intramedullary nail was purely and simply designed for use in the living bone following particular principles, and that its application demanded much experience and practice. The cause of failure is always clearly evident; on the other hand, meticulous work will result in guaranteed success. It is our wish that this book will help the reader to avoid mistakes and failures in the use of Küntscher nailing methods.

We should like to express our thanks to Hans Koenig, M.D. and to his son Thomas Koenig for their competent translation in line with the spirit of the original. Thanks are also due to Benno Lotz for having done so much toward promoting the project and for having been instrumental in enlisting the cooperation of Robert Winquist. We believe that all readers interested in that particular technique will benefit from the additional chapter written by Dr. Winquist on osteotomy describing the saw developed by him. We had the opportunity of convincing ourselves of the excellent performance and value of this instrument.

General Considerations

General Information on Küntscher's Intramedullary Nailing

On March 28, 1940, at the convention of the German Society of Surgery, Gerhard Küntscher provoked sensation and approval as well as controversy with his paper entitled *Intramedullary Nailing of Bone Fractures*. Since that day, Küntscher's name has remained inseparable from intramedullary nails and closed nailing. During the controversial discussion which followed Küntscher's paper, his teacher, Professor A. W. Fischer, prophetically remarked, "I am certain that Küntscher's method represents a great step forward." He was right. After overcoming the many problems and temporary rejections, Küntscher's intramedullary nailing for specific fractures of long bones finally gained worldwide acceptance.

The principle of Küntscher nailing involves the elastic locking of a slotted steel tube with a cloverleaf-shaped profile in a rigid bone canal. Küntscher purposely chose the word "nailing" for his osteosynthesis. The pounding of a nail into wood produces an expansion effect of elastic wood fibers. The fibers have the tendency to return to the original state; this tendency ensures the firm locking of the rigid nail. In the Küntscher nailing technique, the mechanism is reversed. The elastic Küntscher nail as a slotted tube imparts a longitudinal and lateral elasticity to the nail. the engineering principle of using a specific shape to increase the bending strength in a thin metal is utilized in the cloverleaf design. The conical tip of the nail facilitates the driving and ensures the safe positioning of the nail through the use of a guide pin.The Küntscher nail is hollow, because a tubular profile resists bending three to four times more than a solid rod with the same cross-sectional area. This is also the reason that, for each case, the Küntscher nail with the largest possible diameter should be chosen. The rigidity of the nail should at least match that of the fractured bone, so that weight-bearing will not bend the nail at the site of the fracture. Another factor governing the stability of the nail is the necessary thickness of the metal.

The intramedullary canal of long bones has the shape of an hourglass. The cross section is rarely circular and shows irregular narrowing. Therefore, a large enough nail can sel-

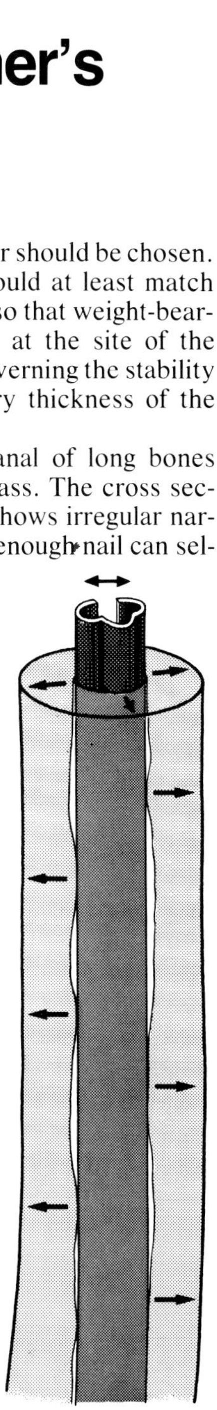

Figure 1 The principle of elastic locking. The compression of the nail slot provides transverse locking as the nail is hammered home. Longitudinal locking is established by curvature of the bone and the irregularities in the medullary canal.

dom be used. The profile of the medullary canal can be fitted to these large nails by reaming. In order to ensure the nail's locking, fractures of long bones must always be reamed. Another advantage of reaming is that jamming of the nail along the narrow isthmus of the medullary canal is avoided. This unfortunately happened occasionally before reaming was commonly practiced.

Even when the intramedullary nailing of fractures in long bones involves only a 2- to 3-cm stab incision, the operation is still considered a major one. Intramedullary nailing should be performed only when a full set of instruments, intramedullary nails of varying lengths and diameters, an image intensifier, and an extension table are available. The surgeon must be familiar with the intramedullary nailing technique. Great demands are placed on him, especially because a major portion of the surgery is done without direct vision. Closed intramedullary nailing can only be monitored by occasional views on the TV screen. For this reason, a good spatial orientation is necessary for the prompt interpretation of the two-dimensional monitor picture. This "blind" approach to intramedullary nailing calls for particular technical skills and knowledge.

No one should attempt to perform an intramedullary nailing without ample preparation and special training.

Indications for Intramedullary Nailing

Only fractures of the long bones of the upper and lower extremities should be considered for intramedullary nailing. Occasionally, though, even the clavicle can be nailed. Fractures of the humerus, radius, and ulna can be nailed, as can fractures occurring in the femur and tibia. A prerequisite for intramedullary nailing is the ability of the nail to lock elastically both the proximal and the distal portions of the fragments. This prerequisite is usually satisfied either in transverse fractures in the middle third of long bones or in fractures having small wedge-shaped fragments, where sufficient cortical support remains, or in fractures of a short spiral nature. The indications can be extended in cases with favorable medullary canals. Comminuted fractures, step fractures, long spiral fractures, and fractures in areas of wide medullary canals can be stabilized with further procedural knowledge using specialized nails, such as Y-nails, trochanter nails, interlocking nails, and compression nails. The timing of the nailing must take into account the general condition of the patient and the condition of the soft tissue of the injured extremity. To avoid contractures or a malposition, the injured extremity sometimes requires temporary skeletal traction or splinting preoperatively.

Intramedullary nailing of growing bones is seldom indicated. Nailing of this type usually is indicated when fractures of the femur or radius or ulna cannot be held correctly without nailing. In order to avoid a disturbance in the growth pattern, reaming should be avoided, and the nail removed as soon as feasible.

Instruments

Relatively few, yet simple, instruments are needed for intramedullary nailing. Basically it is best to use the respective Küntscher instruments matching the specific type of Küntscher nails. For specialized nailing procedures, one should also use the respective special instruments. The use of improper instruments could easily lead to complications. For instance, the threads of an AO-nail may become damaged if implanted with a nail driver of the original Küntscher set. This may complicate the later removal of the nail. A number of nails in various lengths and diameters should be available for each nailing. The original Küntscher nails have four shapes: V-type, straight cloverleaf nails, curved cloverleaf nails, and bent cloverleaf nails. V-type nails are used in bones with very narrow medullary canals, for example, in fractures of the forearm. Tibia and humerus fractures are candidates for the use of bent cloverleaf nails. Ulnar fractures or special types of humeral fractures call for the use of the straight cloverleaf nails in varying diameters. In femoral fractures, straight or curved nails can be used.

The medullary canal is opened by the appropriate awl, which takes the size of the bone cortex into account. The reamer-awl serves to widen the nail's entry portal, particularly in femur nailing. A variety of guide pins are used for reduction, maintenance of the reduced position, and guidance of the cannulated flexible intramedullary reamers and nails. These guide pins are produced in varying lengths with either drill point or ball point, and are used either with or without handles. The guide pins for the intramedullary reamers have a ball end, whereas those used to pierce through the pseudarthrosis covers have a drill bit type head.

The guide pins are manipulated and held either with a T-handle chuck or with an interchangeable guide pin handgrip. Without exception, all reaming should be done with guided flexible reamers. To ream very narrow intramedullary canals, one should use the guided squarehead reamers in varying lengths and in diameters ranging from 4 to 5.5 mm. For all larger intramedullary canals, cannulated flexible reamers with round reaming heads and spiral flutes are available in two different shaft lengths. Reaming head diameters are available in 0.5-mm increments. A nail gauge is used to check the diameters of both the reamer and the nail. The necessary nail diameter is determined by using a Küntscher ossimeter on roentgenograms taken at a 1-m distance.

A 1-lb hammer is used to drive the nail into place. A 2-lb hammer is used only in rare cases. In order to prevent nail deformities while hammering, a nail driver should be used. Various nail drivers are used with different sized nails. The nails are driven either underneath the skin or sunk into the bone with the Küntscher nail set.

With the aid of the nail bender, it is possible to curve manually the smaller intramedullary nails (up to 12 mm in diameter) to match the curvature of the medullary canal. Through this maneuver, however, the nail's resistance to corrosion and stress may be reduced. When a curved nail is indicated, it is therefore recommended to use the pre-curved nails offered by some manufacturers.

Because of its sturdy construction and the fact that it can be driven forward with a hammer, a pseudarthrosis-chisel facilitates the perforation of harder pseudarthrosis covers.

Special instrument sets are available for trochanter nailing, Y-nailing, interlocking nailing, and compression nailing. These instruments are discussed in detail in their respective chapters. An autoclaveable X-ray scale in millimeter and centimeter gradations should be available for all nailing procedures.

The special instruments needed for closed osteotomy are discussed in the chapter entitled *Closed Osteotomy of Long Bones* (p 171).

The following instruments are used for nail removal: extractors in various sizes and slotted hammers. A Rousek extractor set should be used if the extractor hook cannot penetrate the tibial nail slot because of ingrown bone tissue. Nails that have no slot or whose slot has been destroyed may be removed with Griessmann pliers or extractor bushes, or with an extraction instrument that is self-threading. Nails also can be loosened with the aid of a nail catcher. The nail catcher can extract the distal fragment of a broken nail. Using a distractor may also be helpful in the extraction of particularly firmly seated nails.

AO-nails should be removed with the respective instruments.

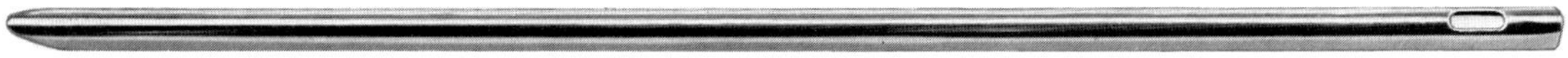

Figure 2 V-type nail.

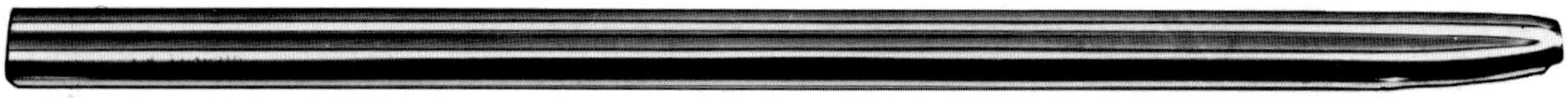

Figure 3 Straight cloverleaf nail.

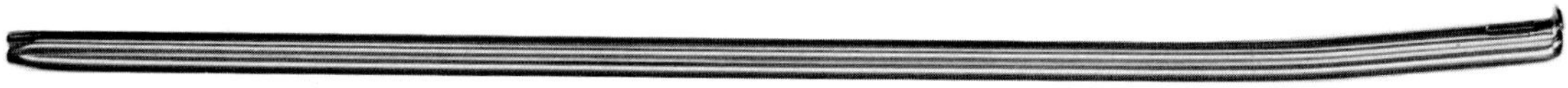

Figure 4 Bent cloverleaf nail.

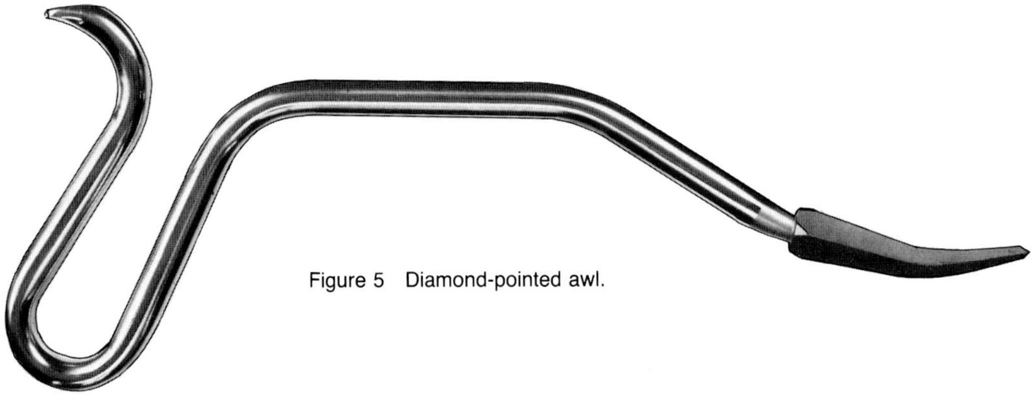

Figure 5 Diamond-pointed awl.

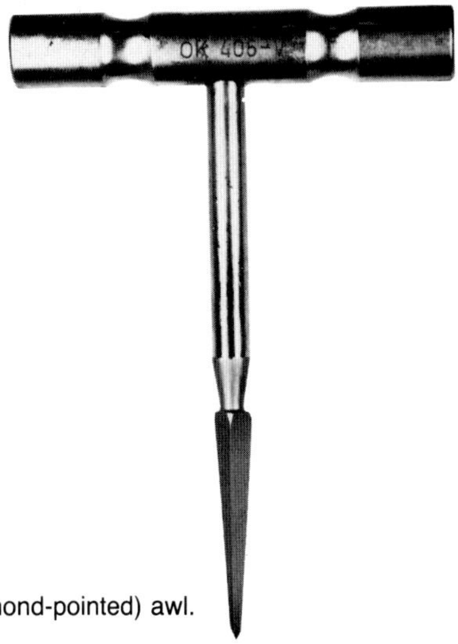

Figure 6 Straight (diamond-pointed) awl.

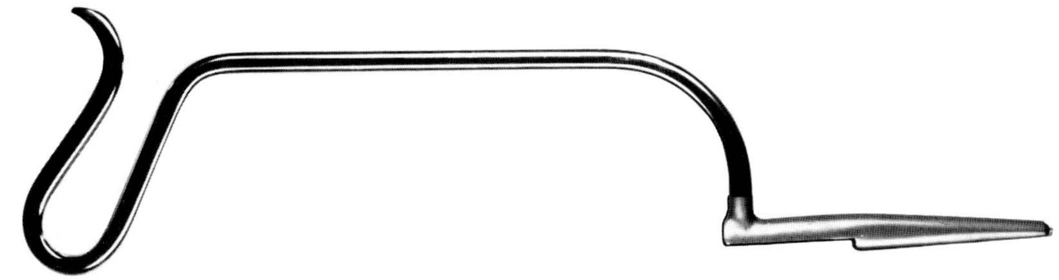

Figure 7 Reamer awl.

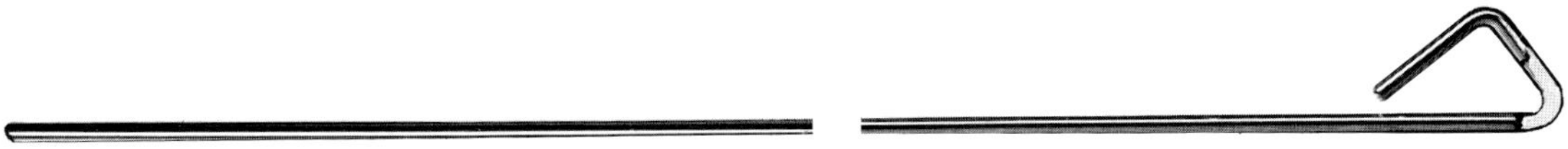

Figure 8 Nail driving guide with handle.

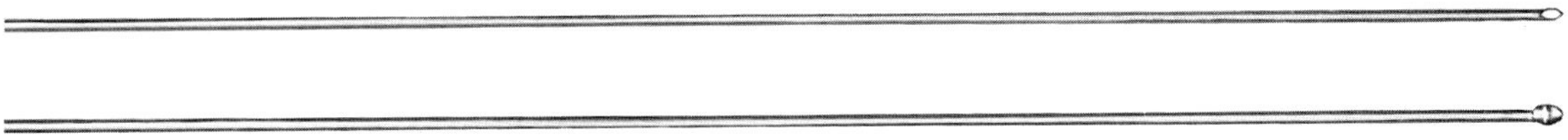

Figure 9 Smooth and ball-point guide pins

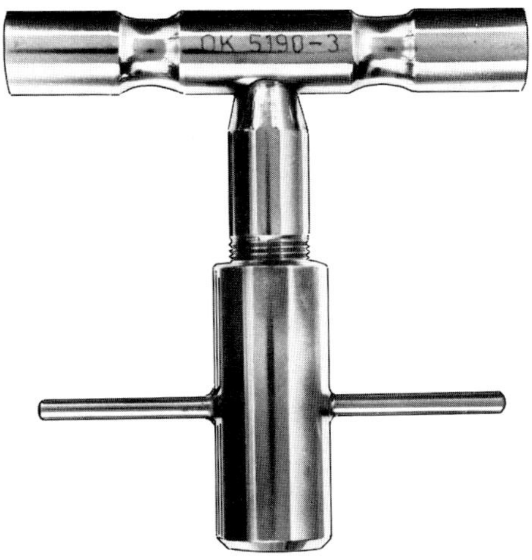

Figure 10 Guide pin handgrip.

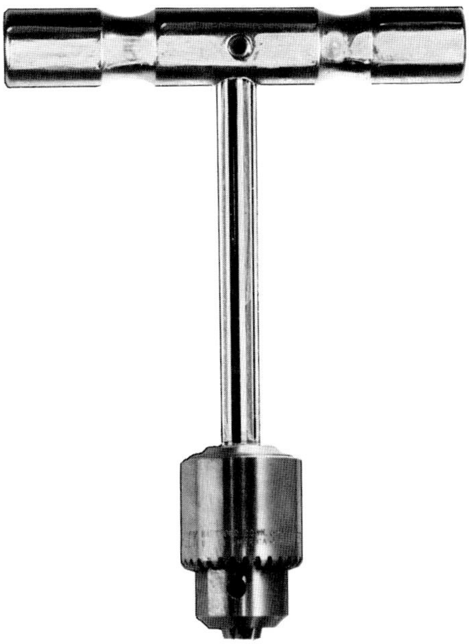

Figure 11 T-handle chuck.

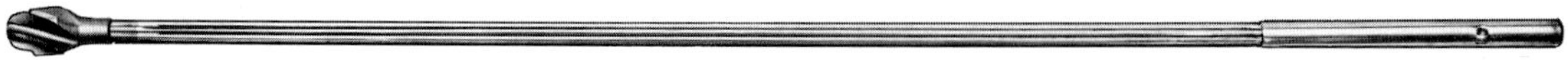

Figure 12 Flexible intramedullary reamer, cannulated for a guide pin.

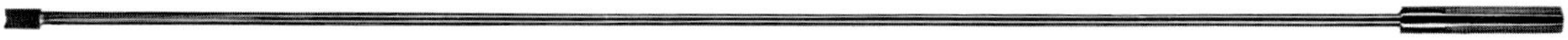

Figure 13 Cannulated squarehead reamer.

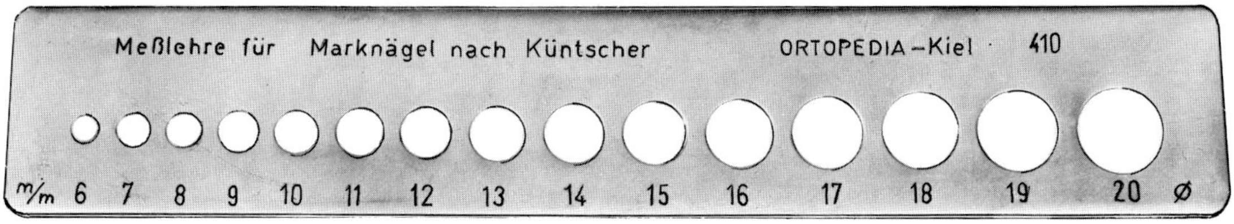

Figure 14 Küntscher nail gauge.

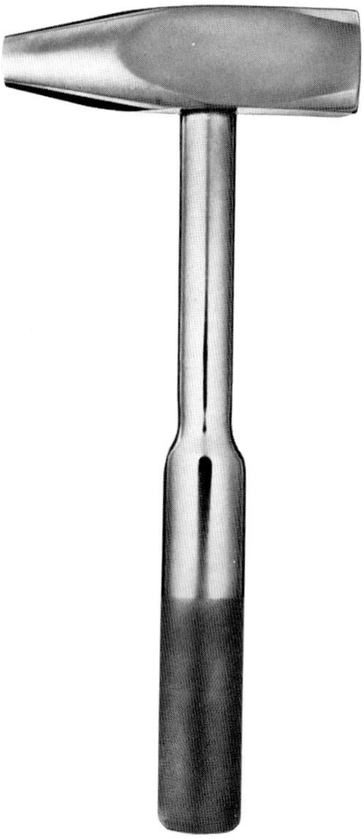

Figure 15 One-pound hammer.

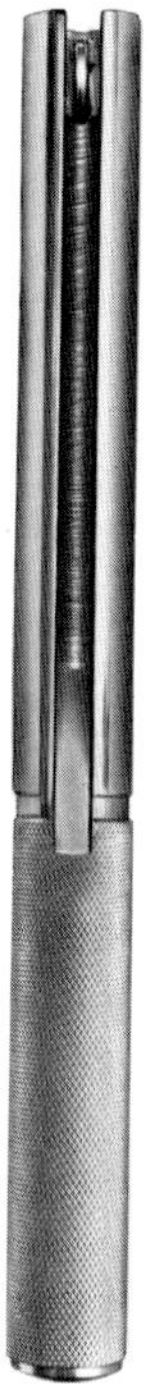

Figure 16 Slotted nail driver.

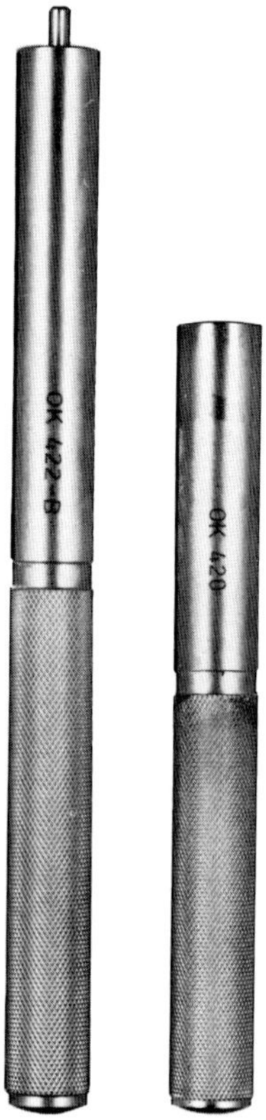

Figure 17 Nail set with and without pin.

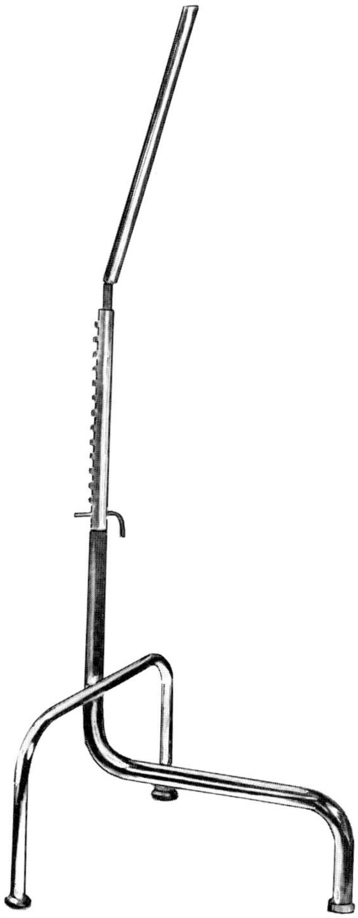

Figure 18 Nail bender with stand.

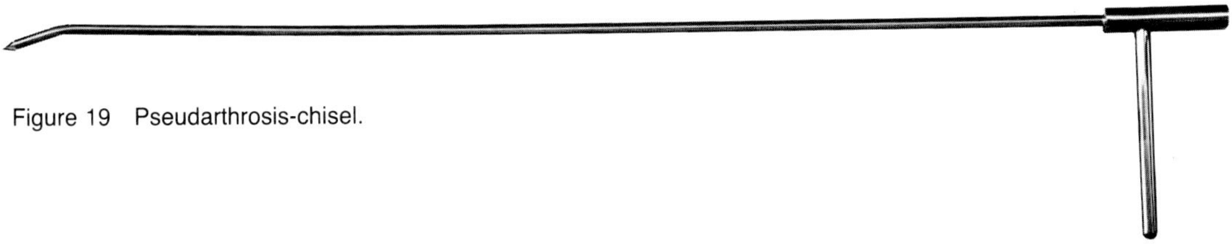

Figure 19 Pseudarthrosis-chisel.

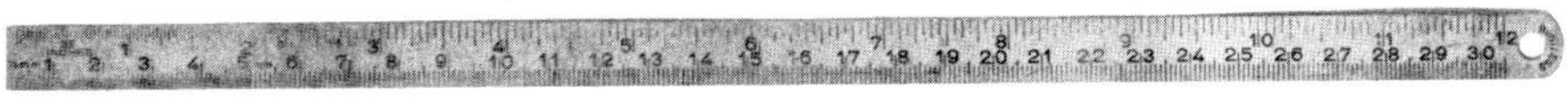

Figure 20 Autoclaveable measuring scale.

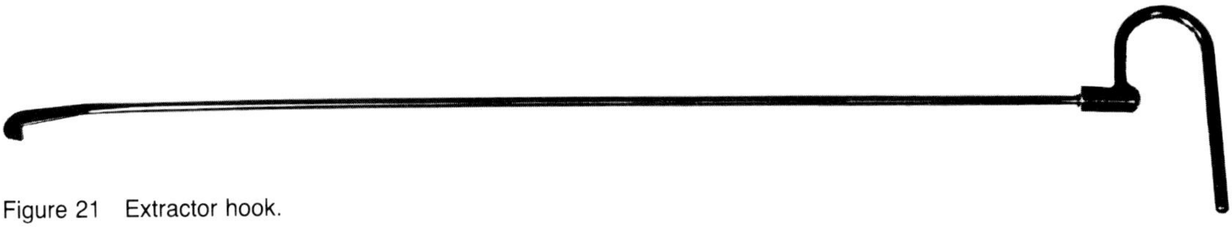

Figure 21 Extractor hook.

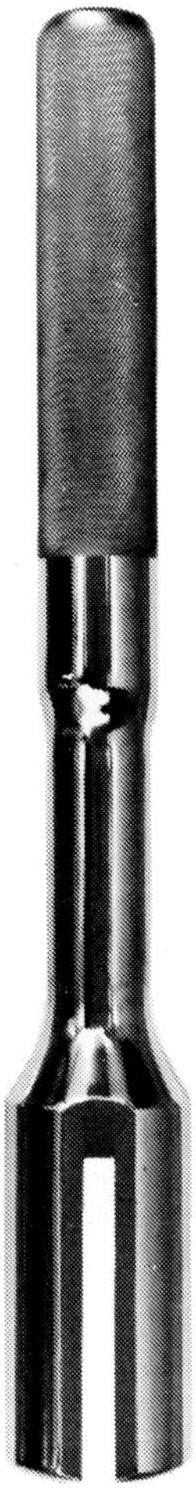

Figure 22 Slotted hammer.

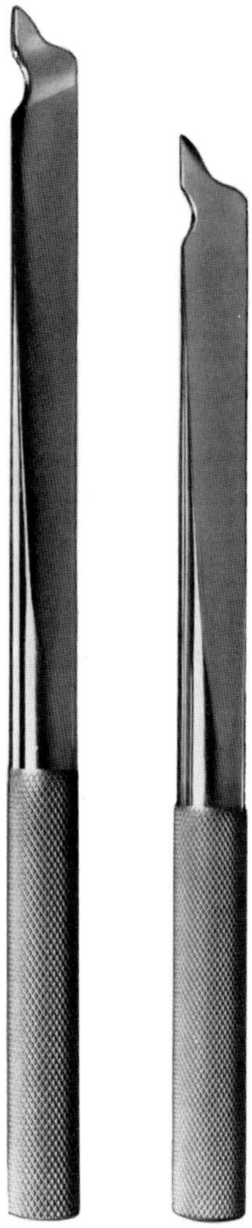

Figure 23 Rousek extractor set.

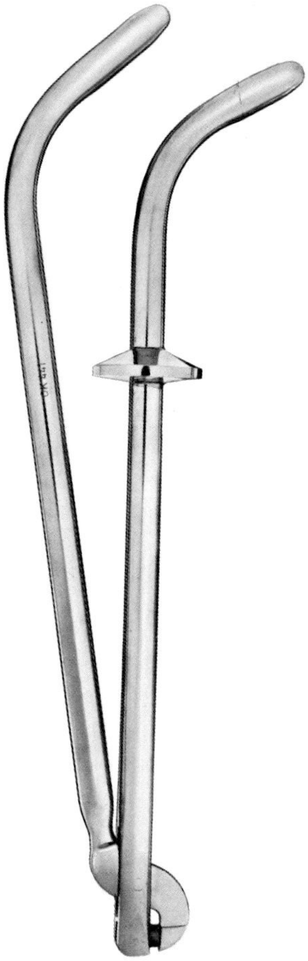

Figure 24 Griessmann pliers, for nail extraction.

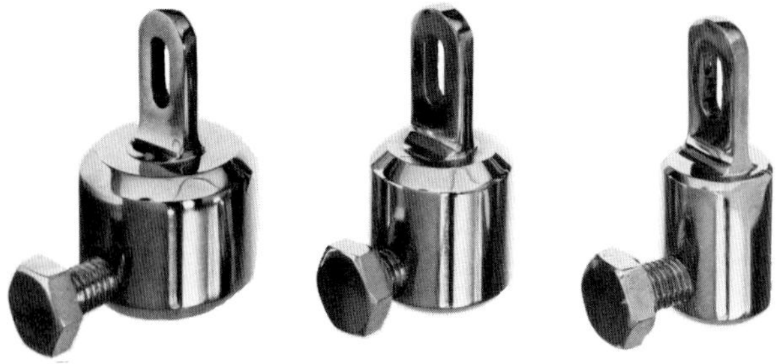

Figure 25 Extractor bushes in varying sizes for the removal of slotless nails.

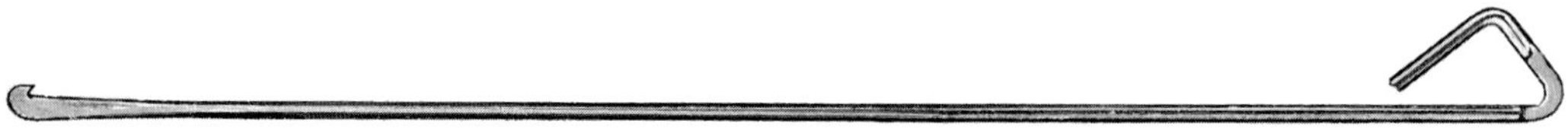

Figure 26 Nail catcher.

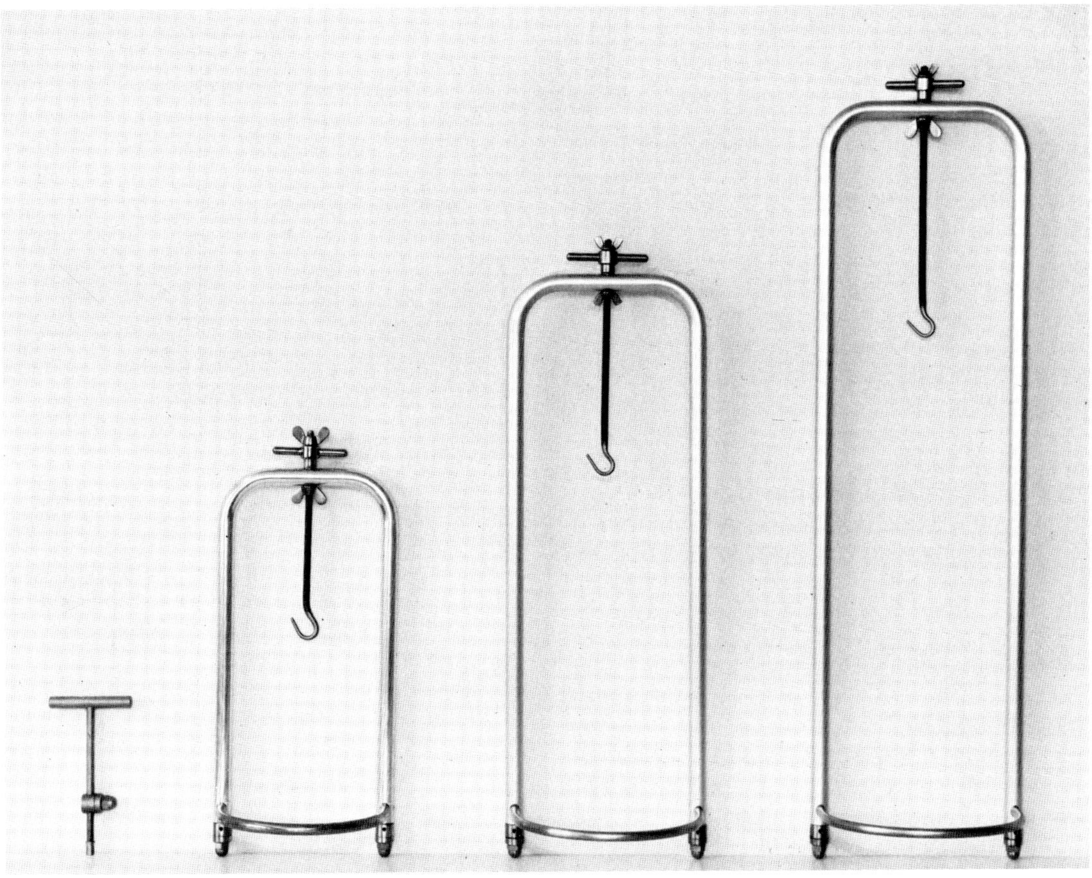

Figure 27 Distractors. Three different sizes with key.

Principles of the Intramedullary Nailing Technique

There is one set of technical rules that must be followed for success in all intramedullary nailings. Before making the stab incision, one must check to see whether the shortening can be overcome and the fracture reduced without much difficulty. If the shortening cannot be overcome, the nailing must be delayed and a distractor must be used for the time being. Küntscher has specified the point of entry for the nailing of each bone. Choosing an entry point other than the one specified by Küntscher may result in complications. One may not ream or nail without previously inserting a guide pin. Otherwise the intramedullary reamer or nail may easily miss the entrance into the distal fragment at the fracture site. One must ream the medullary canal to the maximum extent possible with the guided flexible reamer. The guide pin with the ball point end is used for reaming and facilitates the removal of a broken reamer head. One starts the reaming with the selected head that just passes through the narrowest portion of the canal. The narrowest portion is radiographically determined preoperatively. The canal is then reamed in 0.5-mm increments. The reamer is advanced with only minimal pressure, and at a speed of 100 to 200 rpm. Should resistance increase during the reaming, the reamer is withdrawn and the compacted particles removed from the flanges. Increasing the pressure on the reamer may lead to cracking of the bone cortex. During this reaming procedure, one should periodically fluoroscope in two planes to ensure that the cortex does not become too thin and the bone cortex does not crack. The intramedullary canal is reamed until it is 0.5mm wider than the thickness of the chosen nail. To ensure proper size concordance, it is advisable to check both the reamer and the chosen nail with the Küntscher nail gauge. The length of the nail is determined by inserting the guide pin entirely into the bone and subtracting the length of the protruding portion from the length of the guide pin. The nail driving guide should be large enough so that the nail's tip may be securely guided. The nail is then lightly tapped into the bone with a 1-lb hammer. Short pauses are necessary between the taps; this allows time for the bone marrow to recede and prevents excess fat from becoming compressed into the opened blood vessels. In some cases, when the tip of the nail reaches the distal fragment, extension may be diminished slightly, and some manual pressure may improve the alignment of the fragments. A change in the tapping sound signals a possible complication, in which case the bone should be fluoroscoped in two planes. The nail should be driven into the bone until no more than 2 to 3 mm protrudes at the entry port. The bone dust is not rinsed out of the medullary space. Suction-drainage is contraindicated.

Position

For intramedullary nailing, the patient should be positioned so that two conditions are satisfied: The fracture should be easily visualized by image intensification in two planes, and the typical nailing entry point should be easily accessible. The nailing of the lower extremities necessitates the use of an extension table. A normal operating table with a radiolucent arm support can be used for nailing the upper extremities and clavicle. Fractures of the upper arm and forearm can be positioned on an appropriate fracture table. The positions for the specific fractures are discussed in detail in their respective chapters.

Image Intensification

Preoperative roentgenograms in two planes must be taken of the fractured bones, comprising both adjacent joints. These also serve as radiographic gauges for determining the correct nail length and diameter. These exposures should have a focus to bone distance of 1 m. This configuration yields an image that is magnified by 10 percent, and the magnification must be deducted when calculating the nail length and diameter. Another way to measure the correct nail dimensions is to expose simultaneously the Küntscher x-ray scale in the same plane as the affected bone. Postoperative roentgenograms of the entire bone should be taken in two planes.

Image intensification should be minimized to reduce radiation exposure. Only short exposures are necessary in all instances. An image intensifier with memory aids in decreasing exposure time. As with the roentgenograms, image intensification should always be done in two planes.

Strict adherence to radiation protection procedures is required of all operating personnel. The use of lead aprons and irradiation dosimeters is obligatory. The fluoroscopy exposure time is to be documented.

Tips for Reduction

Reduction devices are seldom necessary in the intramedullary nailing of recent fractures. The best reduction device is the intramedullary nail itself. One can easily oppose the two fragments by using the leverage of a long, thin intramedullary nail, which is inserted into the proximal fragment. After reposition, a guide pin is inserted into the distal fragment through this nail. The nail is then withdrawn, and the fragments are held by the guide pin.

Another aid in reduction is the distractor. It is used in malaligned cases, in old fractures with shortening, and in irreducible pseudarthrosis. It is only rarely used in the positioning of fresh fractures. An effective distraction of an old fracture can be performed by the insertion of a wire extension into the proximal and distal fragments while the extremity is held in a radiolucent distractor (p. 9). The distraction must be done in small daily increments in order to avoid soft tissue damage as well as circulatory or neurologic complications. Distractions should also be monitored by periodic roentgenograms.

Specialized fracture tables, which allow for the addition of auxiliary devices, may also be useful.

Dangers and Complications of Intramedullary Nailing

Because a bone fracture normally poses no immediate threat to life, intramedullary nailing operations should only be undertaken after the accident shock has been successfully treated and has disappeared. Through modern anesthesia and fluid substitutions, the reduction of a fracture and intramedullary nailing are possible without causing shock. Although previously believed to be a complication of intramedullary nailing, fat embolism is now seen as a consquence of inadequate treatment of shock. Owing to the effective treatment of shock that is now available, fat embolism is no longer a cause for concern.

Infection of the bones poses the most severe complication of intramedullary nailing, as it does with all other types of osteosynthesis. Because the soft-tissue incision is relatively small in comparison with the "bony laceration" after the reaming of the medullary canal, the infection of the medullary canal can propagate quickly, although causing relatively late clinical symptoms. If the usual postoperative elevated body temperature does not decrease in two to three days, or if it increases even further, vigorous antibiotic treatment should be instituted immediately. One should be alert for the signs of osteomyelitis. The symptoms are increasing bone pains, swelling of the soft tissue, and sustained fever. Therefore, the temperature curve becomes septic and the incision becomes inflamed. A rise in the white blood count with a shift to the left is also noted. No radiographic changes can be seen at this early stage. The incision should be opened at the first sign of infection, even though the incision itself may not yet be directly involved. Only the prompt reopening of the incision can hinder the propagation of the infection. Specimens should be obtained for culture and sensitivity testing. Only in acute cases is the systemic antibiotic treatment indicated. Suction-drainage, according to Willenegger, is necessary and supplements the antibiotic treatment. A firmly seated intramedullary nail must not be removed at this stage (p. 153).

Once the exact width measurements of the medullary canal have been determined radiographically, the reaming of the canal easily avoids the jamming of the intramedullary nail. If the nail jams as a result of an operative mistake, one has to decide whether the jamming occurs in the proximal or the distal fragment. If the jamming occurs in the proximal fragment, the nail might be hammered retrograde or removed with extraction devices (pp. 8, 160 and 161). If this is not possible, the nail can be sawed off at the entry point of the bone. The rest of the nail will loosen itself in time by bone resorption and can later be removed like a nail without a slot. If the nail jams in the distal fragment, the osteosynthesis is nearly always solid. If the nail cannot be easily retrieved, it is sawed off close to the entry port. After a solid healing of the fracture and resorption around the nail, the nail is removed like a nail without a slot (p. 158).

Trying to advance a jamming nail may lead to a cracking of the bony tube. A solid osteosynthesis with a regular Küntscher nail is then rendered impossible. The osteosynthesis thereafter can only be accomplished with a special nail or by a different method such as AO-osteosynthesis. The bone can be cracked if an incorrect nailing entry point is used.

Furthermore, another cause for cracking the bony tube is using too thin a guide pin, which does not correctly lead the tip of the nail into the distal fragment. Therefore, one should check that the guidance of the nail on the driving guide is firm and that the guide is securely held within the confines of the nail tip. Using a nail with insufficient diameter will lead to a broken nail because the nail is weaker than the bone. Thus, the fracture fails to heal and pseudarthrosis ensues. Even though a nail with too small a diameter may not break, no firm osteosynthesis exists, and the intramedullary nailing leads to pseudarthrosis.

Using too large a reamer and applying pressure may crack the bony tube. A reamer head that becomes filled with bone dust acts like an oversized reamer. For this reason, reamers should be withdrawn periodically and cleansed of bone dust.

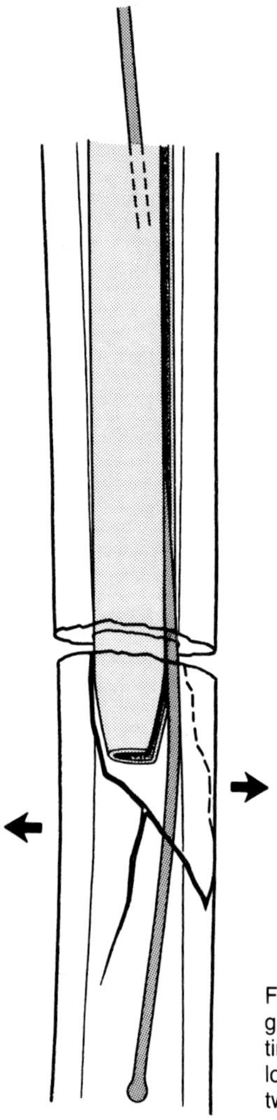

Figure 28 The nail is not guided by the guide pin. Splitting of bone caused by the locking of the guide pin between the nail and the bone.

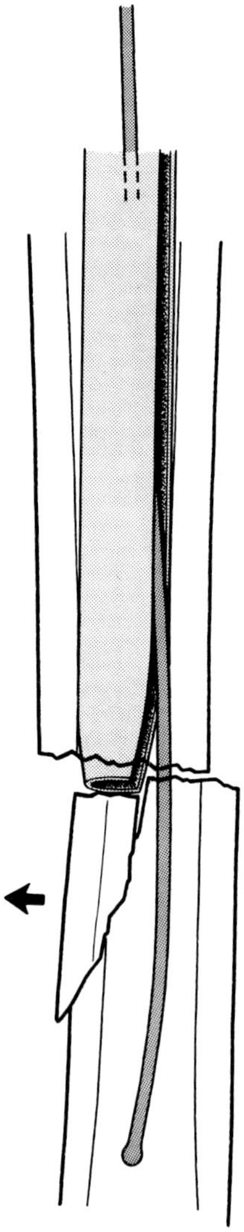

Figure 29 The nail is not guided by the guide pin. Splitting of the bone caused by the impact of the nail onto the corticalis.

Detailed Section

Closed Intramedullary Nailing of Fractures

Intramedullary Nailing of the Femur

Indications

All transverse fractures having satisfactory cortical support, including those with wedge-shaped fragments, lend themselves to intramedullary nailing, as do short spiral fractures occurring in the middle third of the femur. One should adhere to the following rule: the intramedullary nail must be longitudinally locked in both fragments. The nail must also have a sufficiently large diameter. Only medullary canals of uniform width inherently allow for elastic locking; medullary canals with irregular widths must be reamed.

Positioning and Reduction

The patient is positioned on the fracture table with his injured side up. The hip joint of the injured extremity should be flexed 45 to 90 degrees relative to the perineal support (Fig. 30). This position, along with adduction, renders the tip of the trochanter prominent and easily palpable. Traction to the injured extremity is applied either with the knee joint extended via a boot attached to an extension device (Fig. 30), or flexed via supracondylar skeletal traction attached by a Kirschner wire tractor to the extension device (Fig. 31). The lower leg must be supported in the latter case.

Should the shortening not be overcome by traction, a distractor must be used preoperatively. One is always able to overcome any shortening by using a distractor. The positioning of the distractor is the same as previously described (Fig. 245).

Image Intensification

A correct assessment of the fracture requires preoperative roentgenograms, taken in two planes, of the femur and adjacent joints. These films may serve as gauges in determining the proper length and diameter of the intramedullary nail. The image intensifier must be positioned in such a way that the femur can be fluoroscoped in two perpendicular planes. Roentgenograms showing the entire femur in two planes should also be taken at the conclusion of the operation.

Operative Techniques

A stab incision, 3 cm long, should be made over the trochanter tip, and its medullary canal should be opened with the proper awl. The unencumbered hand of the surgeon is positioned on the thigh. The awl is inserted into the medullary canal to a depth of 2 to 5 cm, generally directed toward the curved axis of the femur. The insertion point is just medial to the greater trochanter and posterior to the central axis of the femoral neck in the region of the obturator fossa. The awl is exchanged for a guide pin, to which is attached the guide pin handgrip. The guide pin is then advanced in a rotating motion. Careful light taps with the slotted driver may free a guide pin if it becomes trapped in cancellous bone. The guide pin's position in the proximal fragment is checked in two planes by image intensification.

The entry portal is enlarged by inserting

the reamer awl over the guide pin. If a smooth guide pin was initially used, it must now be exchanged for a long ball-point guide pin for reaming. The reamer awl is then removed. The final reduction is now done if necessary by using a ball-point guide pin whose tip is slightly angulated. The guide pin is advanced into the epiphysis of the distal fragment and verified in two planes by the image intensifier. Ream the medullary canal with a flexible cannulated reamer using a ball-point guide pin. One starts the reaming with the end-cutting 8-mm reamer, which just passes through the narrowest portion of the medullary canal. Ream the medullary canal until the desired width is attained. When reaming is completed, the appropriate nail driving guide is inserted, alongside of the ball-point guide pin. Only thereafter should the ball-point guide pin be removed. The nail-driving guide centers the distal end of the nail in the canal and reduces the chance of impingement on the distal cortical segment. The chosen intramedullary nail is then carefully tapped over the inserted nail guide. The nail's passage through the fracture site should be monitored in two planes by fluoroscopy. When the tip of the nail passes the fracture site by 4 to 5 cm, the guide pin is removed. The nail is driven with a Küntscher nail set for the last few centimeters until it is flush with the trochanter tip. Suture the incision.

Should the femur fracture lie in the distractor, one should do the following: The patient with a distractor applied can be positioned on the fracture table, either in supine position or with the fracture side up. Once the awl has opened the medullary canal, the long ball-point guide pin is introduced into the distal fragment. The distractor may be removed once the guide pin is correctly positioned in both fragments, as determined by fluoroscopy. The operation then continues as already described.

Common Mistakes

If one forgets to verify that the shortening has been corrected, closed intramedullary nailing becomes impossible.

One knows that the guide pin has perforated into the soft tissues if it can be advanced without resistance or bone friction. The guide pin cannot enter the distal fragment if the fracture has not been adequately reduced. The aforementioned reduction aids must be used.

The nail cannot be securely guided if the nail driving guide pin is too small, because the guide pin will leave the tip of the nail through the slit. Should this mistake not be corrected, a locking of the nail's tip with the pin and the distal cortex will result at the fracture site. It is even possible to crack the distal fragment if one attempts to drive the nail any further.

If the nail can be driven easily over the guide pin and little resistance is met, no elastic locking can occur. The diameter of the nail is too small and the possibility of postoperative rotational maladjustment exists.

Aftercare

If no major additional injuries exist, the patient may bear weight as tolerated on the first postoperative day. If other injuries hinder early weight-bearing at least exercises of the nailed extremity should be initiated immediately. Physiotherapy promotes early mobilization.

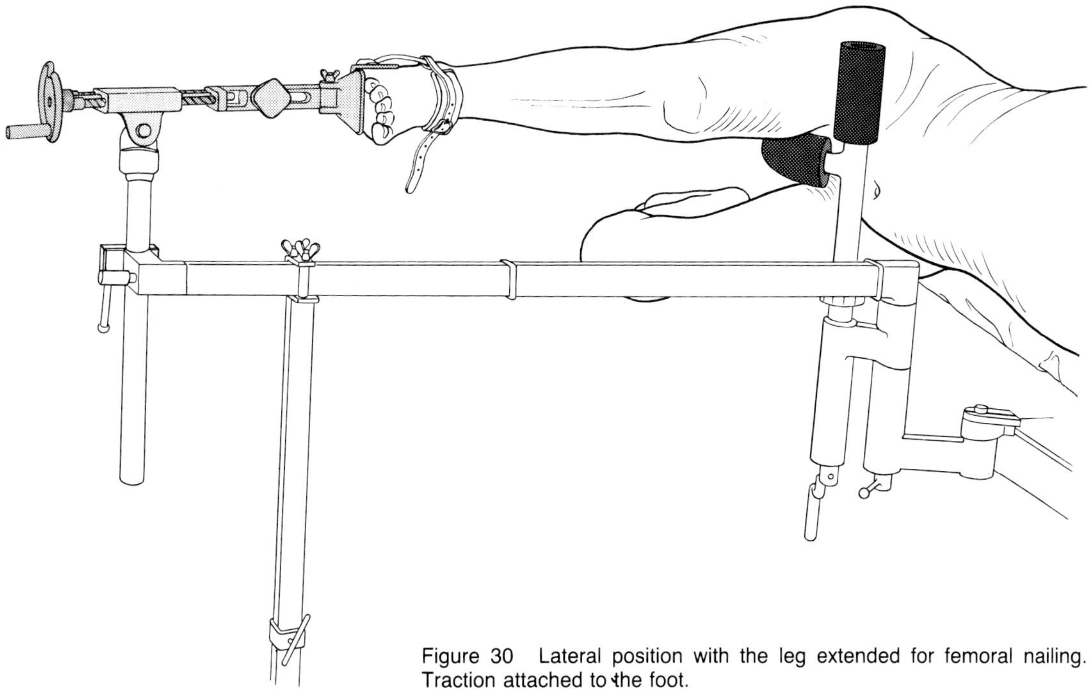

Figure 30 Lateral position with the leg extended for femoral nailing. Traction attached to the foot.

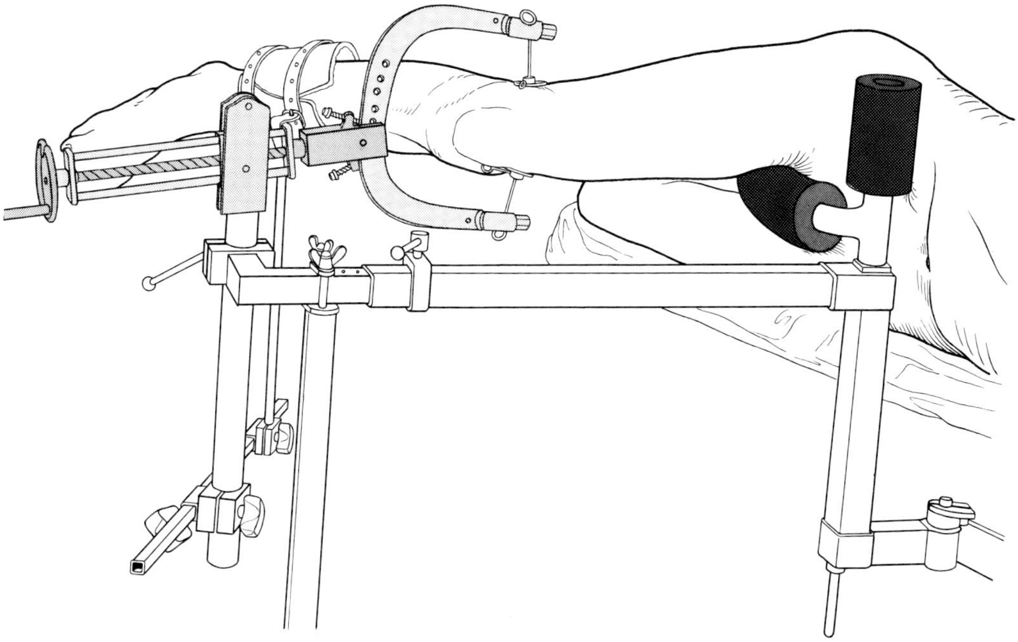

Figure 31 Lateral position with the knee flexed. Supracondylar skeletal traction.

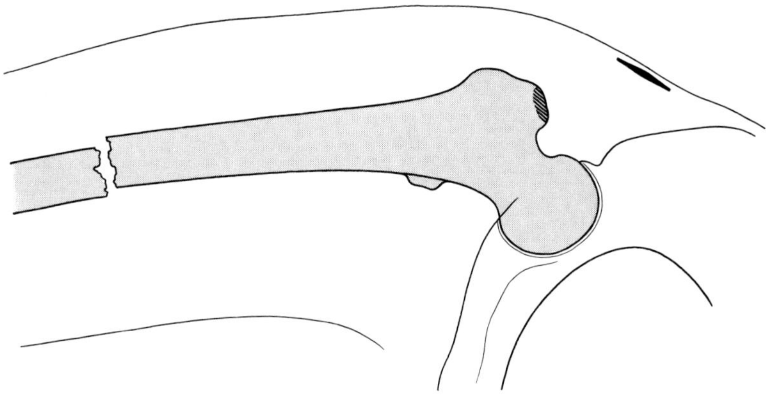

Figure 32 Stab incision and nail entry point at the trochanter tip for femoral nailing.

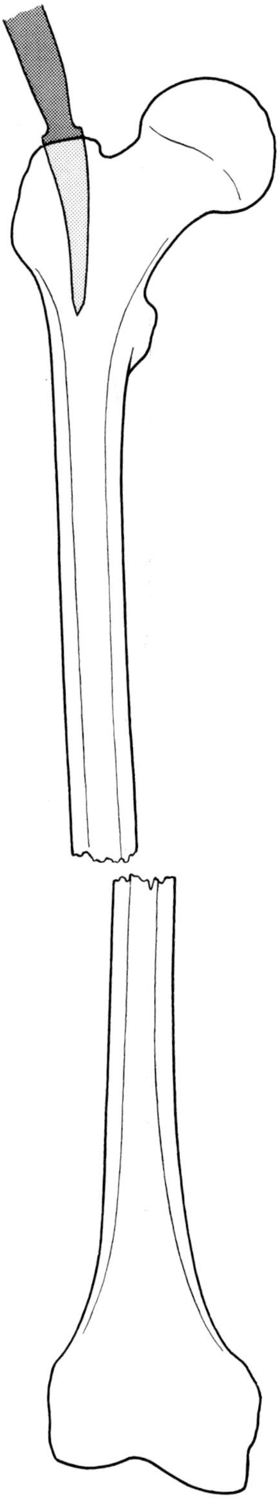

Figure 33 Opening of the medullary canal by the femoral awl.

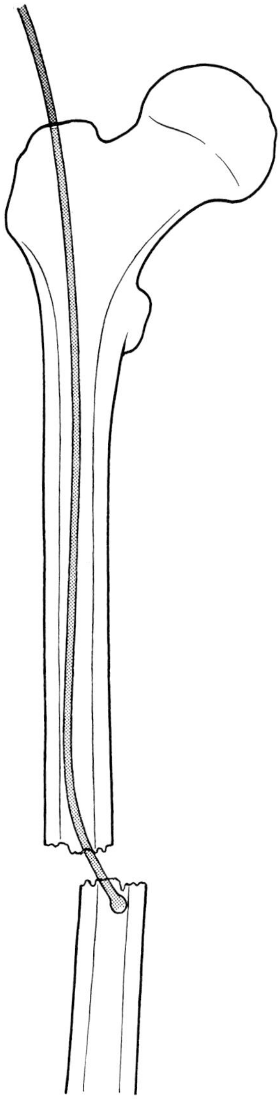

Figure 34 Reduction of the fracture by a bent ball-point guide pin.

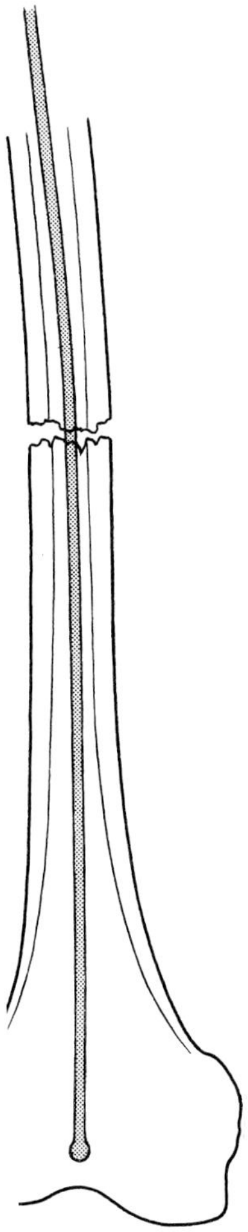

Figure 35 Reduced fracture, the guide pin in the distal fragment.

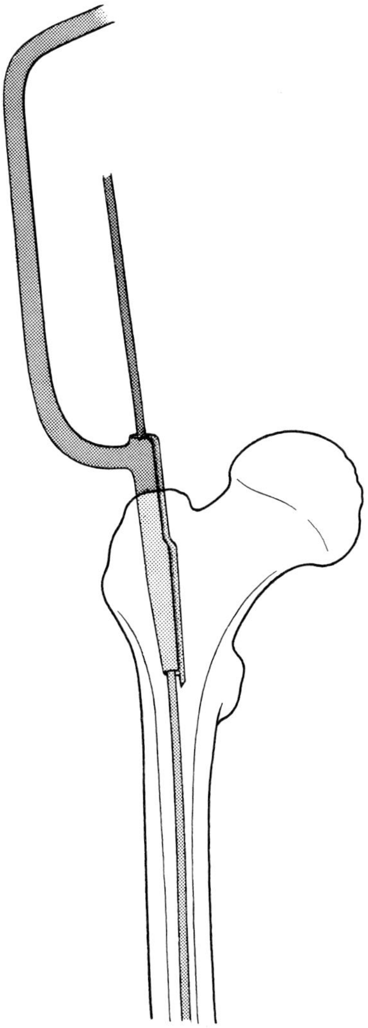

Figure 36 Enlargement of the nail entry port by the reamer awl.

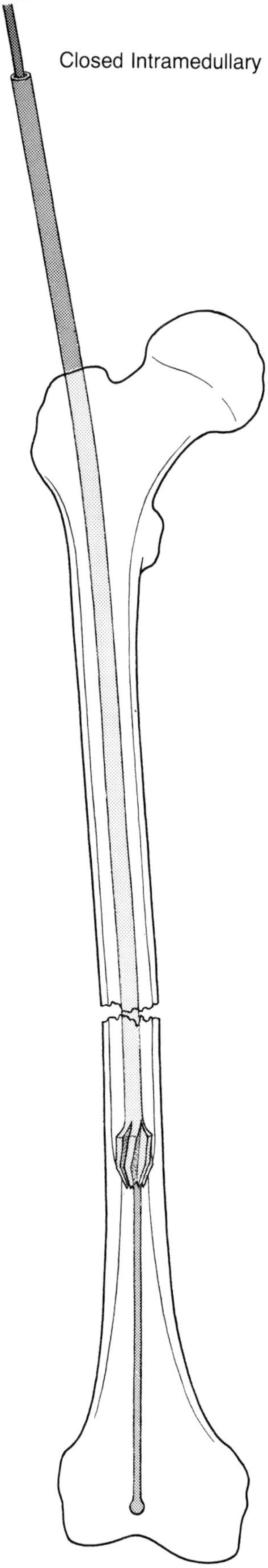

Figure 37 Reaming of the medullary canal over the correctly positioned guide pin.

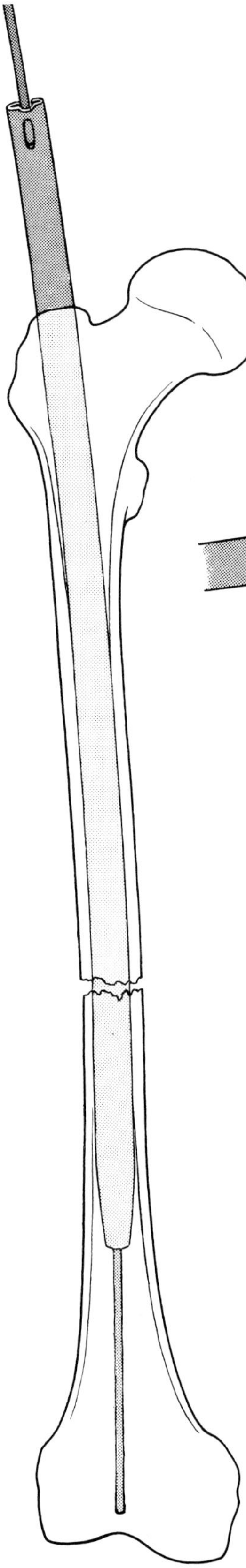

Figure 38 Driving the nail over the correctly positioned nail driving guide.

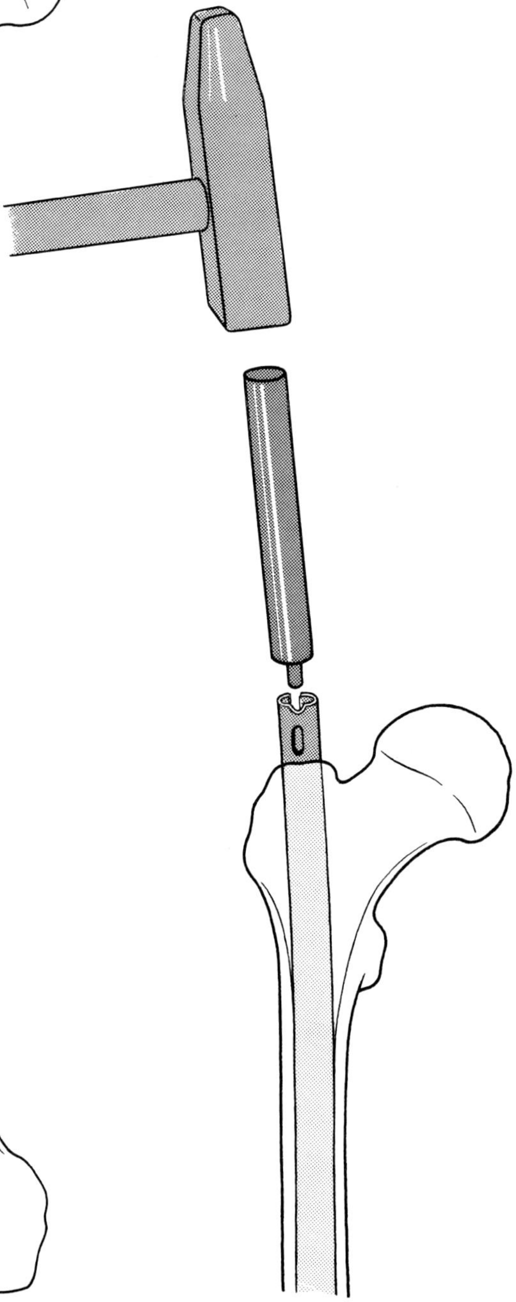

Figure 39 Final setting of the nail with a nail set.

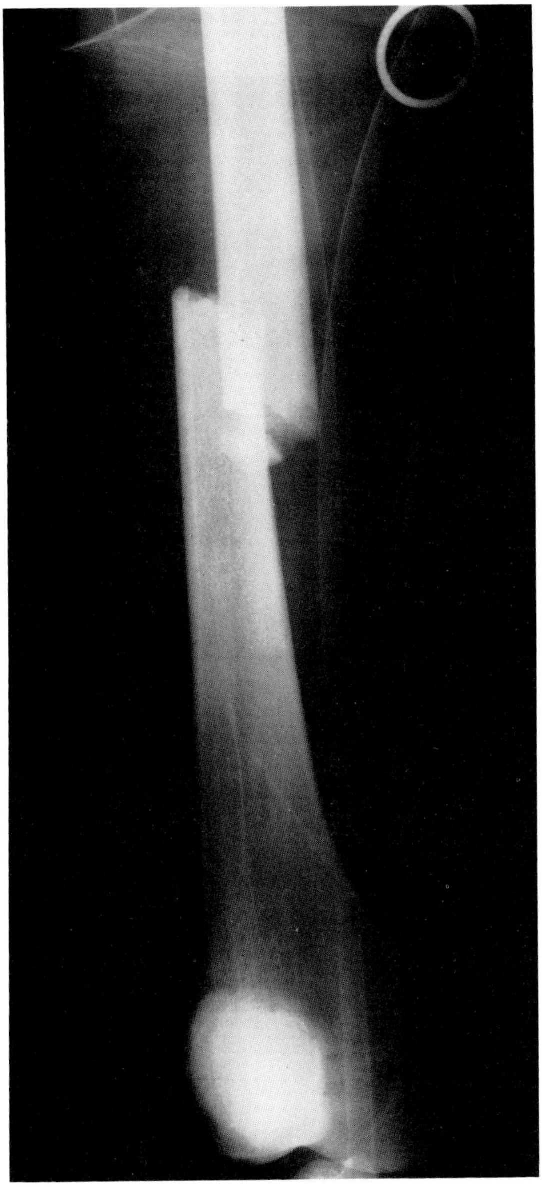

Figure 40 Fresh femoral fracture, AP, in an inflatable splint.

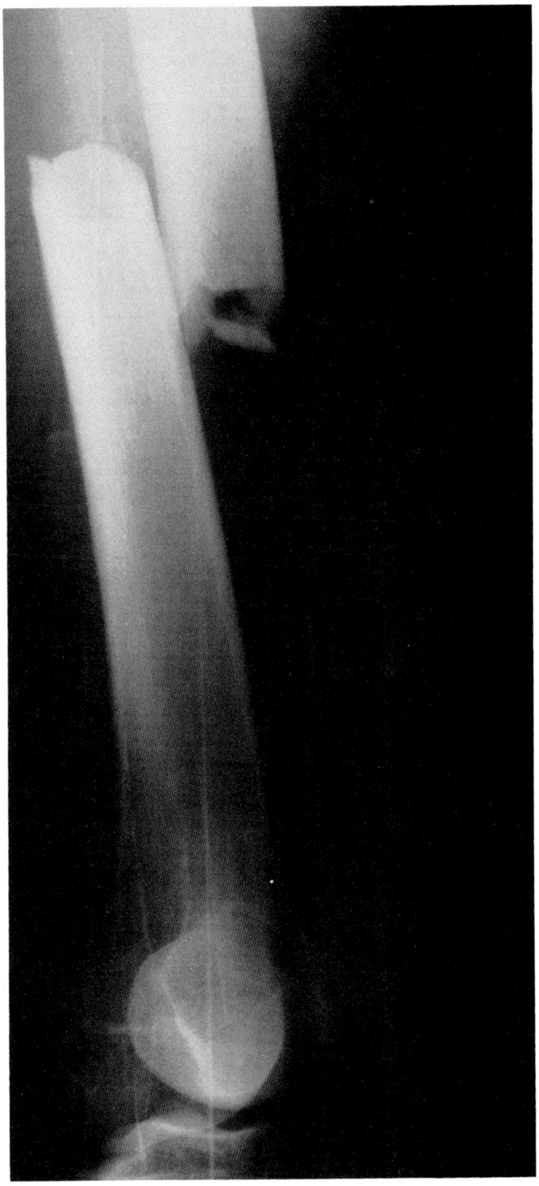

Figure 41 Lateral view of the fresh femoral fracture.

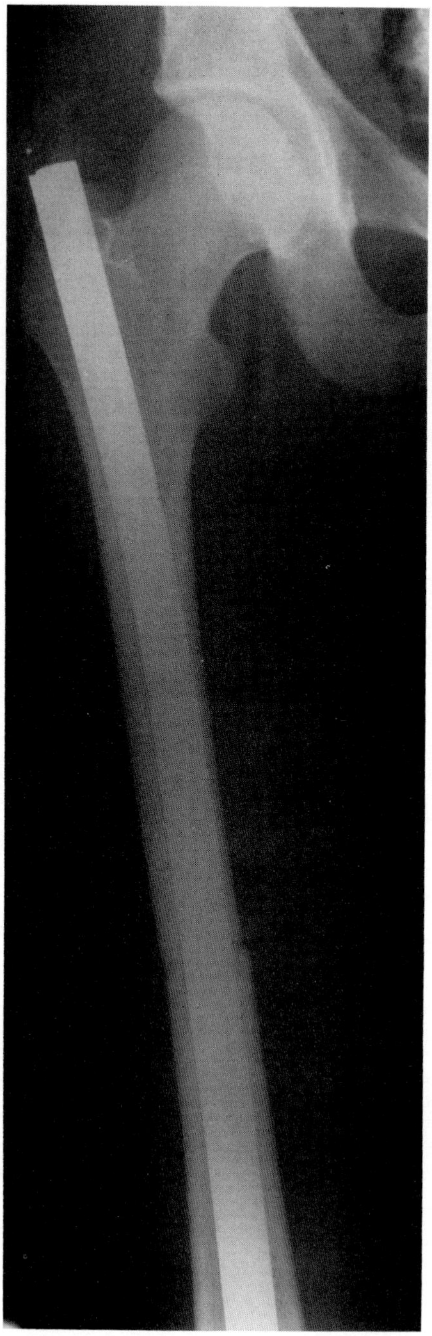

Figure 42 Same fracture after the intramedullary nailing, AP view. The large Küntscher nail follows the curvature of the bone, providing additional longitudinal locking.

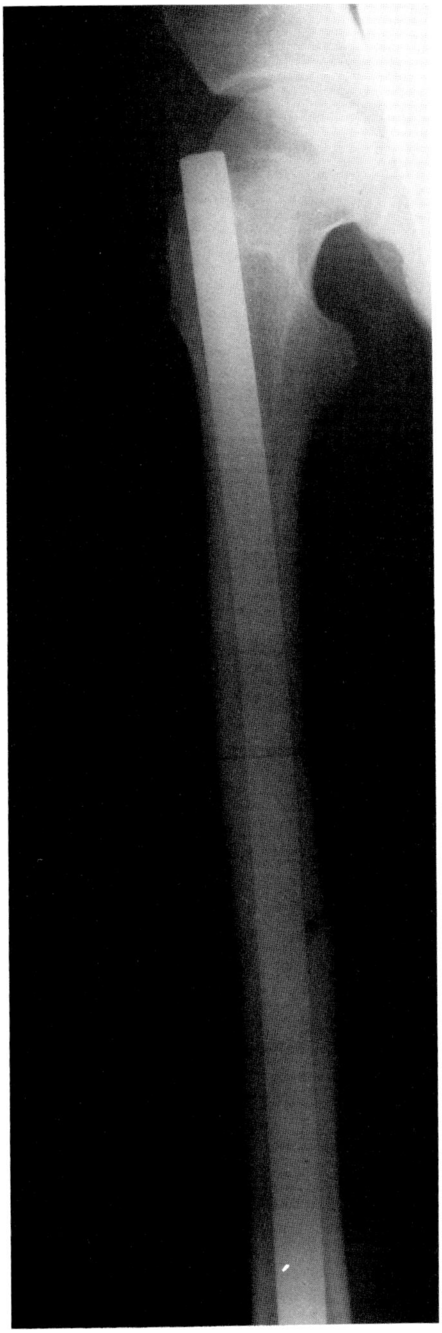

Figure 43 Lateral view, after femoral intramedullary nailing.

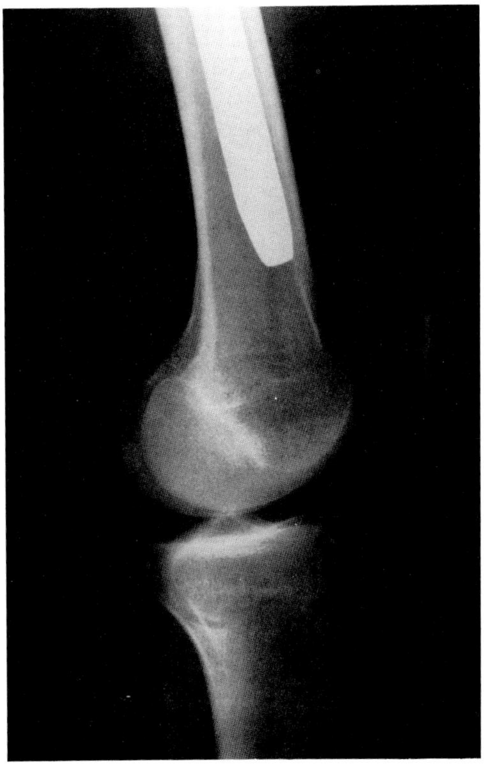

Figure 43A Correct position of the nail tip, lateral view.

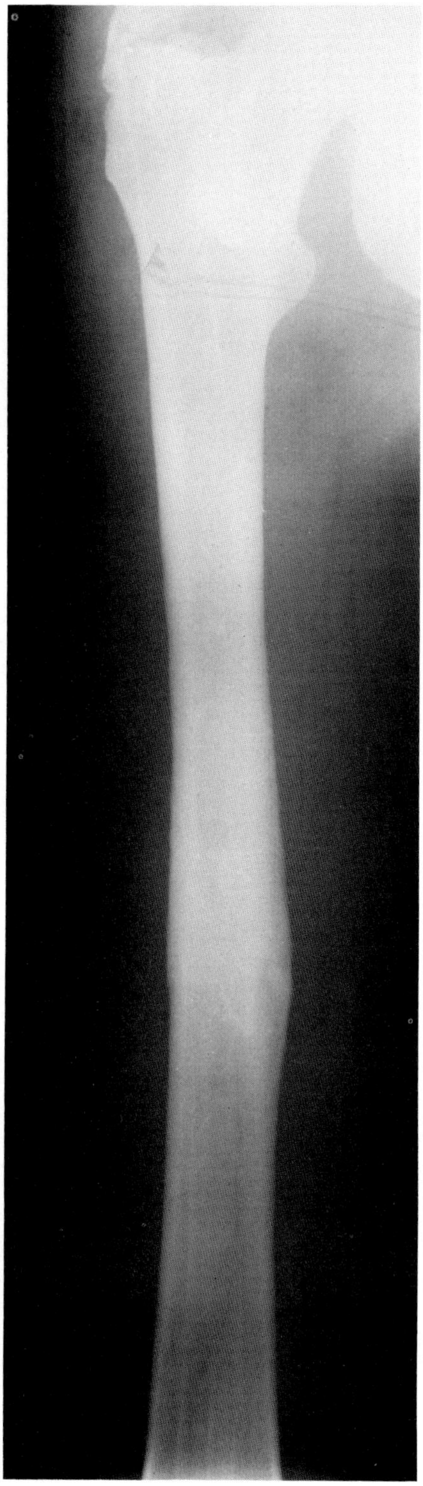

Figure 44 Twenty-one months postoperatively, and following nail removal, AP view.

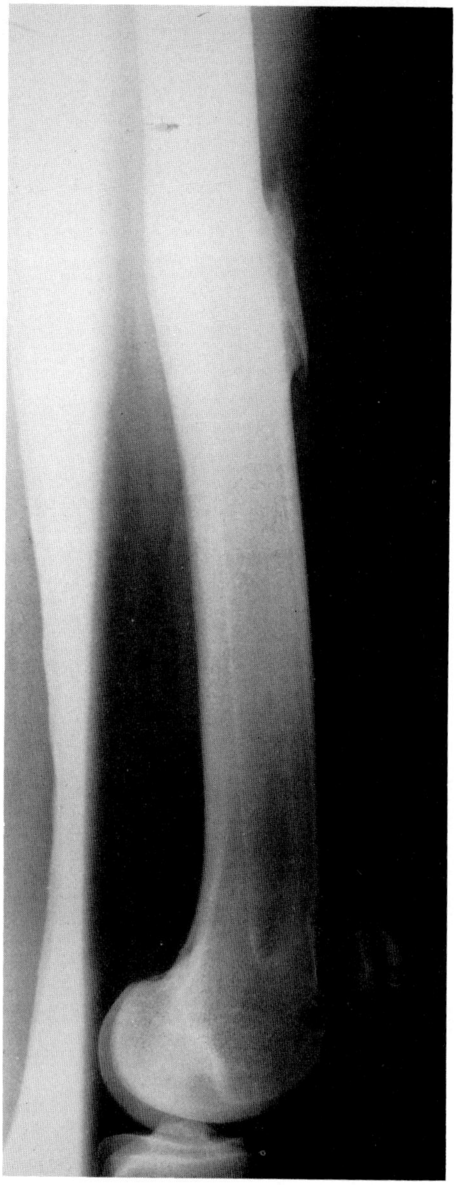

Figure 45 Lateral view following nail removal.

Intramedullary Nailing of the Tibia

Indications

Only the tibia is nailed in fractures of the lower leg. Fibula fractures are ignored, except for the fractures of the lateral malleolus. Indications for tibia nailing include all transverse fractures, even those with small wedge-shaped fragments if sufficient cortical support exists, and small spiral fractures occurring in the middle third of the long bone. The intramedullary nail must be amply locked lengthwise in both fragments. If this condition is met, the indications may be widened to include fractures occurring in the proximal or distal third of the long bone.

Positioning and Reduction

The patient is supine on the fracture table, and the hip of the injured extremity is flexed approximately in a right angle. The knee joint is flexed between 90 and 115 degrees (i.e., knee extension equals zero) over an upholstered radiolucent support, and the foot is attached by a boot or skeletal traction through the os calcis to the extension device. Ample traction is always attainable in this position. The positioning of the uninvolved leg is determined by the options of the fracture table in use. Free movement of the image intensifier must be possible. The thin layer of the soft tissue immediately over the tibia demands special attention during the repositioning of the fracture. In order to avoid any soft tissue interposition, one must always apply traction before any rotational correction. The rotational position of the foot is always compared with that of the uninvolved foot. If no deformities of the lower extremity exist, the middle of the patella lies in the same line as that of the second toe of the foot. After reduction, the tibial crest of both fragments should be aligned. Obstacles to the reduction, such as soft tissue interposition or separated bone pieces, can be overcome by interchanging traction with relaxation and careful angulation and rotation maneuvers. The additional reduction aids described on pages 11 and 174 are seldom necessary.

Image Intensification

Preoperative roentgenograms of the tibia, including the knee and ankle joints, must be taken in two planes, preferably at a distance of 1 m in order to serve as radiographic gauges for the determination of the correct dimensions of the nail and reamers. The image intensifier is positioned on the side of the uninjured extremity. Fluoroscopy of the injured tibia must be possible in both planes without jeopardizing the asepsis. After the nailing of the tibia is completed, roentgenograms in two planes of the entire bone are indicated.

Operative Technique

The entry point of the tibia lies proximal to the tibia tubercle in the midline behind or slightly medial to the patellar ligament and is easily palpable. The anatomy of the medullary canal and of the entry point call for a specially shaped nail which is slightly bent at its proximal end and is guided only at the nail tip by a guide pin. The skin incision is approximately 3 cm long and is carried from the proximal end of the tibia tubercle close to the apex of the patella. Through the split patellar ligament or just medial to it, the tibial awl is used to generously open the medullary canal directly proximal to the tibia tubercle. The tip of the awl is brought close to the anterior cortex by lowering the handle of the awl and is advanced as deep as the instrument allows. Withdraw the awl. It is now recommended that the short (25 cm long) flexible reamers (7 mm through 9 mm in diameter) be used to enlarge the entrance to the medullary canal. A guide pin is not necessary for this maneuver. A pin handgrip or a T-handle chuck is now attached to a long ball-point guide pin, which is introduced into the medullary canal. The guide pin is advanced to the fracture site by light hammering taps and slight rotational movements. The transition of the guide pin from the proximal into the distal fragment is monitored by the image intensifier in two planes. The guide pin is then advanced into the wide portion of the distal medullary canal. Ream the medullary canal in increments of 0.5 mm until the desired width is obtained. Insert the smooth nail driving guide into the distal fragment and remove the ball-point guide pin. Drive the selected nail over the nail driving guide. Fluoroscopy should be used repeatedly during the nailing procedure, especially during the passage of the nail at the fracture site. If a gap exists in the fracture, reduce the traction. The nail is driven until it is flush with the proximal edge of the tibia tubercle. Withdraw the guide pin. If the guide pin is bent, sometimes rotational movements and light tapping with the slotted driver against the handchuck are necessary. Do not remove blood or bone dust from the medullary canal before closing the incision.

If the fracture of the tibia is positioned in a distractor, position the fractured tibia with the distractor on the fracture table, as already described. In this case, the wire tractor of the distractor is attached to a traction device of the fracture table. The operative procedure is identical to the one already described up to the point where the guide pin is introduced into the distal fragment. At this time, the proximal Kirschner wire and the wire tractor of the distractor are removed without endangering the successful reduction. The wire tractor through the os calcis is attached to the traction device of the fracture table. Thereafter, the tibia nailing is identical to that already described.

Common Mistakes

If the entry point is too far distal, the nail cannot normally enter the medullary canal. Instead, it encounters the inner dorsal cortex at a steep angle and splits the bone. The entry point is not as easily found if the knee is not flexed 90 to 115 degrees. The guide pin may exit the tip of the nail if proper guidance of the pin at the tip of the nail is not checked before the introduction of the guide pin. In this case, the nail can either deadlock with the bone and the guide pin at the fracture site or the nail can meet the cortex of the distal fragment. If the nail is driven forward in this position, the bone can crack. Excessive distraction of the fragments can also lead to this complication. If the fragments can be exactly opposed by reducing the traction, the nail can be driven distally even if the guide pin is too small. This is only possible if there are no interpositioned bony pieces, which hinder the re-entry of the guide pin into the nail. If a bony piece locks in the nail slit, one must first remove the guide pin and then the nail. Removing the nail before removing the pin can split the proximal fragment. A larger nail driving pin is then introduced into the distal fragment and the chosen nail is driven over this guide. If the nail cannot be driven forward with the same amount of force or the sound changes while tapping, a jamming of the nail is imminent. Use of a guide that is too small or inadequate reaming of the medullary canal can cause this complication. If a nail is either too short or too small, the elastic locking is inadequate, and the osteosynthesis is not stable enough for rotation and weight-bearing. The protruding end of a nail that is either too long or not driven deep enough can cause soft tissue irritation around the patellar ligament.

Aftercare

If no major additional injuries exist, the patient may bear weight as tolerated on the first postoperative day. If other injuries hinder early weight-bearing, exercises of the nailed extremity should be initiated immediately. Physiotherapy promotes early mobilization.

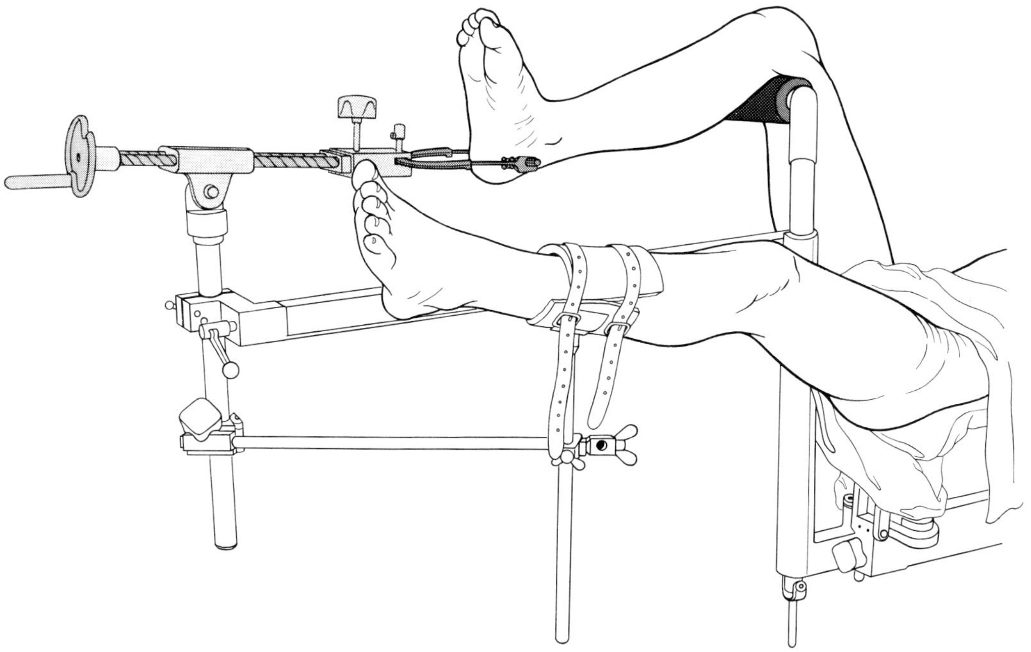

Figure 46 The correct position on the fracture table for tibial nailing.

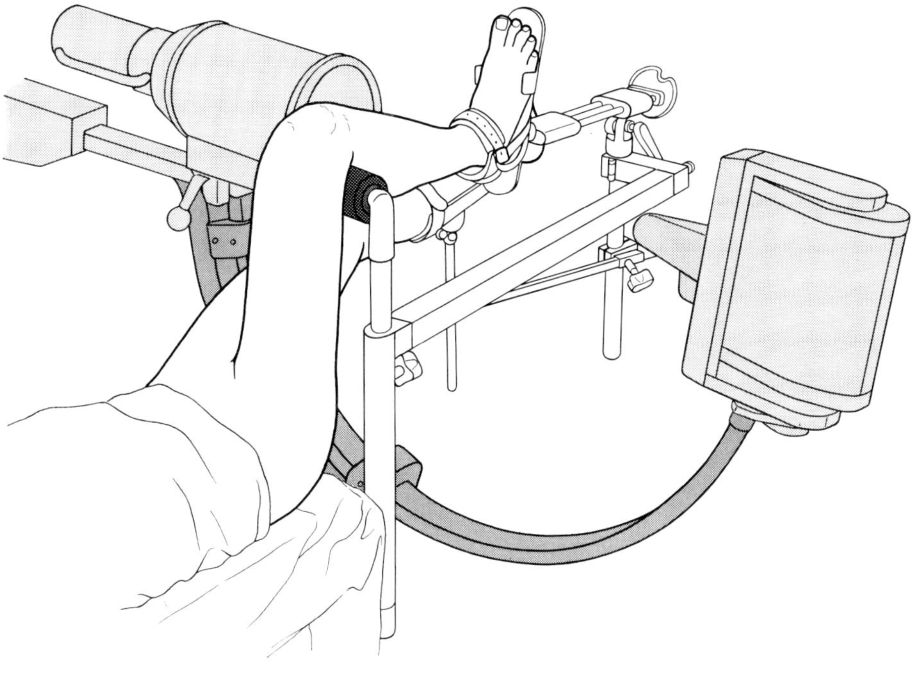

Figure 47 The position for the tibial nailing with image intensifier for lateral fluoroscopy.

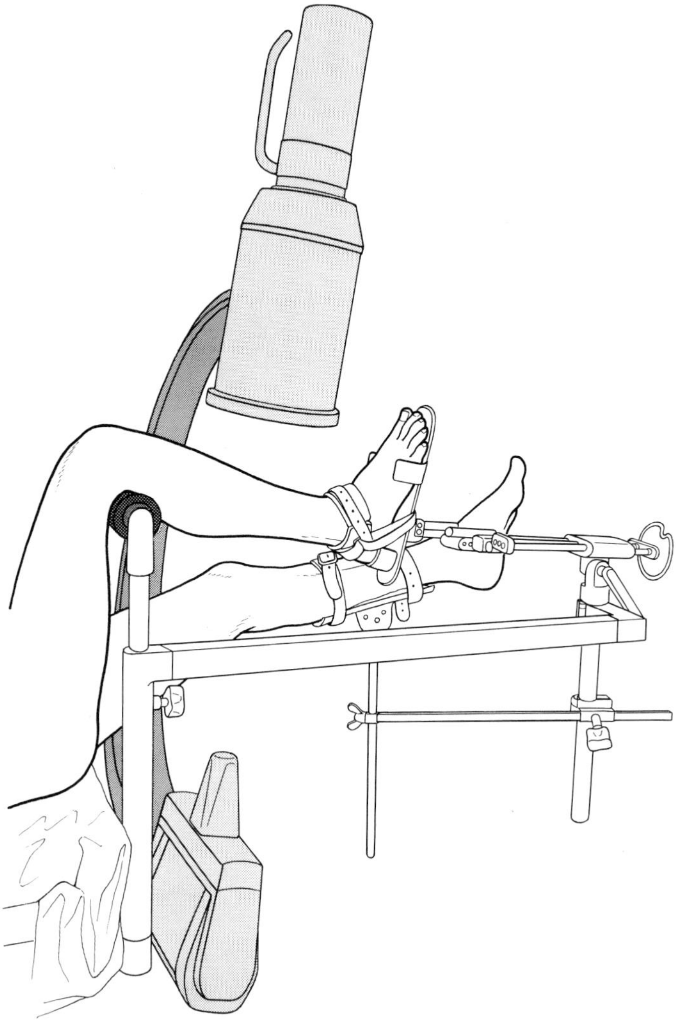

Figure 48 The position for tibial nailing with the image intensifier for AP fluoroscopy.

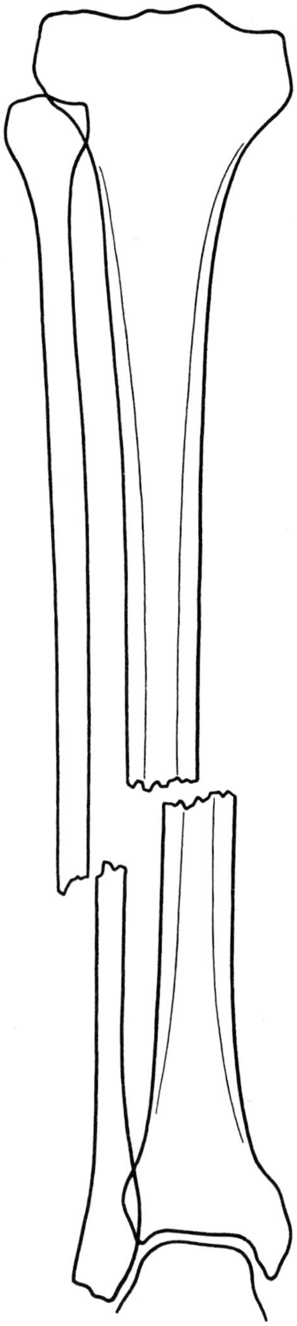

Figure 49 Displaced lower leg fracture, AP view.

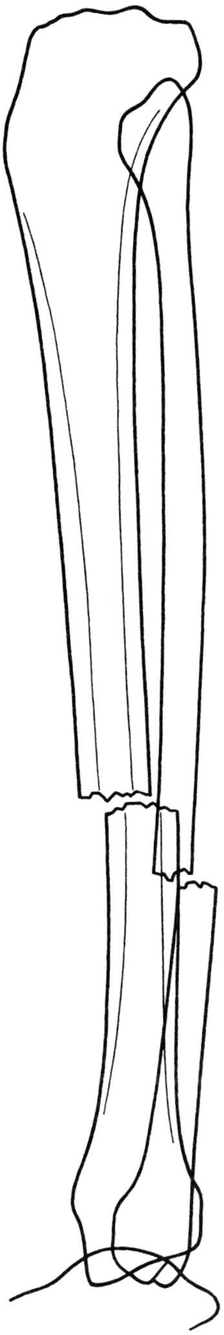

Figure 50 The same fracture, lateral view.

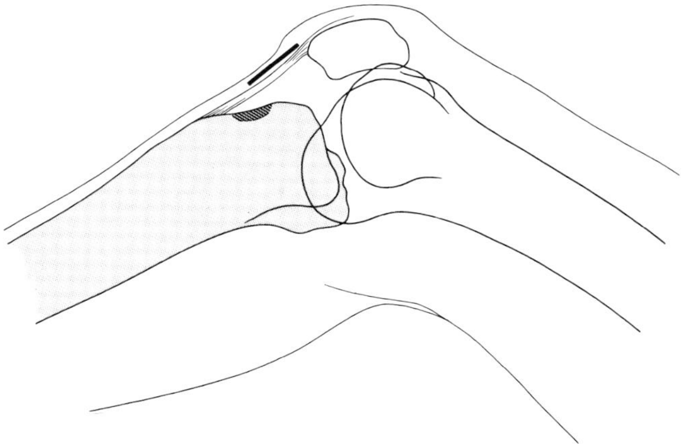

Figure 51 Stab incision and the nail entry point for tibial nailing.

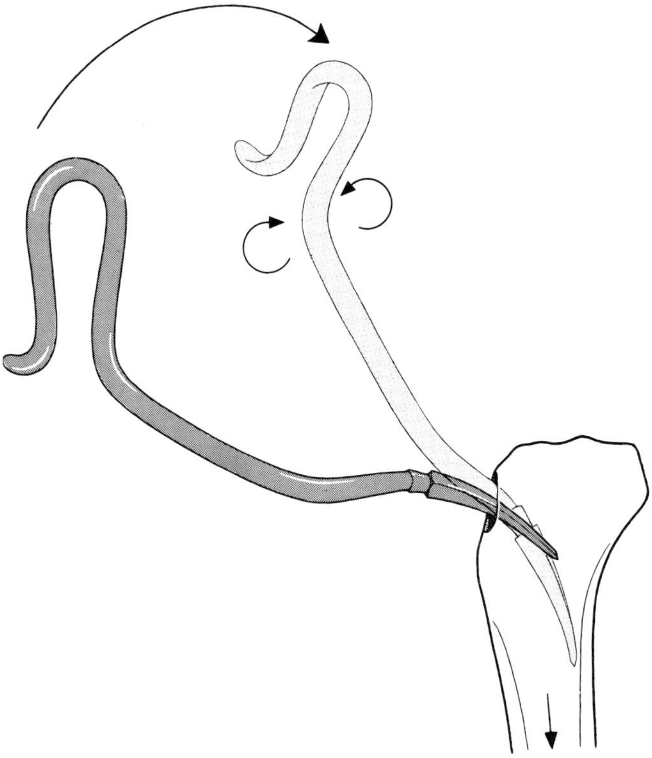

Figure 52 Opening of the medullary canal with the tibial awl for the tibial nailing.

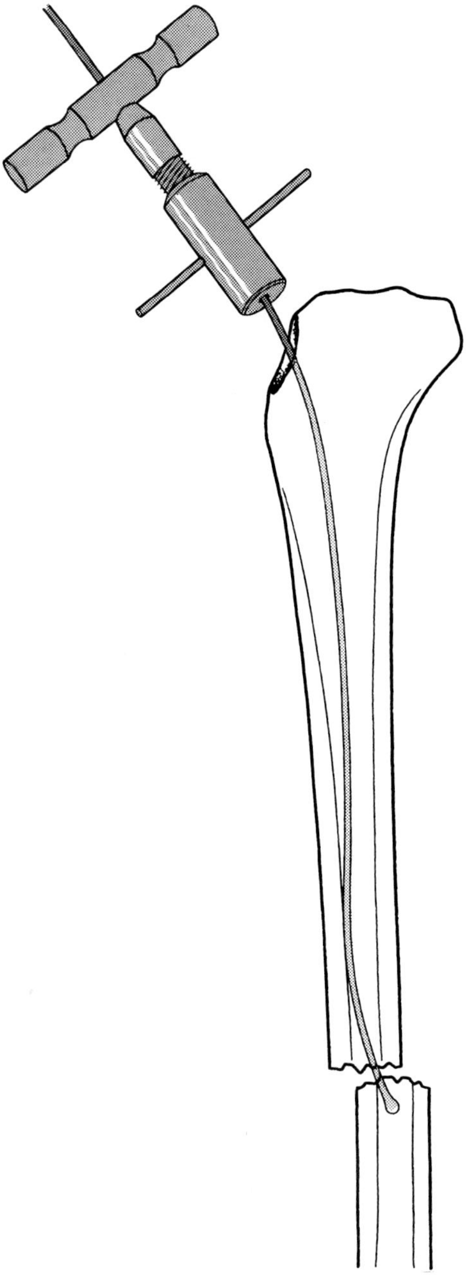

Figure 53 Final reduction of a tibial fracture with a ball-point guide pin.

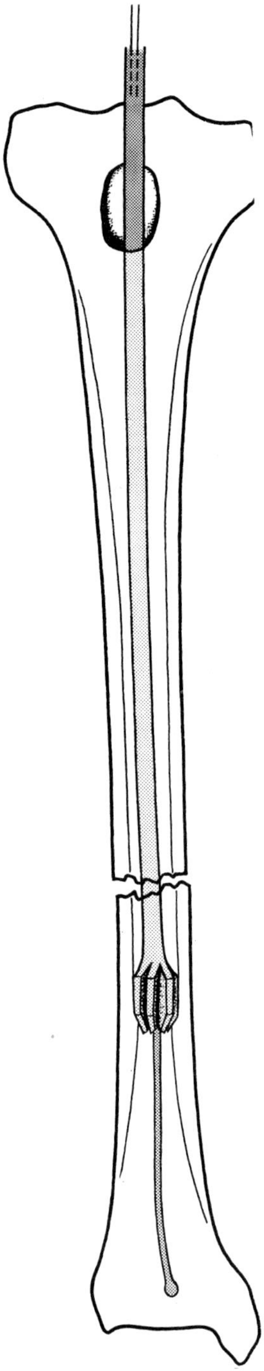

Figure 54 Reaming of the medullary canal, using the guided flexible cannulated reamer over the guide pin, AP view.

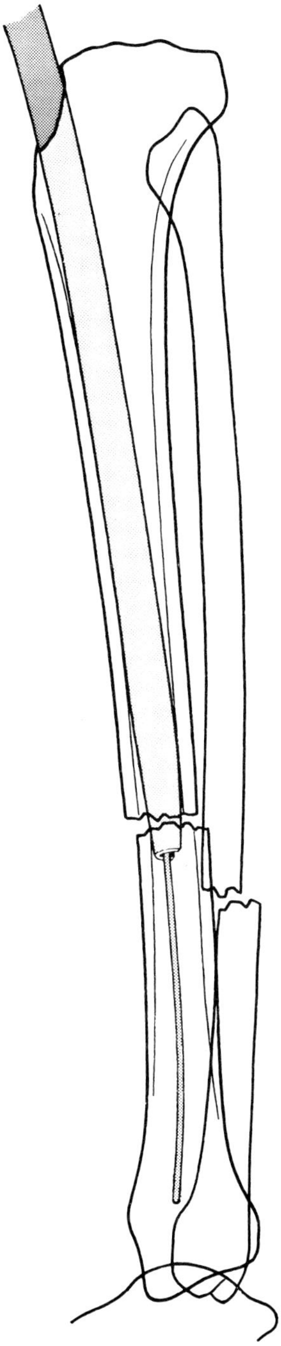

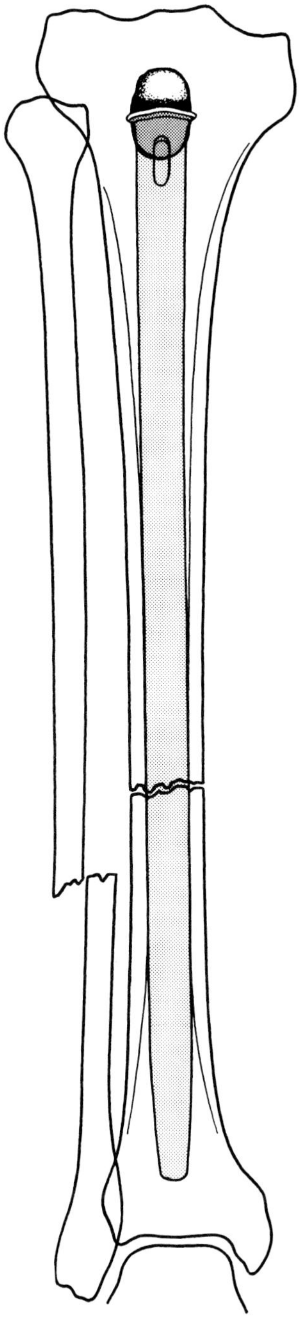

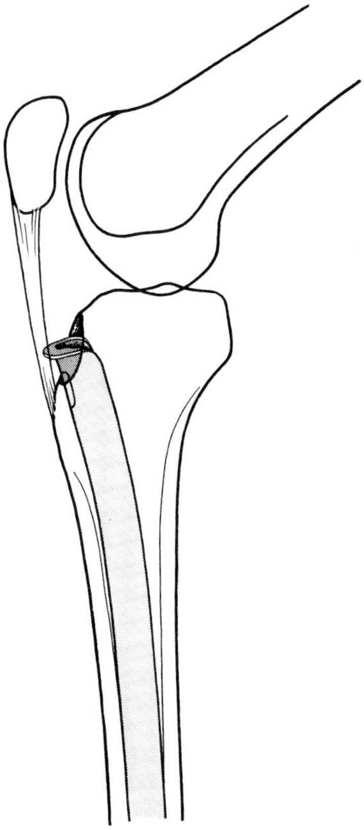

Figure 57 The sinking of the nail lip under the patellar ligament.

Figure 55 Driving the tibial nail over the guide, lateral view.

Figure 56 Completed tibial nailing.

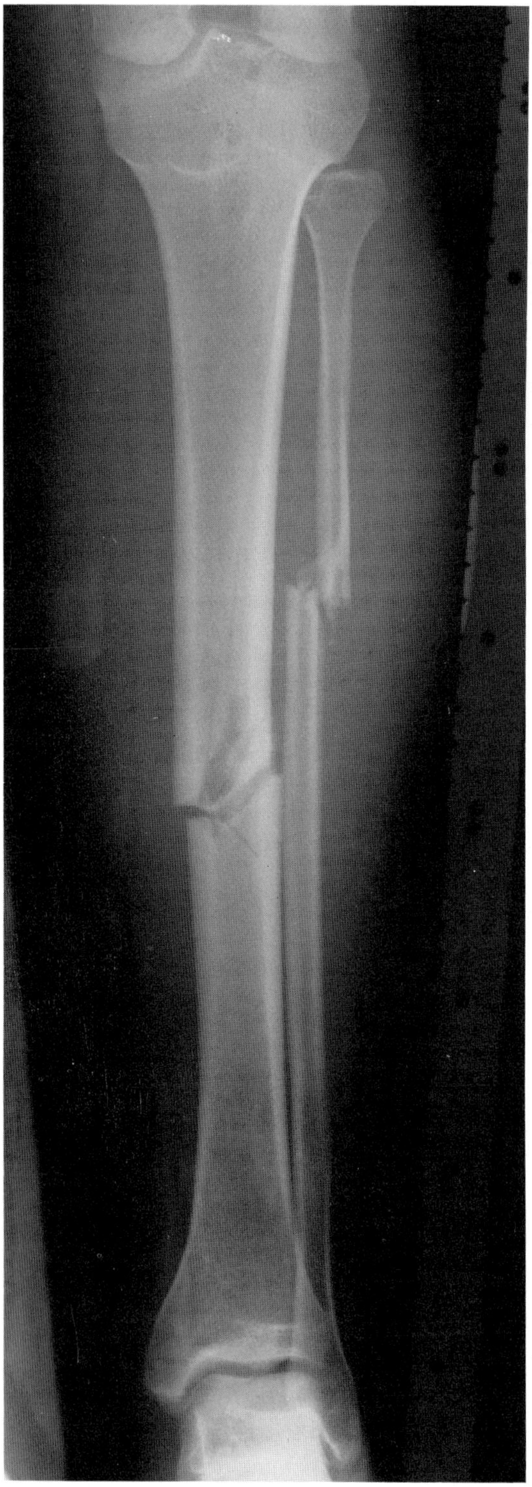

Figure 58 Fresh shaft fractures of the tibia and fibula, with a small wedge-shaped fragment of the tibia. AP view with the x-ray scale exposed in the same plane for the determination of the correct nail dimensions.

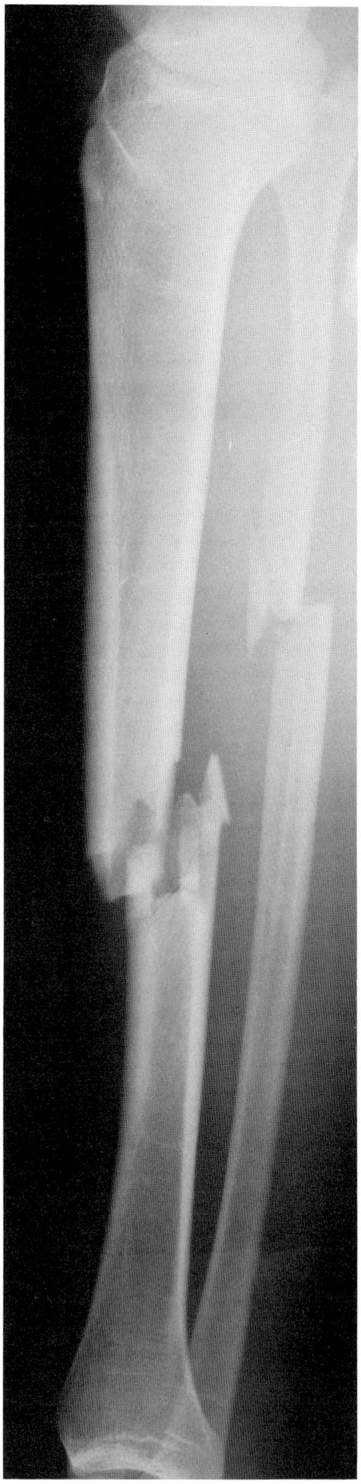

Figure 59 The same fractures in lateral view; the x-ray scale is simultaneously exposed in front of the tibia.

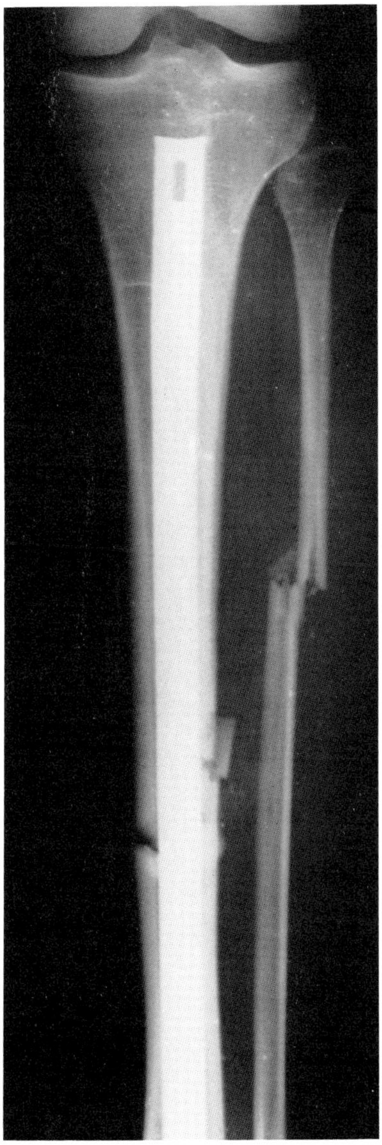

Figure 60 The same fractures after Küntscher tibial nailing, AP view.

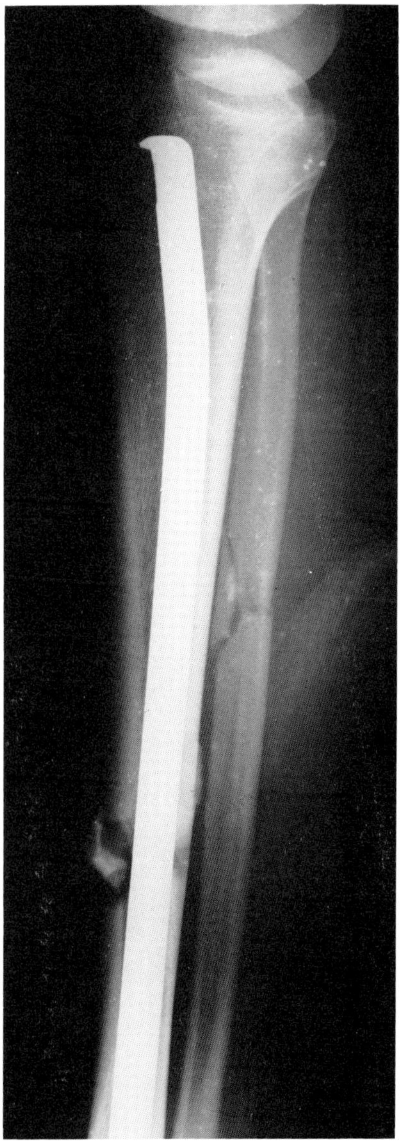

Figure 61 The same fractures in lateral view after tibial nailing. A wedge-shaped fragment of the tibia is rotated. This is of no significance if sufficient soft tissue coverage exists.

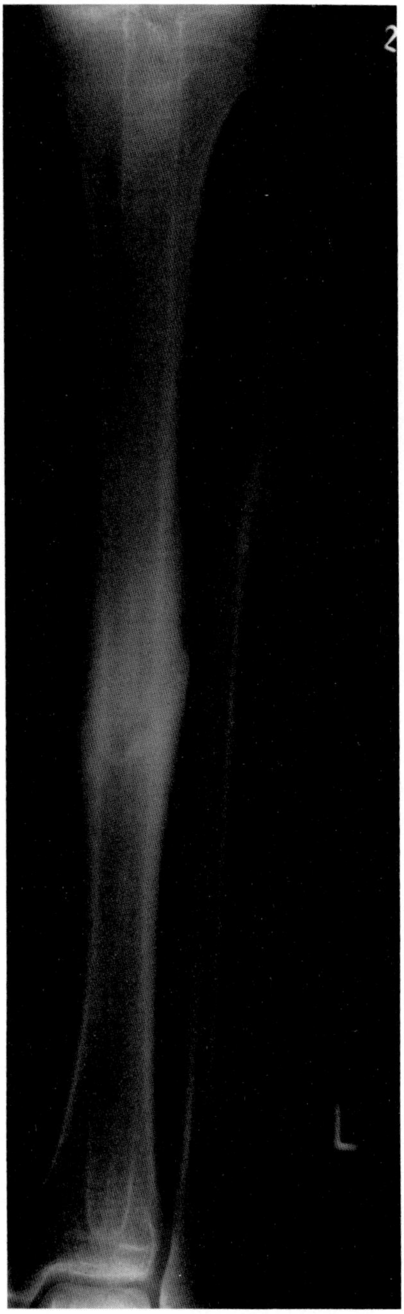

Figure 62 The same fractures, eight months post-operatively, following nail removal, AP view.

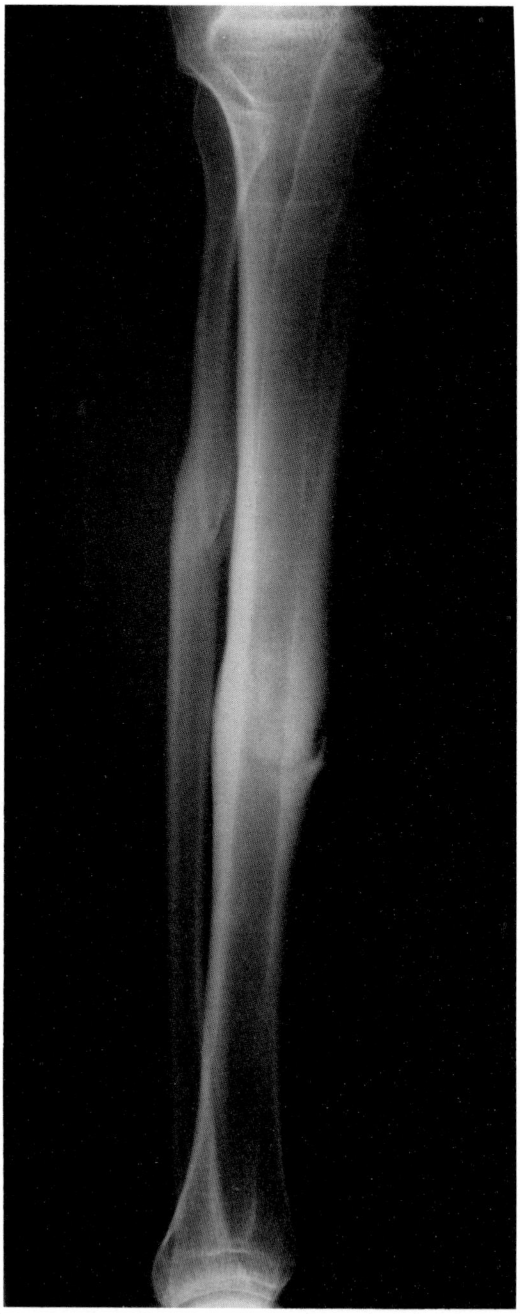

Figure 63 Lateral view after bony healing and nail removal. The rotated tibial fragment is fused with the callus.

Intramedullary Nailing of the Humerus

Indications

The intramedullary nailing of the humerus is indicated in transverse fractures, either with or without small wedge-shaped fragments in the area of the diaphysis. It is important to ensure that the width of the medullary canal allows for locking on both sides of the fracture. The two possible entry points for humerus nailing are (1) the proximal entry point, at the head of the humerus, and (2) the distal entry point, at the dorsal aspect, proximal to the fossa olecrani at the end of the medullary canal. One should always choose the entry point farthest away from the fracture.

Positioning and Reduction

The nailing of the humerus from the proximal entry point can be done with the patient supine on a regular operating table. The shoulder of the injured arm must be positioned as far over the edge of the table as needed to make fluoroscopy of the arm possible. The hand of the injured arm must be laid on the uninvolved shoulder. Pull the flexed elbow with countertraction on the armpit to reduce the fracture. The upper arm is held beyond the edge of the table for fluoroscopy.

The nailing of the humerus through the distal entry point can also be done with the patient positioned on his healthy side on the fracture table. The reduction is accomplished via skeletal traction through the olecranon and countertraction on the armpit. Fluoroscopy in two planes must be possible. The reduction of fractures of the humerus is seldom problematic.

Image Intensification

Preoperative roentgenograms in two planes comprising the entire humerus should be taken at a 1-m distance for gauging purposes. With the patient supine, the image intensifier is positioned on the injured side of the patient perpendicular to the operating table. The image intensifier is positioned parallel to the longitudinal axis of the patient if he is positioned on his healthy side. Postoperative roentgenograms of the entire humerus in two planes should be taken.

Operative Technique from Proximal

A stab incision is made laterally over the humeral head, just distal to the acromion, while the patient's involved hand is positioned on his uninvolved shoulder. The medullary canal is opened in this position by the proper awl, inserted at the major tubercle near the anatomic collar of the humerus. The awl is withdrawn and exchanged for a guide pin. The surgeon's unencumbered hand ventrally secures the involved humerus. The guide pin is aimed at the middle of the elbow joint. The guide pin is then advanced with rotational and, if necessary, tapping movements up to the fracture. The guide pin's position in the proximal fragment is verified by fluoroscopy in two planes. After the fracture is reduced, the guide pin's advance into the distal fragment is monitored by fluoroscopy in two planes. The entry point can be enlarged by the reamer awl positioned over the guide pin. If a smooth guide pin (i.e., without a ball-point) was used for the reduction, a ball-point guide pin should be inserted into the distal fragment, and thereafter the original smooth guide pin should be withdrawn. This maneuver should be monitored by image intensifier. Ream the medullary canal with flexible guided reamers in 0.5-mm increments until the desired width is reached. The chosen nail should be 0.5 mm smaller than the largest reamer head used. Proper guidance of the nail tip over the smooth guide pin should be checked prior to insertion. The humeral nails are identical to the tibial nails. Carefully drive the nail over the guide. The passage of the nail tip into the distal fragment must be monitored by fluoroscopy in two planes. The intramedullary nail is driven until the end of the nail is flush with the bone at the entry portal. The guide pin is removed, and the incision is closed.

Operative Technique from Distal

The distal entry point lies just proximal to the fossa olecrani on the dorsal aspect of the humerus. The skin incision is 3 cm long and the triceps tendon is split longitudinally. Expose the humerus. Drill a hole at the distal end of the medullary canal in midline with a 3.2 mm (1/8″) twist-drill bit, held perpendicularly to the long bone. The drill hole is enlarged by tilting the drill toward the elbow. After the fracture is reduced, a guide pin is advanced through the distal fragment under image intensification. Ream the medullary canal with a guided flexible reamer in 0.5-mm increments until the desired diameter is reached. Carefully drive the nail over the guide. The nail must be pushed toward the distal fragment during the driving process in order to avoid splitting the bone. The passage of the nail tip into the proximal fragment is verified by fluoroscopy. The nail is driven in as deeply as possible. No ill efeects are caused if the end of the nail protrudes a few millimeters out of the entry site. Remove the guide and close the incision.

Special Technique for the Elderly

Because the intramedullary nail can be permanently left in place in the elderly, proximal fractures are nailed with a straight nail, affording an atypical entry point. The patient is positioned supine, as already described. The skin incision is made over the middle of the humeral head, directly ventral to the acromion. Drive a sharp guide pin through the middle of the humeral head and advance the pin into the distal fragment under image intensification. The entry point is widened by the reamer awl, and a wedge-shaped fragment is cut out from the ventral edge of the acromion. Reaming of the medullary canal is unnecessary in the elderly. Drive the chosen nail, which should just pass through the narrowest portion of the medullary canal, over the nail driving pin. Withdraw the guide. The nail should be driven with a nail set until it is flush with the humeral head and does not protrude. Close the incision.

Common Mistakes

If the entry point is distal to the major tubercle, the reamer eats the lateral cortex away, and the nail hits the contralateral cortex, causing the bone to crack. If the wrong entry point is chosen, intramedullary nailing through the proximal entry point is impossible. The situation is rectified by making the correct entry point. If the nail directly hits the contralateral cortex, despite the correct entry point, the tip of the nail must be slightly bent with a nail bender in order to avoid splitting the bone. If the nail is driven in from the distal entry point, the bone may split if the entry point is not sufficiently oblique.

Aftercare

Special aftercare is unnecessary. Active exercises can be started either immediately postoperatively or in a few days, depending on the condition of the soft tissue.

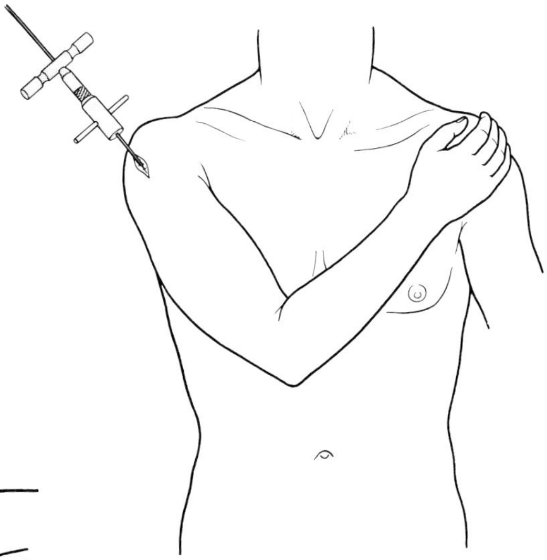

Figure 65 The correct position of the patient and the stab incision for the humeral nailing from proximal entry.

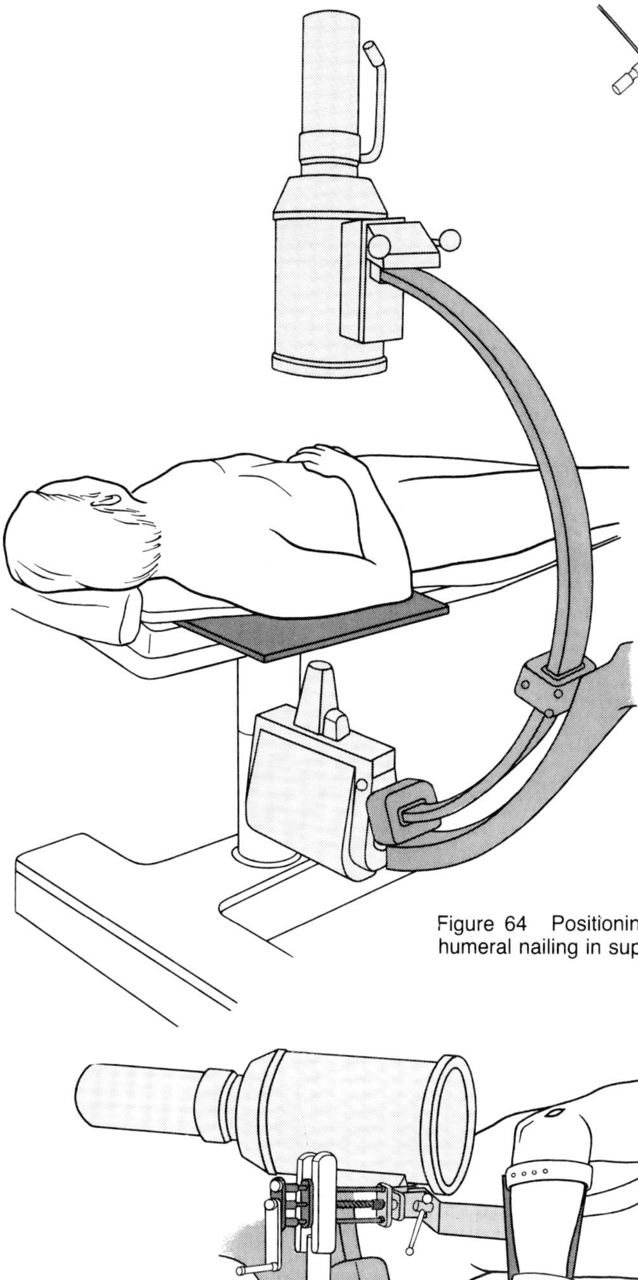

Figure 64 Positioning of the patient and the image intensifier for the humeral nailing in supine position.

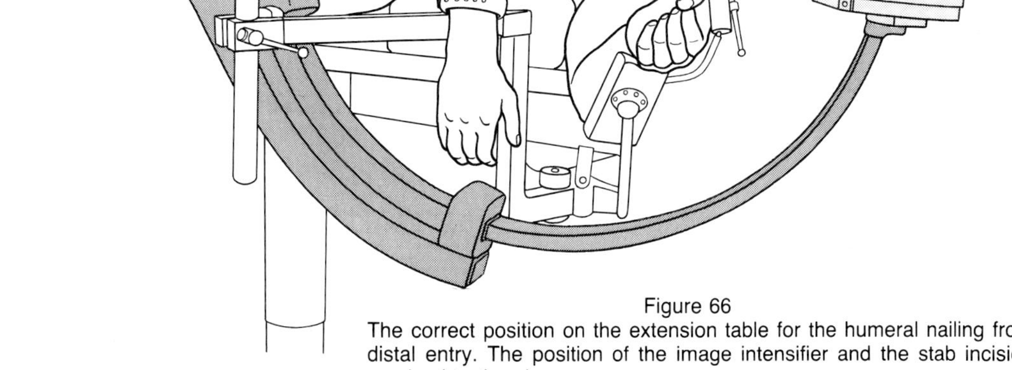

Figure 66
The correct position on the extension table for the humeral nailing from distal entry. The position of the image intensifier and the stab incision proximal to the olecranon.

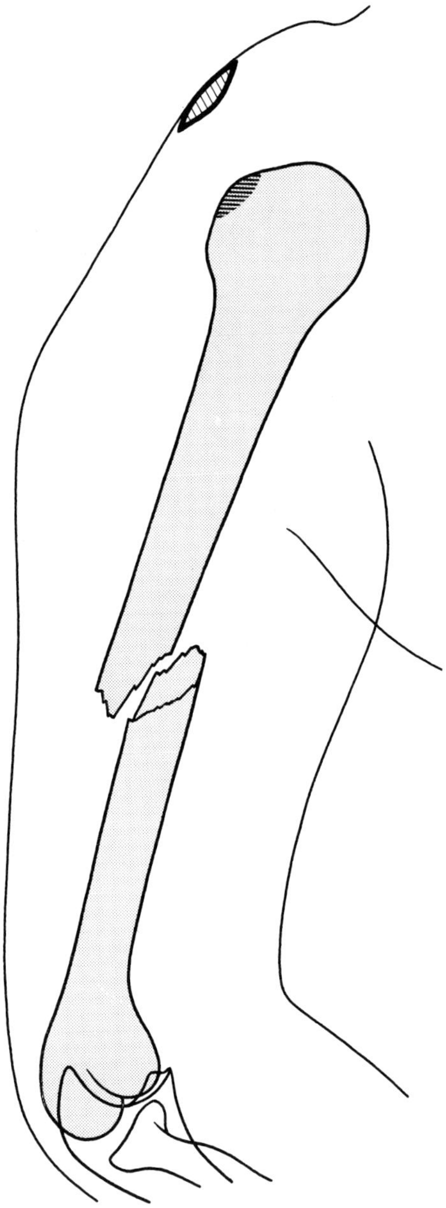

Figure 67 Fracture of the humeral shaft. Stab incision and nail entry point.

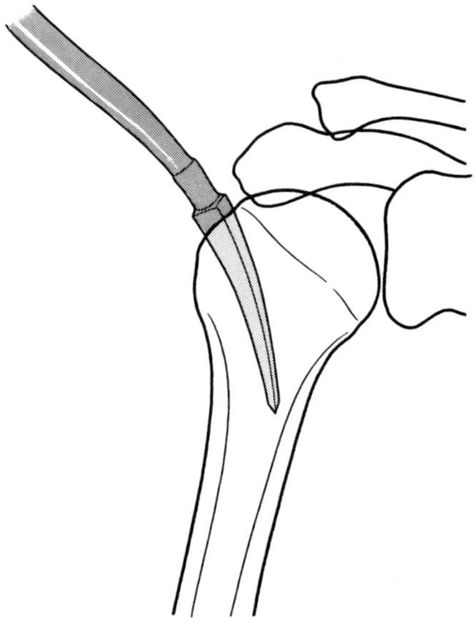

Figure 68 Humeral fracture. The opening of the medullary canal with an awl for the nailing from proximal.

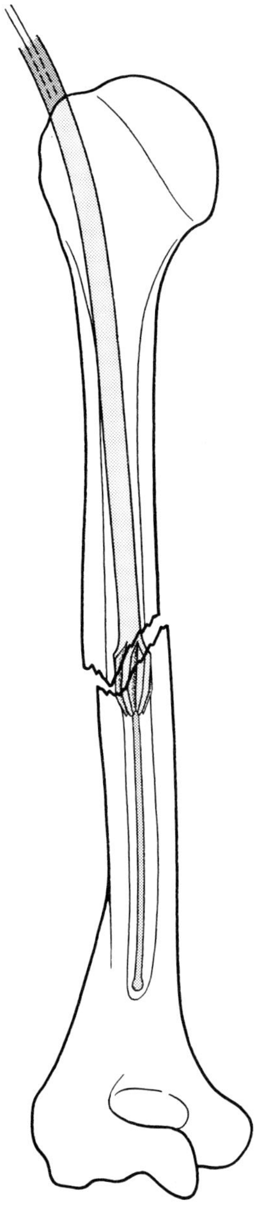

Figure 69 The reaming of the medullary canal over the ball-point guide pin from proximal.

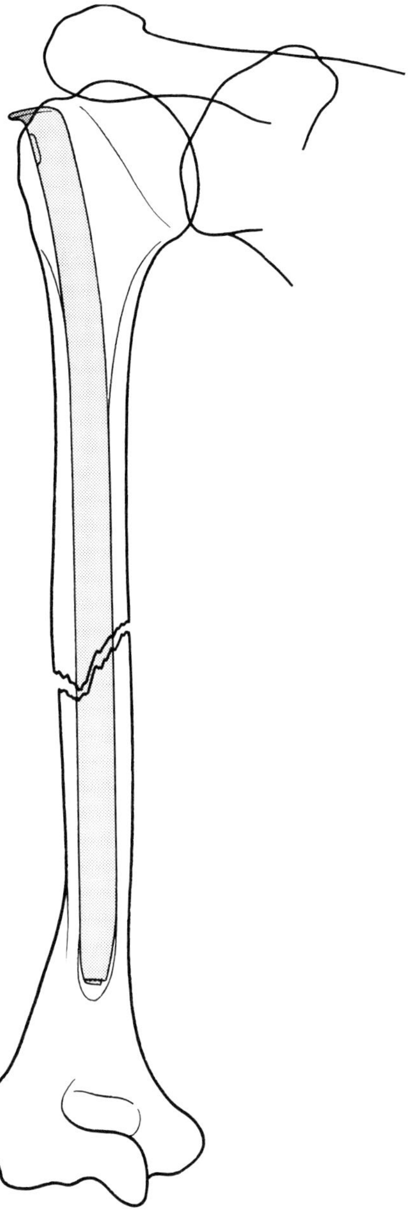

Figure 70 Completed humeral nailing from proximal, AP view.

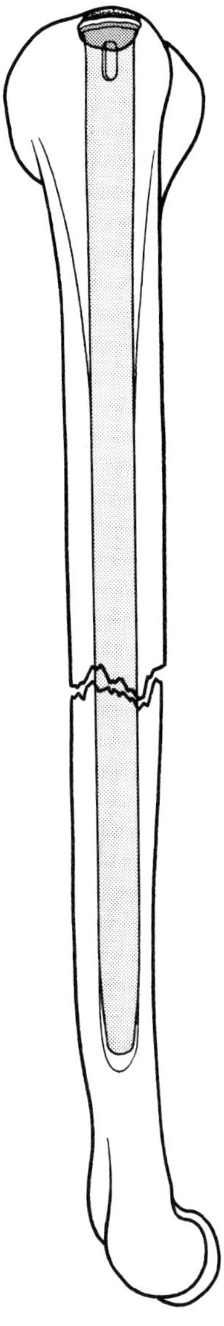

Figure 71 Completed humeral nailing from proximal, lateral view.

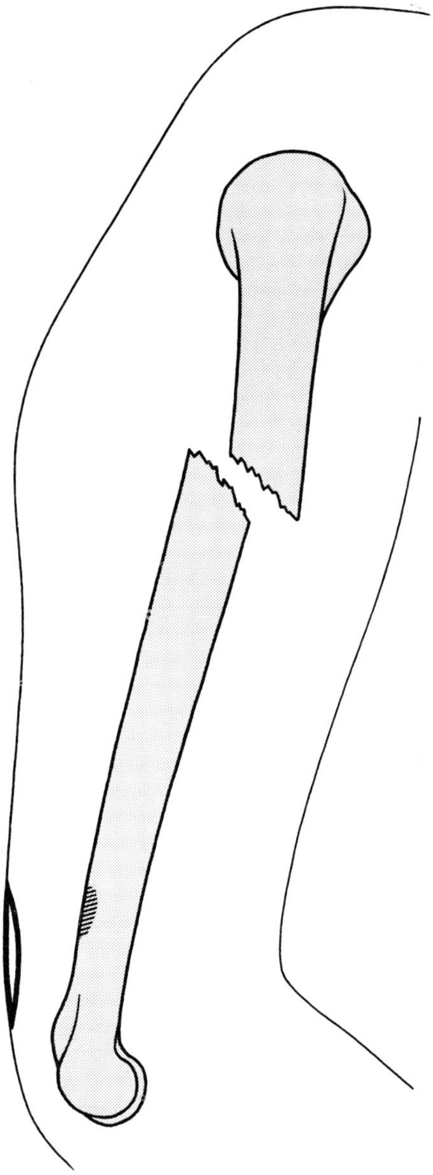

Figure 72 Humeral fracture, proximal third. Stab incision and nail entry point for the nailing from distal.*

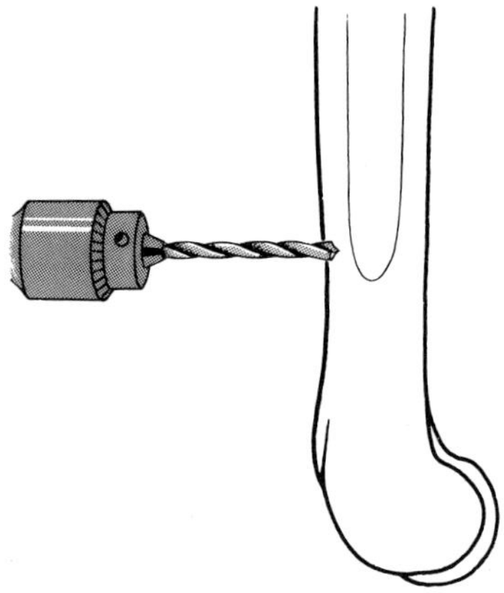

Figure 73 Drilling a starter hole at the nail entry point for the nailing from distal entry.

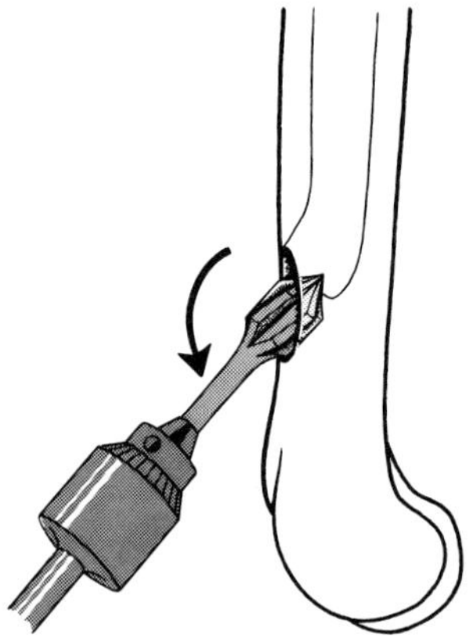

Figure 74 Enlarging the nail entry point with a tapered cortical reamer for the nailing from distal.

*Note: The original thesis recommended the entry point to be made at the proximal end of the fossa olecrani. H.K.

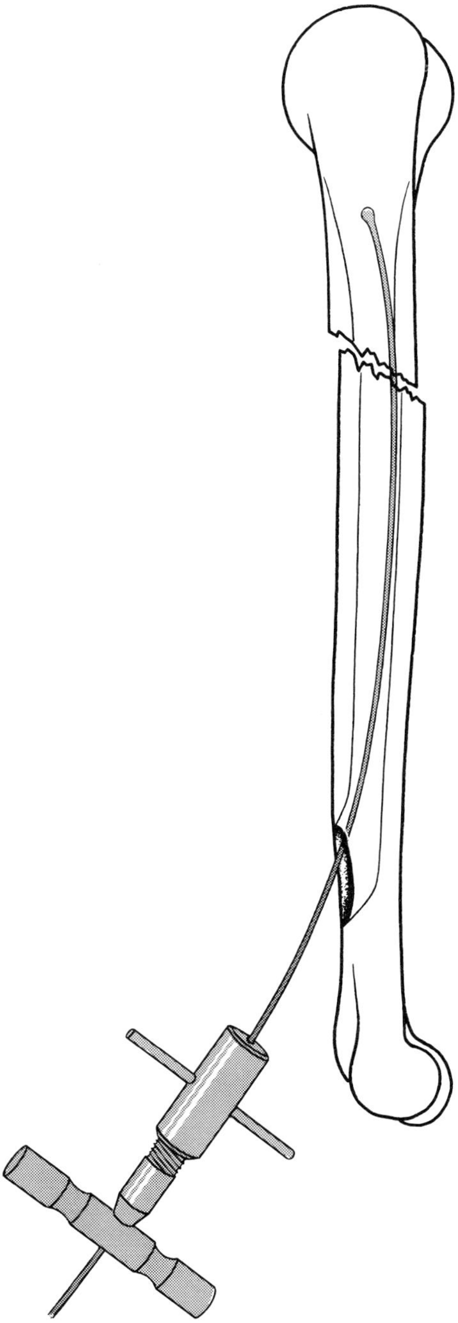

Figure 75 Humeral fracture, proximal third, after reduction and the positioning of the guide pin from distal into both fragments.

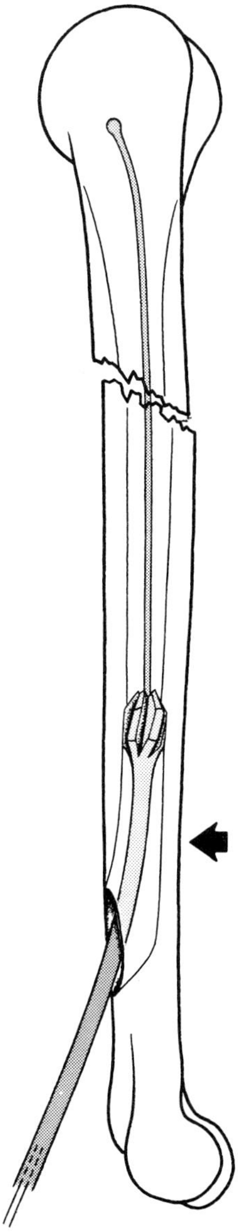

Figure 76 The reaming of the medullary canal from distal over the positioned guide pin. Note the indicated point of possible bone splitting, if the nail entry portal is too narrow.

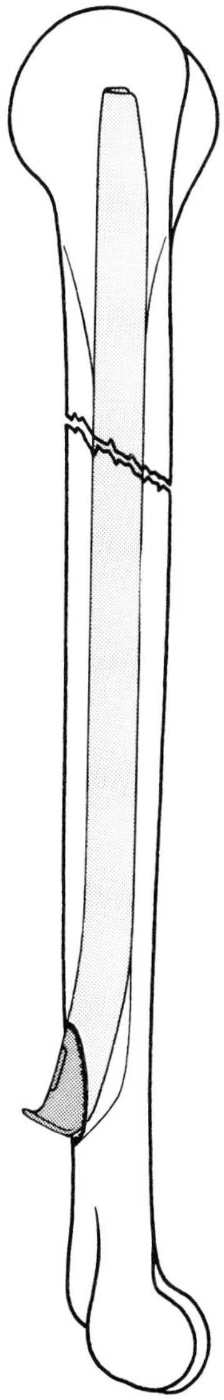

Figure 77 Completed humeral nailing of the fracture in the proximal third from distal, lateral view.

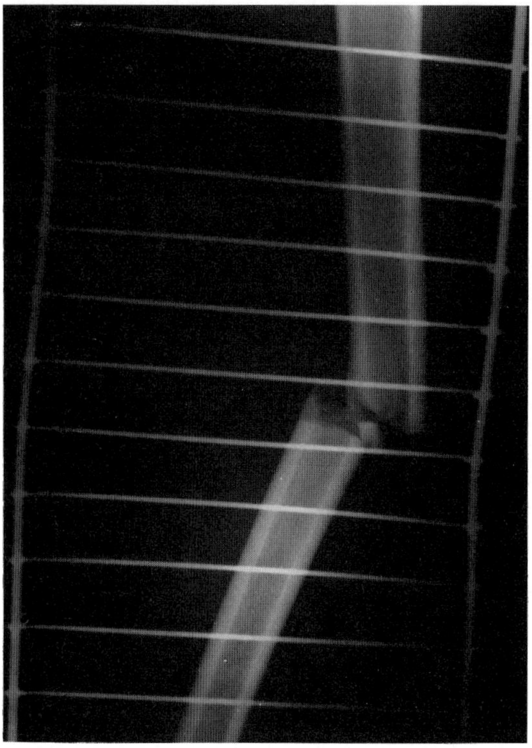

Figure 78 Fresh fracture of the humerus, cropped, AP view.

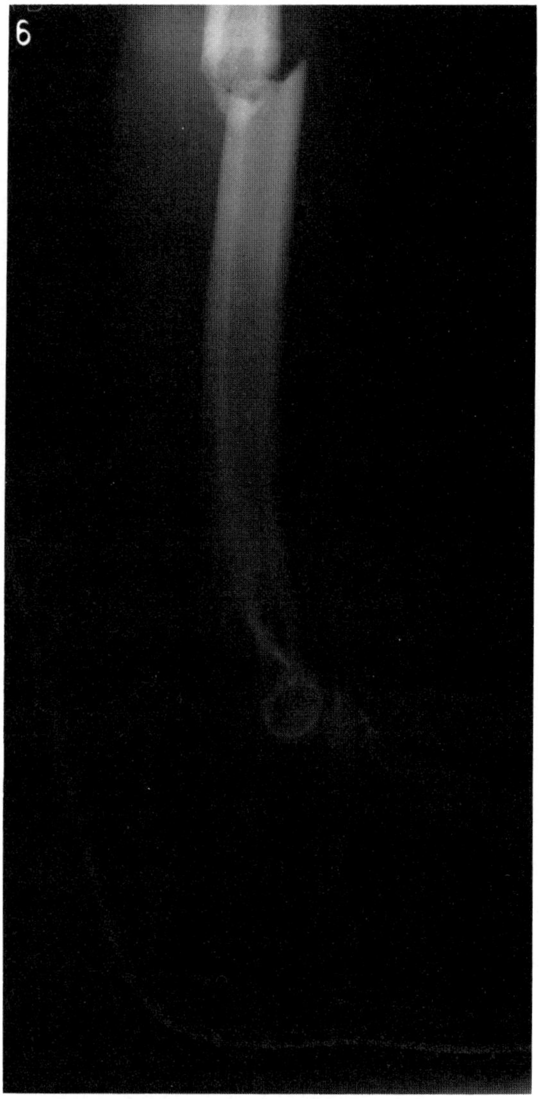

Figure 79 Lateral view of the fresh humeral fracture.

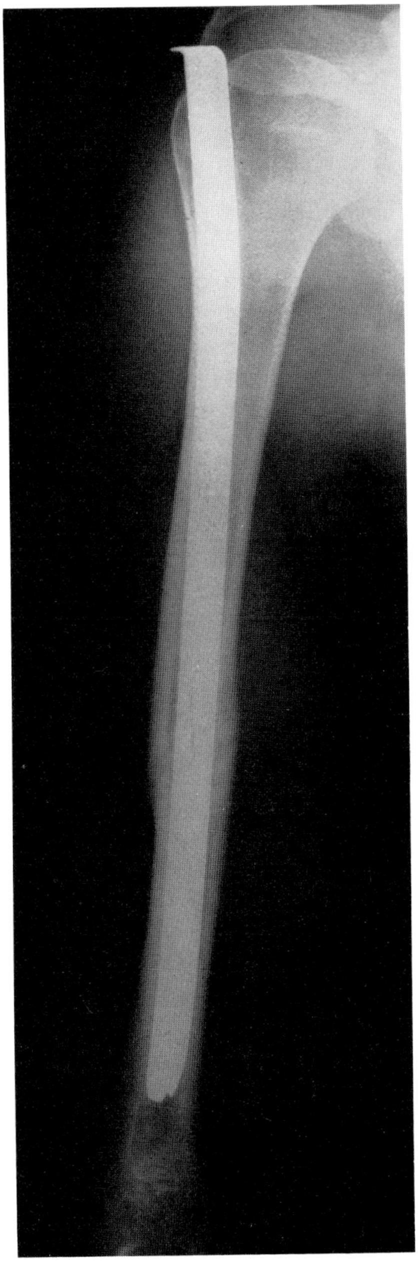

Figure 80 The same humeral fracture, five months after the accident, and the nailing from proximal, AP view. Bone healing completed.

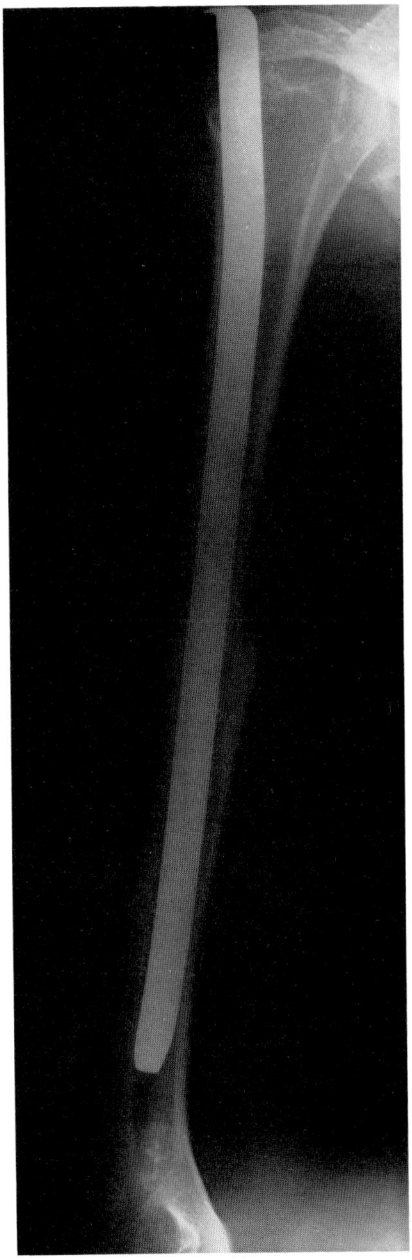

Figure 81 Lateral view, five months after the nailing from proximal.

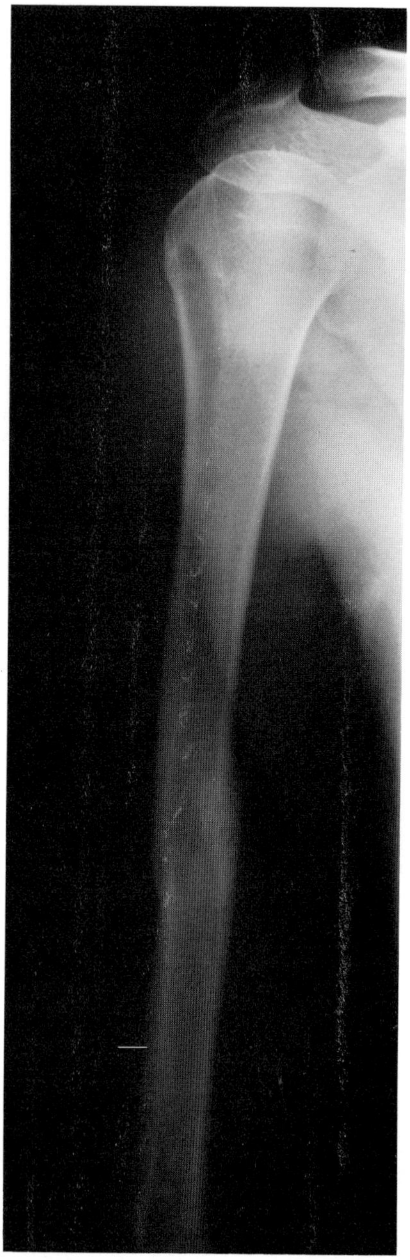

Figure 82 Completed bony healing after nail removal, seven months after the accident, AP view.

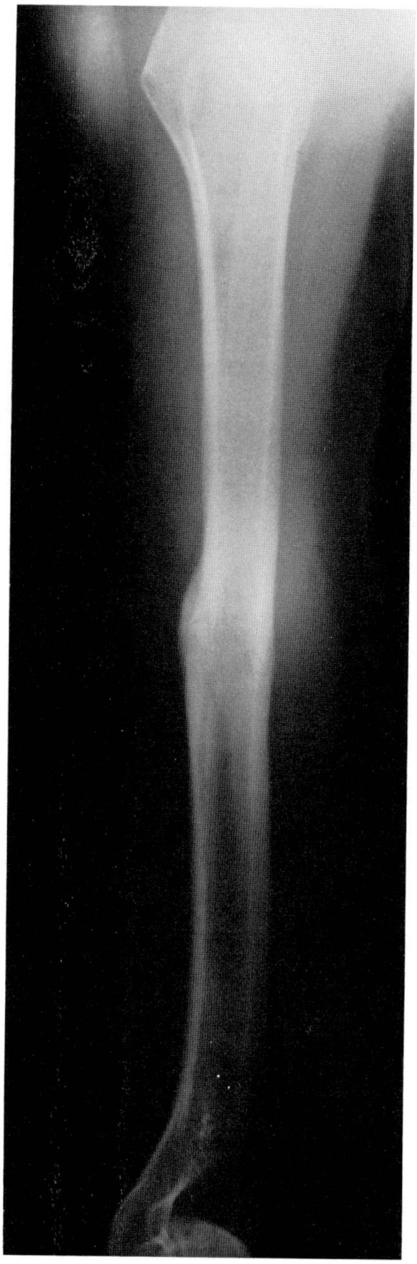

Figure 83 Lateral view after nail removal.

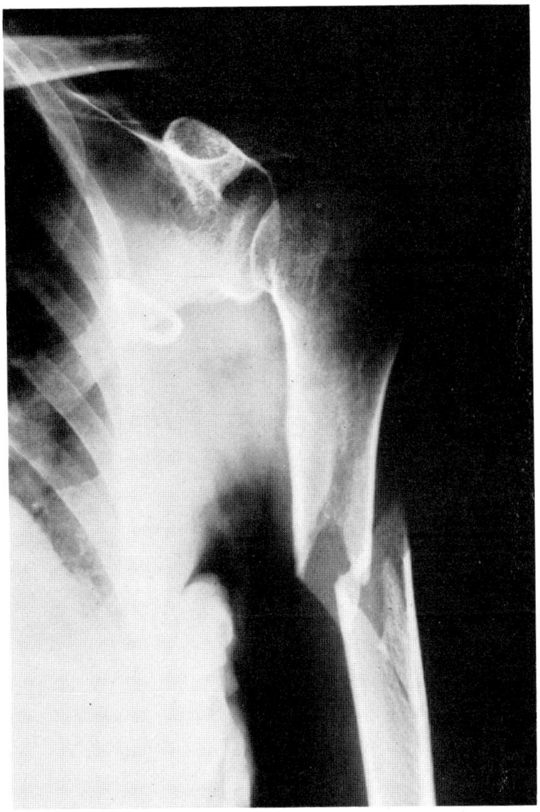

Figure 84 Humeral fracture, proximal third, AP view.

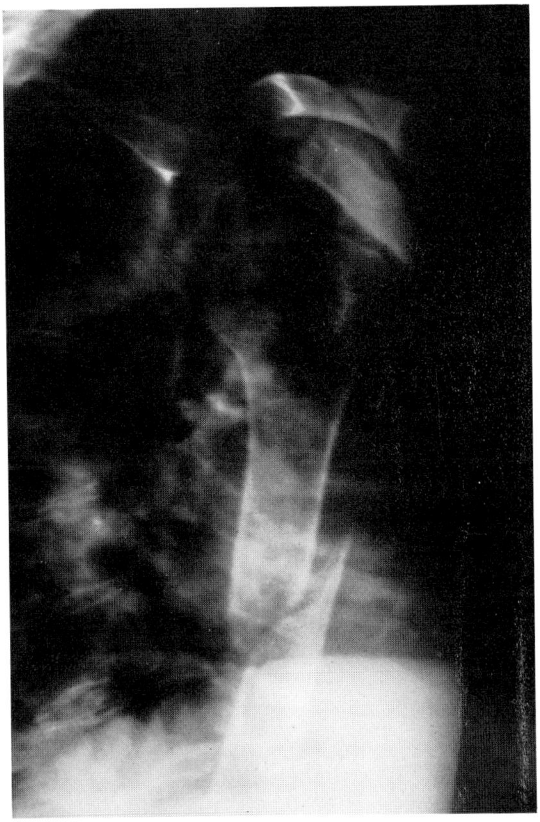

Figure 85 Lateral view of the proximal humeral fracture, exposed through the chest.

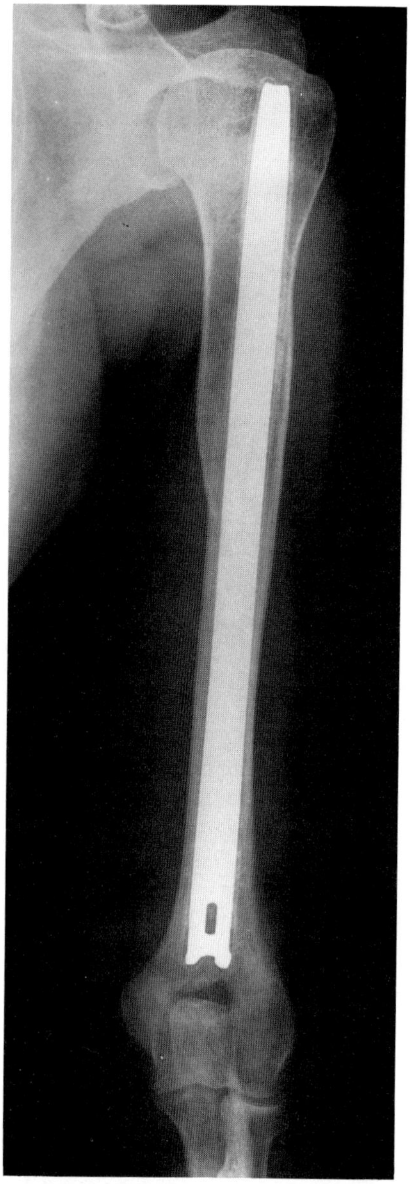

Figure 86 The same nailed humeral fracture, bony healing completed after 18 months, AP view.

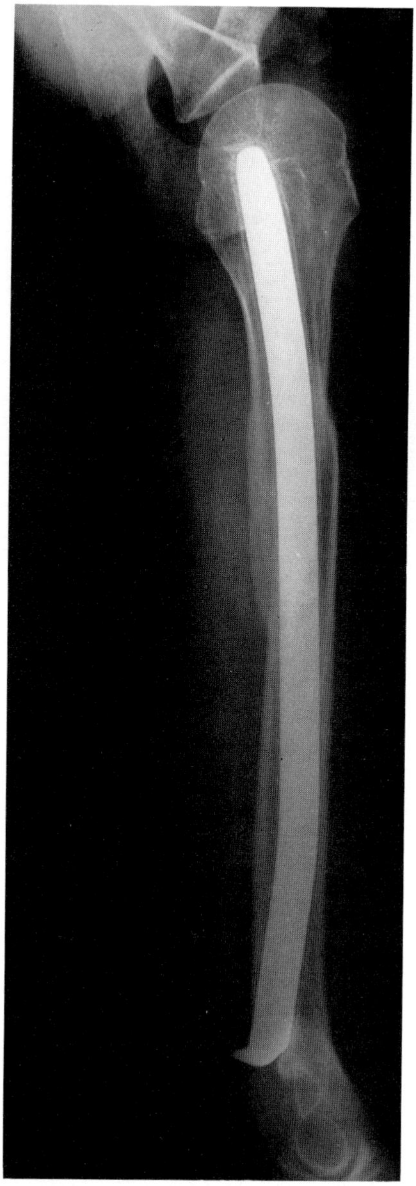

Figure 87 Lateral view of the humeral fracture, proximal third, nailed from distal, after 18 months.

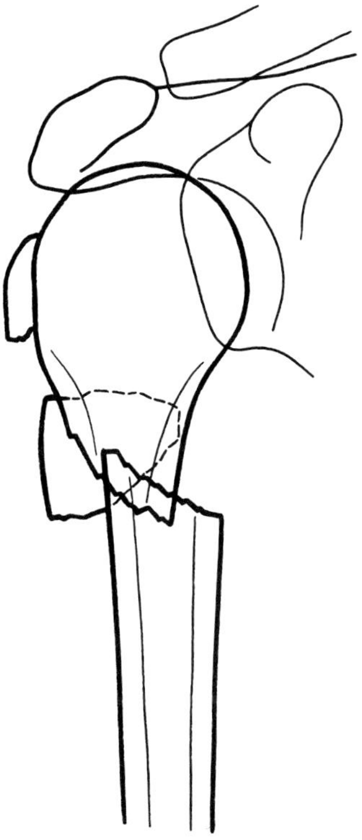

Figure 88 Comminuted subcapital fracture of humerus, AP view.

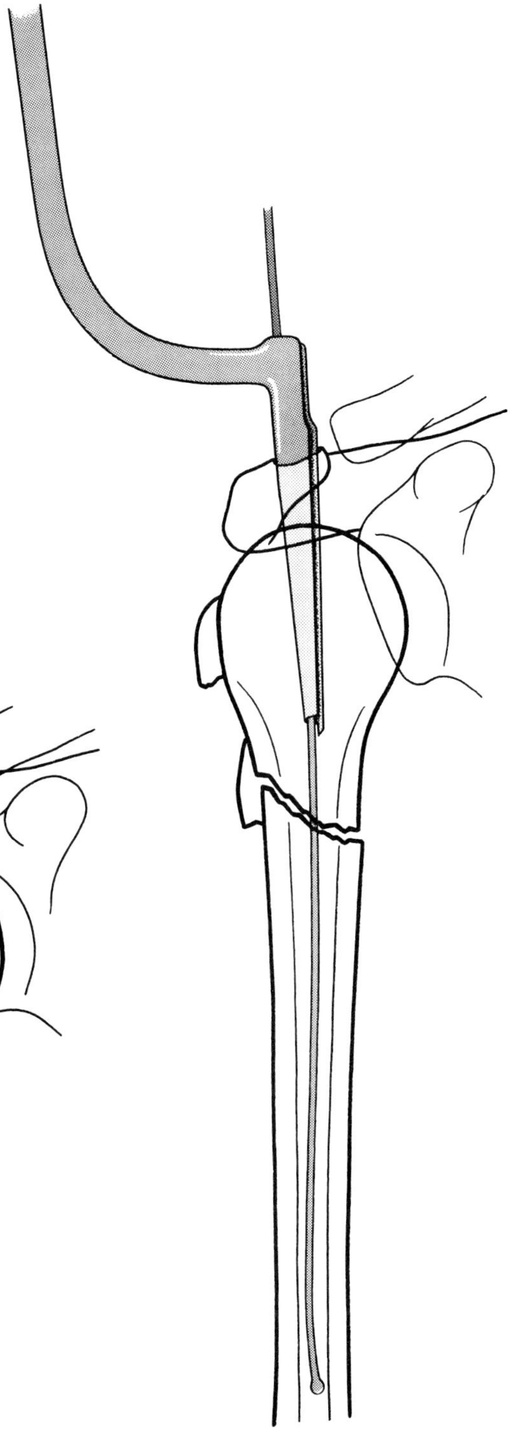

Figure 89 The condition after the reduction of the comminuted subcapital humeral fracture. The non-typical nail entry portal is enlarged with a reamer awl over the guide pin through the acromion into the center of the humeral head.

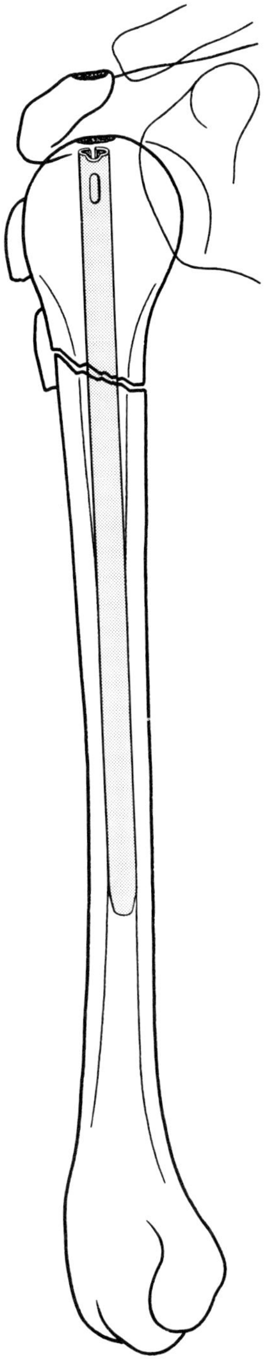

Figure 90 Completed nailing of the comminuted subcapital humeral fracture with a buried straight nail.

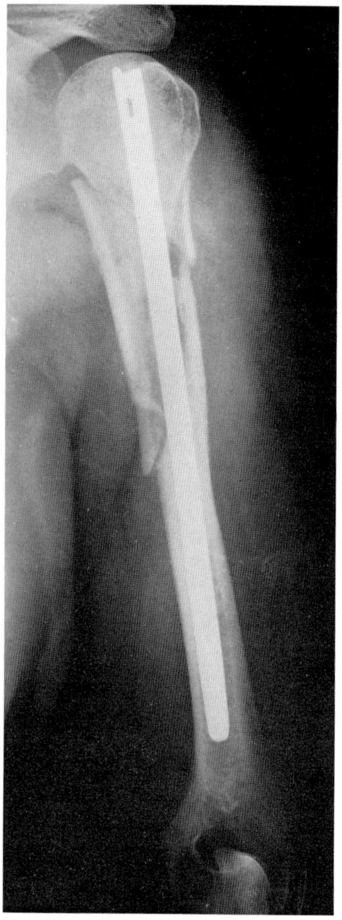

Figure 91 Comminuted subcapital humeral fracture in a 75-year-old patient after the straight nail is buried, AP view.

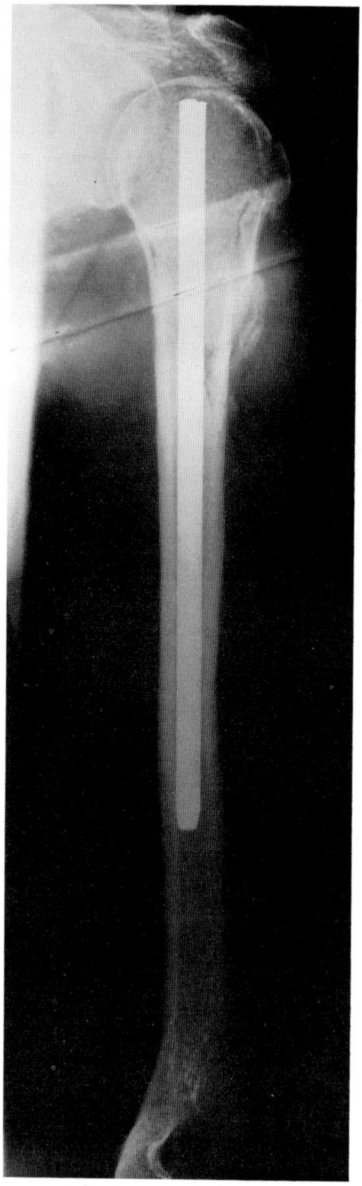

Figure 92 The same fracture showing bony healing one year later.

Intramedullary Nailing of the Forearm

Intramedullary Nailing of the Radius

Indications

Intramedullary nailing is indicated in all transverse and short spiral fractures, excluding those in the proximal fourth and the distal third of the radius.

Positioning and Reduction

In all forearm nailings, the upper arm is abducted at a right angle from the trunk, and the forearm is positioned on a radiolucent extension of the normal operating table or on an auxiliary table.

The reduction of a displaced radial fracture can usually be accomplished by traction at the hand and elbow, possibly with pronating and supinating movements. Should the reduction not be possible despite these maneuvers, a distractor should be applied for a few days. The proximal skeletal pin should be inserted perpendicularly through the ulna, 3 to 4 cm distal to the olecranon. The distal skeletal pin should pierce the distal radius in an AP direction. The wrist joint must be extremely palmar flexed and angulated toward the ulna. The styloid process of the radius becomes easily palpable in this position.

Image Intensification

Preoperative roentgenograms should be taken of the forearm and its adjacent joints in two planes at a 1-m distance. These films can serve as gauges for the determination of the correct nail and reamer dimensions. The image intensifier is moved under the arm extension from the side. Postoperative roentgenograms should be taken of the entire forearm in two planes.

Operative Technique

A stab incision is made over the styloid process of the radius at the radial edge. At this point the awl is used to open the medullary canal. A small ball-point guide pin, which is usually slightly angulated at its tip, is inserted into the distal fragment. After reduction, the guide pin is advanced into the proximal fragment under fluoroscopy. The guided flexible reamer enlarges the medullary canal to the predetermined width in 0.5-mm increments. One should exchange the ball-point guide pin for a thin smooth nail driving guide by inserting the smooth guide first and then withdrawing the ball-point guide pin. If the radius is nailed in the distractor, the distractor can be removed after the introduction of the small smooth nail driving guide. Once the nail tip of the chosen V-nail has been bent slightly toward the guide pin, drive the nail over the guide pin into the distal fragment. The end of the distal nail is then bent into the shape of the distal radius. Withdraw the guide and close the incision.

Common Mistakes

(See the Intramedullary Nailing of Fractures in the Forearm [Radius and Ulna].)

Intramedullary Nailing of the Ulna

Indications

Transverse and short spiral fractures of the ulna from the coronoid process up to the distal fourth of the ulna are indications for this procedure. The two possible entry points are (1) the proximal entry point, in the middle of the olecranon, and (2) the distal entry point, directly medial to the styloid process of the ulna. The entry point of choice is the one farther from the fracture site.

Positioning and Reduction

The positioning and reduction of the ulnar fractures are as described for radial fractures. Once again, the reduction, on rare occasions, may not be immediately possible, and a distractor must be used for a few days. The distractor is positioned as described for radial fractures.

Image Intensification

Image intensification is the same as for radial fractures.

Operative Technique

Nailing through the proximal entry portal is performed through a longitudinal skin incision over the middle of the olecranon. The medullary canal is opened with an awl. After reduction, a small ball-point guide pin is inserted through the proximal fragment under fluoroscopy into the distal fragment. Ream the medullary canal in 0.5-mm increments until the desired width is reached. If a V-nail is used, the ball-point guide pin should be exchanged for a smooth nail driving guide pin by first inserting the smooth guide pin and then withdrawing the ball-point guide pin.

The chosen V-nail is then driven into the medullary canal. A cloverleaf nail with a small diameter may also be used in the nailing of ulnar fractures. In this case, a changing of the guide pin is unnecessary. Withdraw the guide pin and close the incision.

Nailing through the distal entry point is accomplished by palmar flexing the wrist maximally and making the stab incision directly over the styloid process. Thereafter, the same operative technique is used as described for the nailing through the proximal entry portal. However, the distractor, if used, should be removed after the guide pin has been inserted.

Common Mistakes

(See the Intramedullary Nailing of Fractures in the Forearm [Radius and Ulna].)

Intramedullary Nailing of Fractures in the Forearm (Radius and Ulna)

Indications

Transverse and short spiral fractures occurring in the middle third of the radius and ulna can be nailed simultaneously. If the radial fracture is in the middle third of the shaft, the ulna can be nailed with the same operative technique as described for the isolated ulnar fracture, if the ulnar fracture is between the coronoid process and the distal fourth. If the proximal medullary canal of the radius has a favorable shape, a more proximal radial fracture may still lend itself to the intramedullary nailing. Extending the nailing indication more distally for the radius is not advised.

Positioning and Reduction

Positioning and nailing of forearm fractures is identical to the nailing of isolated ulna and radius fractures.

The earlier the nailing is done, the easier is the reduction. Reduction is accomplished by angulating the elbow in a right angle and applying traction to the hand and the firmly held elbow. If the reduction cannot be accomplished, a distractor should be applied as described on page 47. All inveterate fractures of the forearm and those not reducible by previously described methods necessitate inserting the distal distractor wire transversely through the distal ends of the radius and ulna (see the chapter entitled *Pseudarthrosis of the Forearm*, p. 127).

Image Intensification

Preoperative roentgenograms are to be taken for all fractures of the forearm in two planes at a distance of 1 m. These films will serve as gauges for determining the nail and reamer dimensions. The image intensifier is positioned as already described for the isolated radius and ulna nailing (i.e., on the side of the injured arm). Postoperative roentgenograms must be taken in three planes.

Operative Technique

The skin incision is made as described for the isolated nailing of the radius and ulna. The radial fracture is reduced first because the radius maintains the length of the forearm. All shortening is usually overcome after the reduction of the radius. After the medullary canal of the radius is opened and the fracture is successfully reduced, the ball-point guide pin is inserted into the medullary canal.

Thereafter, the ulna is reduced. The proper entry point is chosen, depending on the localization of the fracture site. The guide pin is then introduced into either the distal or the proximal entry portal. If the fracture of the forearm was previously placed in a distractor, remove the distractor after insertion of both guide pins. The nailing of the radius is then done as previously described. Thereafter, the ulna is nailed.

Common Mistakes in Forearm Nailing

If the nailing entry point into the radius is too far proximal to the styloid process, or too far dorsal or palm-ward, the nail will hit the contralateral cortex, even if its tip was bent. This may cause splitting of the bone.

If the proximal entry point to the ulna is not in the middle of the olecranon tip, the guide pin can miss the medullary canal and enter the elbow joint.

When nailing the ulna through the distal entry portal, any shift of the entry portal, either proximal or V-ulnar-ward, of the styloid process, can lead to deadlocking in the contralateral cortex. This may also lead to cracking of the bone.

Applying too much pressure to the reamer may also lead to splitting of the bone. The same can happen if the bone dust is not periodically cleansed from the reamer head.

Because of its special profile, a V-nail's tip must be bent satisfactorily toward the guide pin. Failure to do so may cause the V-nail to be insecurely guided by the guide pin, and may result in the nail missing the opposite medullary canal. For this reason, one should repeatedly fluoroscope. If the ulna is nailed first, the radius nail may jam owing to unsatisfactory reduction. Large protrusions of the nail from the radius or ulna may irritate the soft tissue and delay wound healing.

Aftercare

The type of aftercare is dependent on the gravity of the soft tissue involvement. Active exercises are started as soon as the swelling has decreased. Heavy lifting should be postponed until the fractures have healed. Minor decreases in mobility from the distal entry point are common and disappear after the removal of the nails.

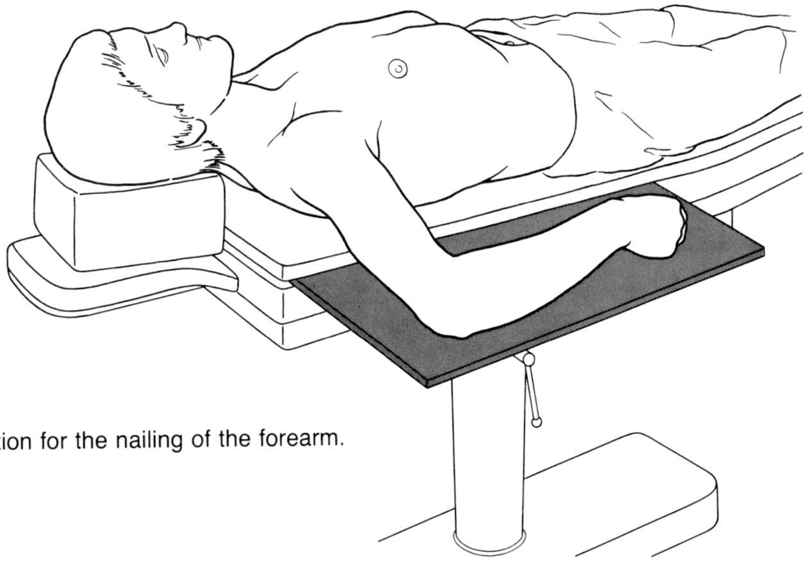

Figure 93 The correct position for the nailing of the forearm.

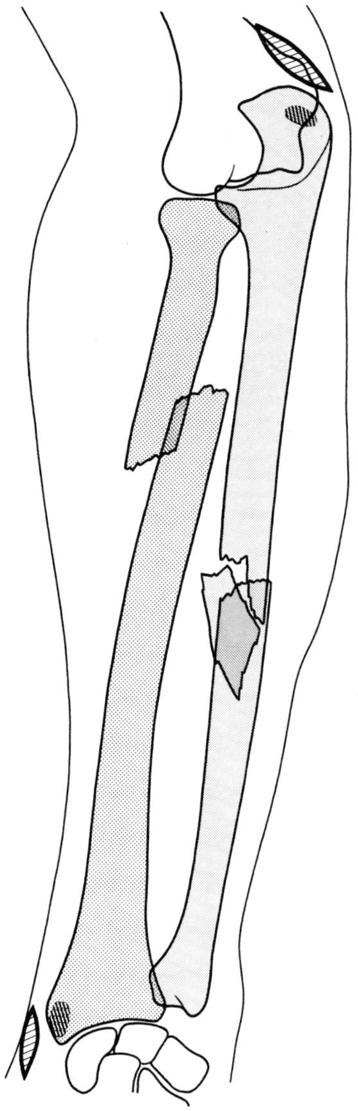

Figure 94 Fractures of the radius and ulna. The stab incisions and nail entry portals, at the olecranon for the ulnar nailing and at the styloid process of the radius for the radial nailing.

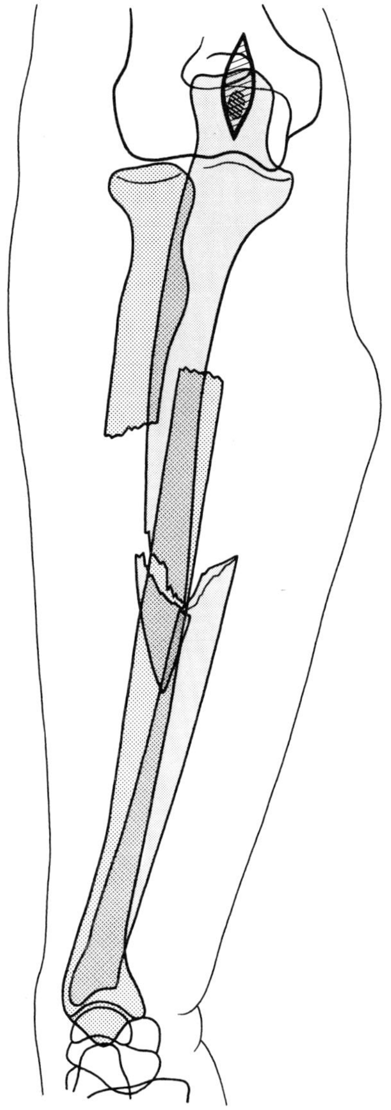

Figure 95 Fractures of the forearm, lateral view. Stab incision and nail entry portal at the olecranon.

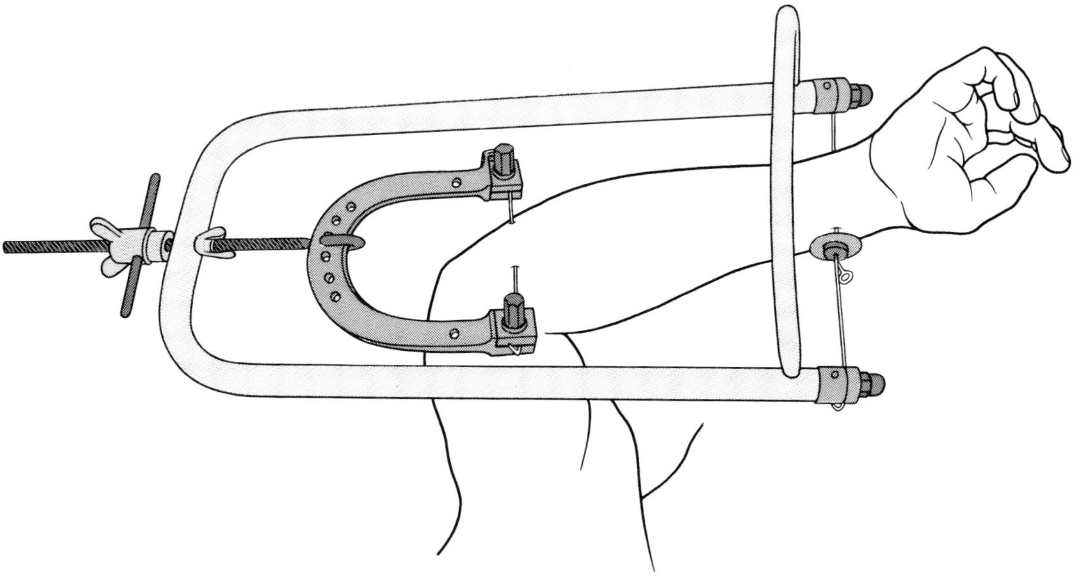

Figure 96 The distractor for the forearm. Proximal Kirschner wire through the ulna, distal to the olecranon. Distal Kirschner wire in AP direction through the distal radius.

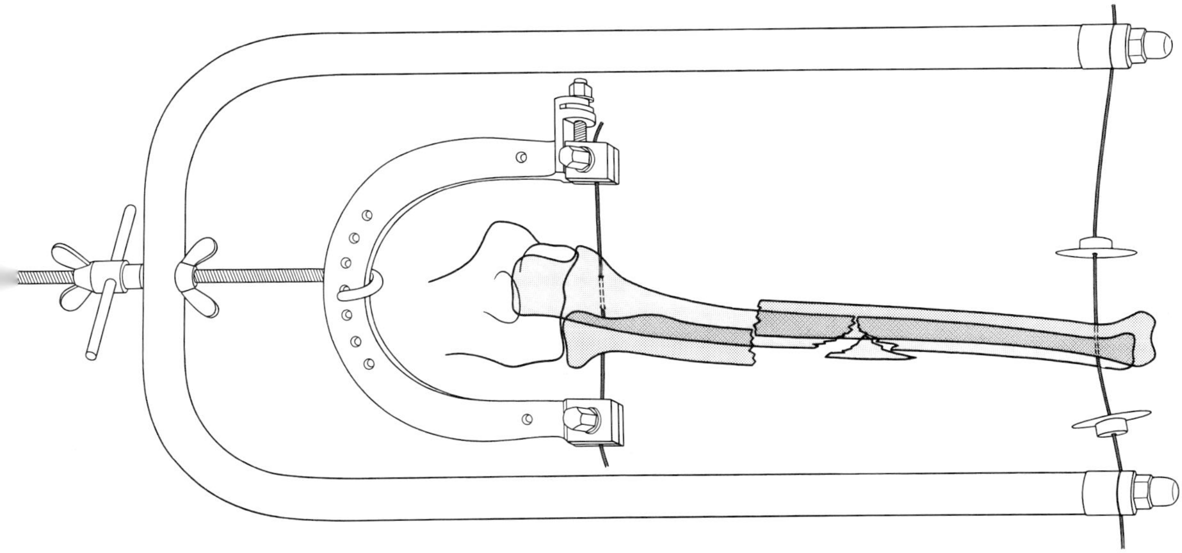

Figure 97 Fracture of the forearm in the distractor. Position of the Kirschner wires.

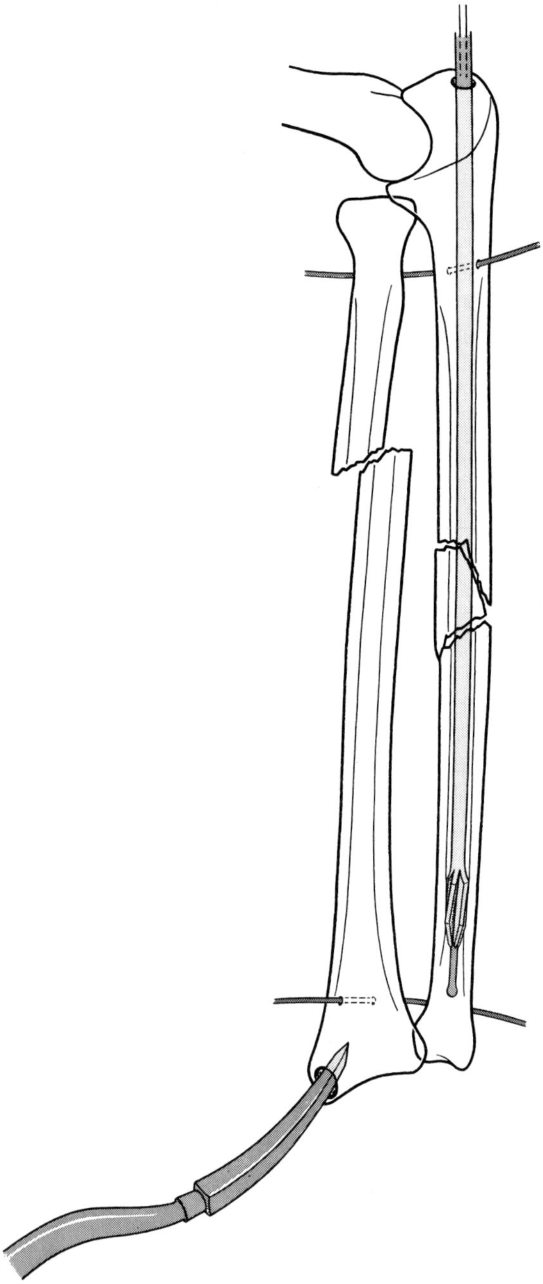

Figure 98 Fracture of the forearm in the distractor. Reaming of the ulnar medullary canal over the guide pin. Opening of the medullary canal with an awl for the radial nailing.

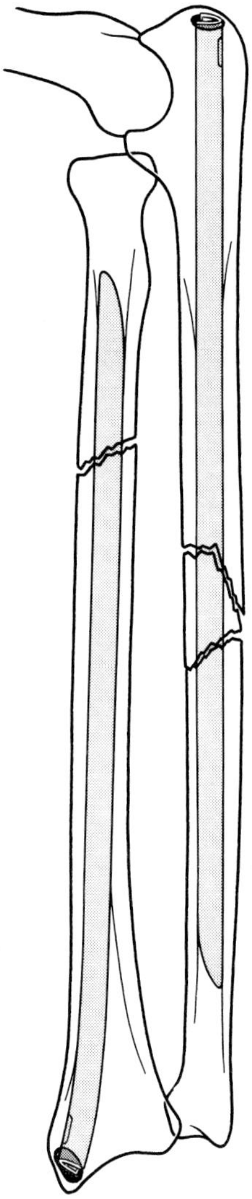

Figure 99 The same position of the forearm, after the nailing of both bones.

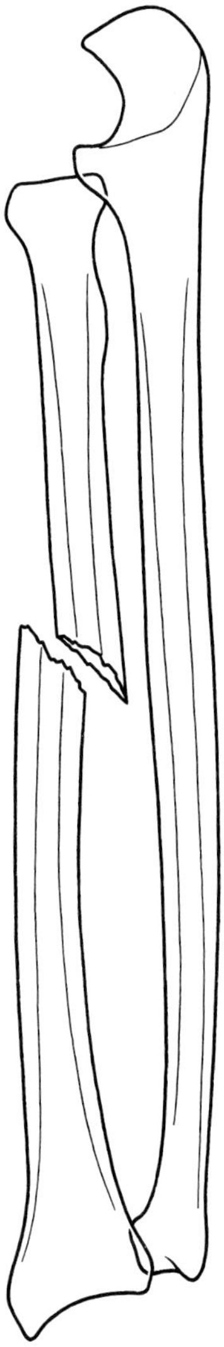

Figure 100 Fracture of the radial shaft.

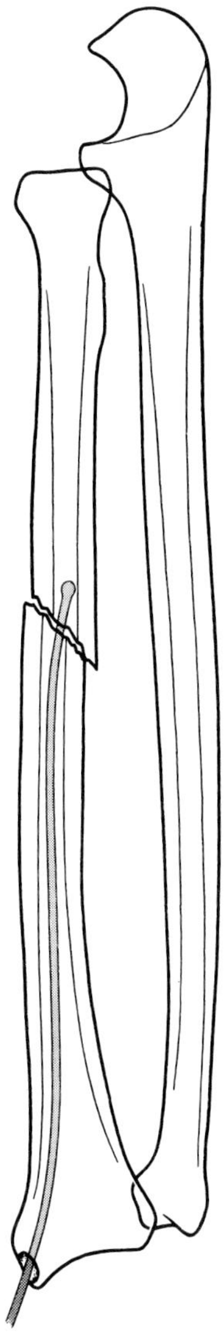

Figure 101 Reduction of the radial fracture with a guide pin.

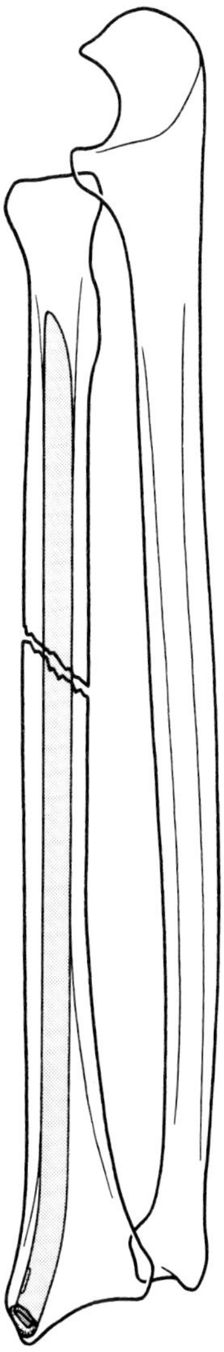

Figure 102 The completed nailing of the same radial fracture.

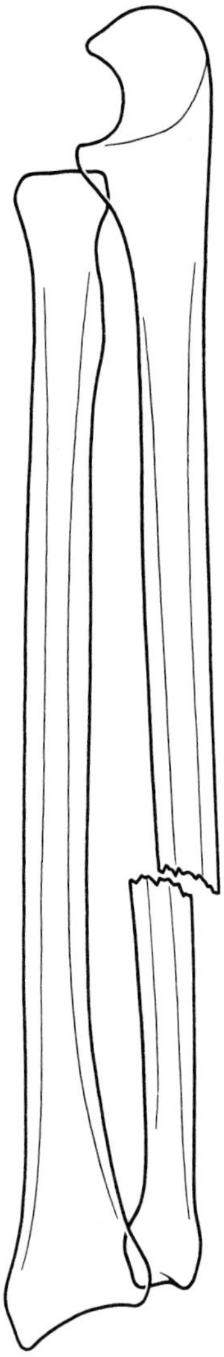

Figure 103 Fracture of the ulna, distal third.

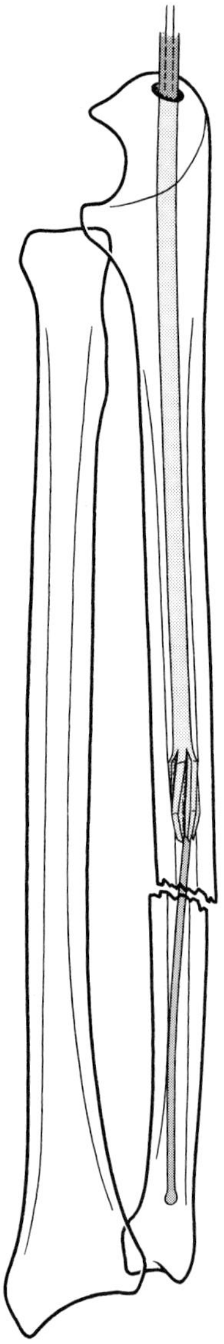

Figure 104 Reaming of the medullary canal over a guide pin in an ulnar fracture of the distal third.

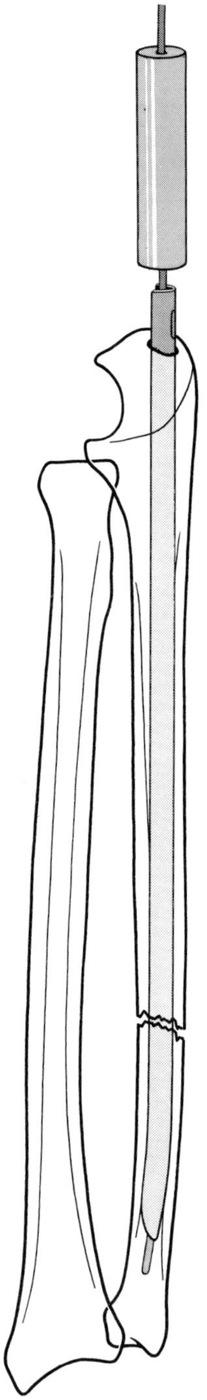

Figure 105 Driving of a V-type nail with the aid of a nail set.

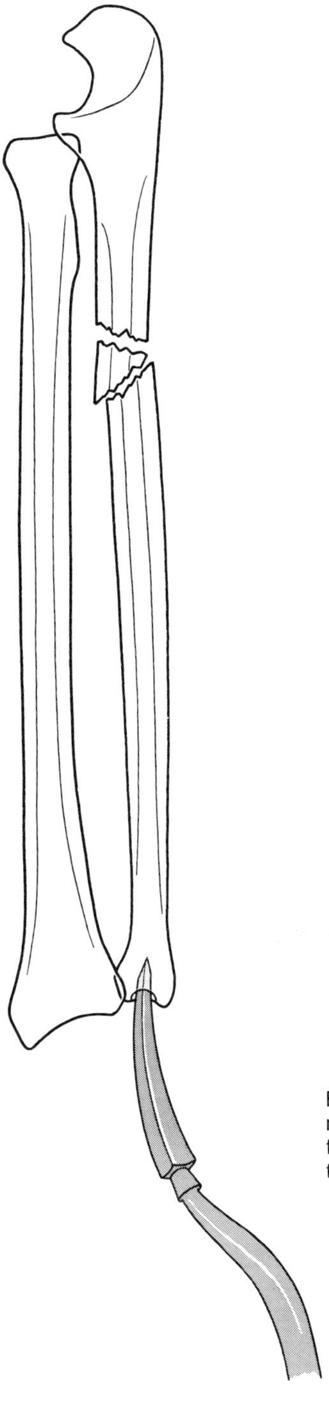

Figure 106 Ulnar fracture in the proximal third. Widening of the nail entry port with an awl at the styloid process of the ulna.

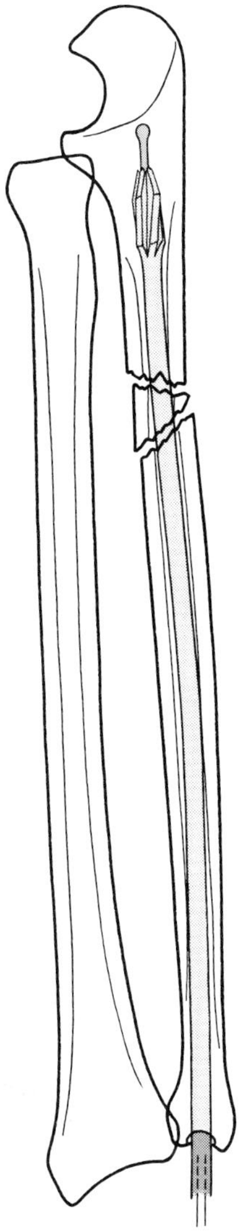

Figure 107 The reaming of the medullary canal over a guide pin from distal entry, in an ulnar fracture of the proximal third.

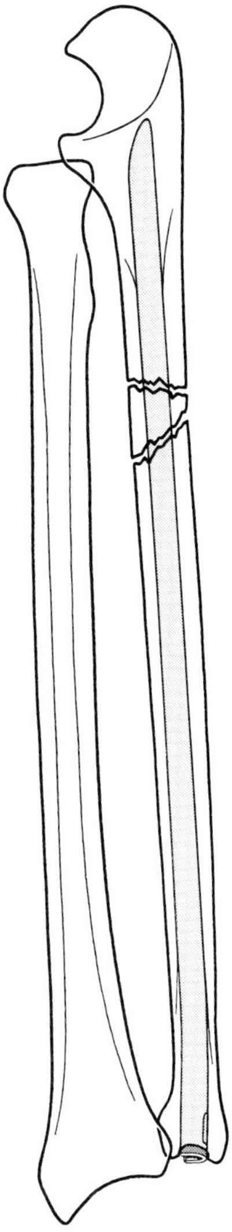

Figure 108 The completed nailing of an ulnar fracture in the proximal third from distal entry.

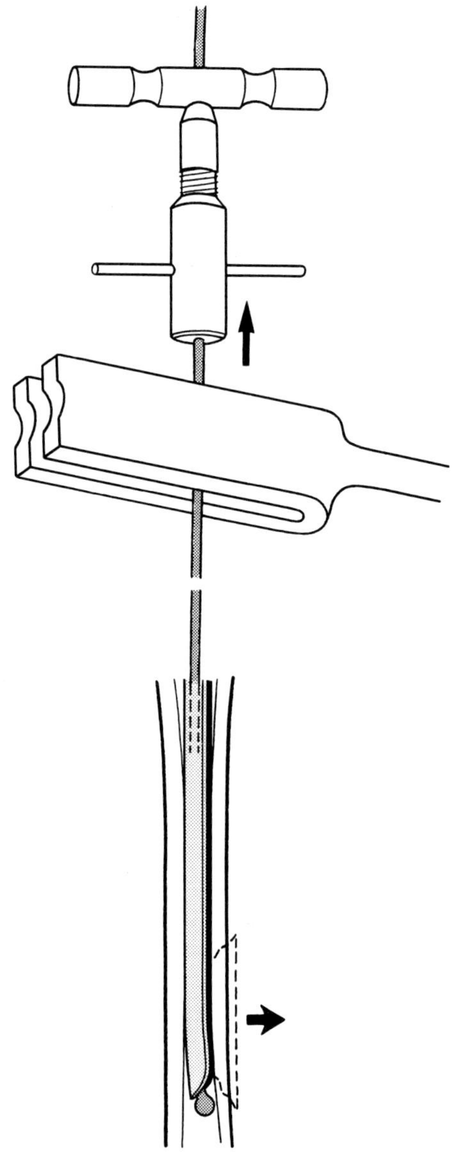

Figure 109 The ball-point guide pin was not exchanged for a smooth guide pin before the insertion of the V-type nail. The bone splits when the ball-point guide pin is extracted while the nail is in place.

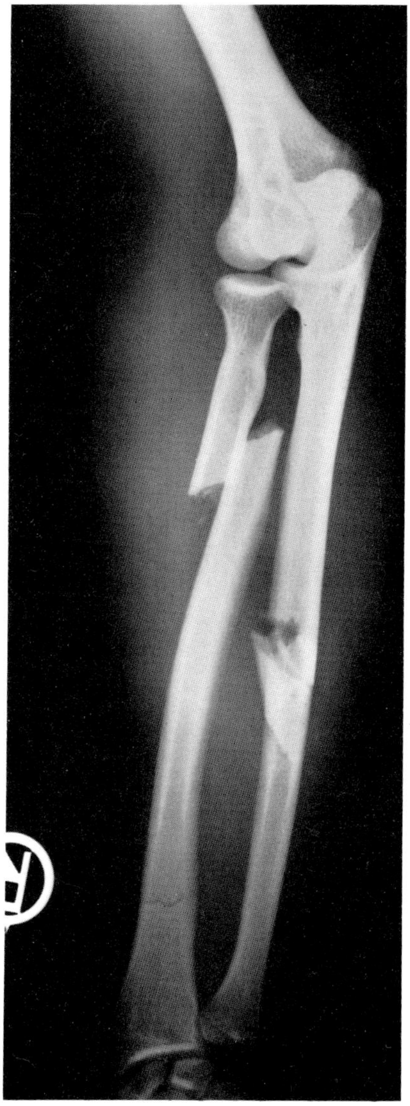

Figure 110 Fresh fracture of the forearm with shortening, AP view. The radius shows a second undisplaced fracture in the distal third.

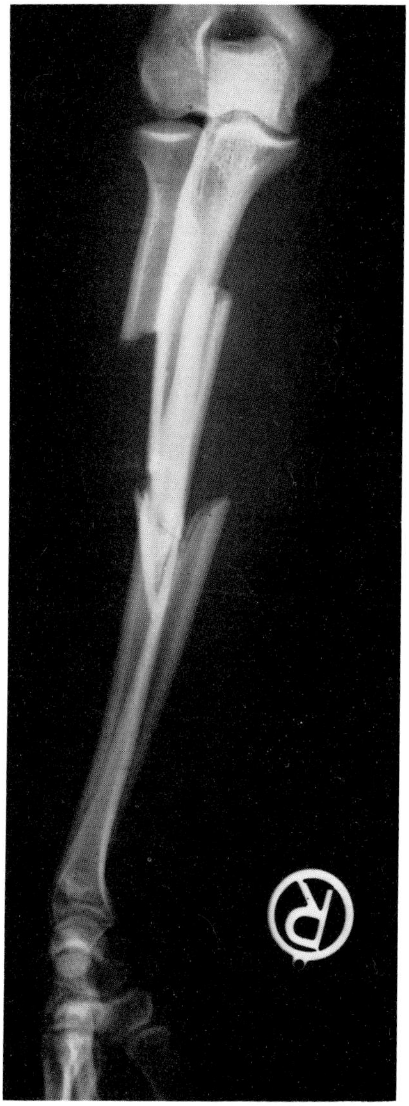

Figure 111 Lateral view of fresh fracture of the forearm.

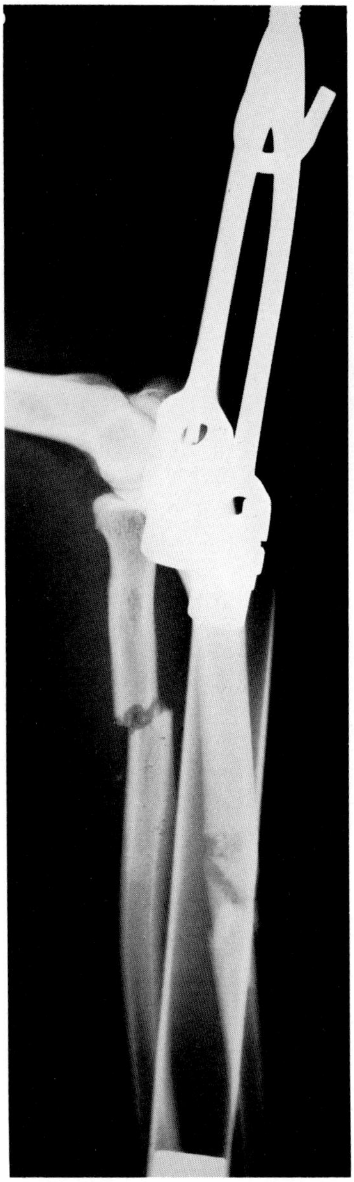

Figure 112 The fracture of the forearm was placed in a distractor for reduction. In the oblique view, an aluminum tube of the distractor is superimposed over the ulna; the wire tractor is superimposed over the elbow joint.

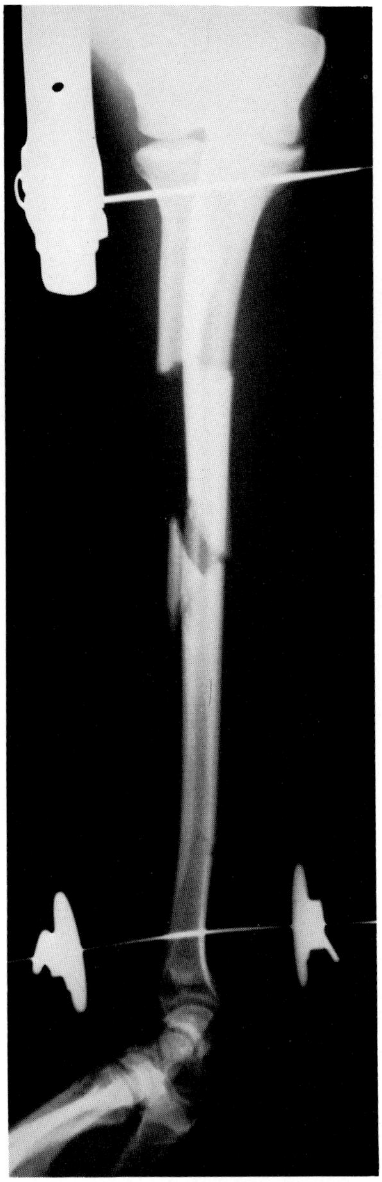

Figure 113 Lateral view of the fracture of the forearm in the distractor. The proximal Kirschner wire is inserted through the ulna; the distal Kirschner wire is inserted in an AP direction through the distal radius.

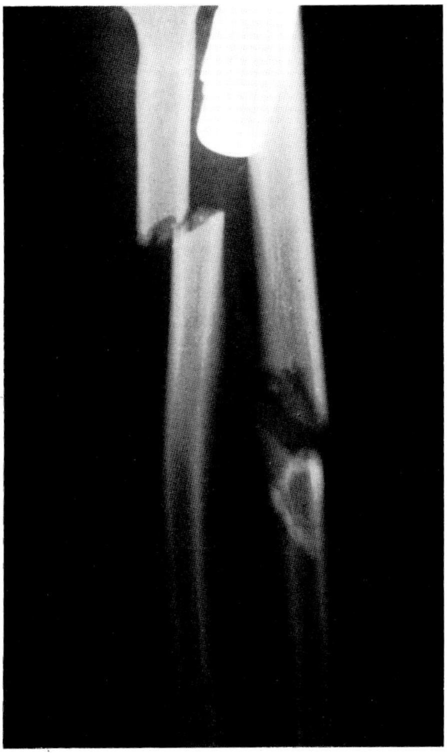

◀ Figure 114 After six days of slowly increased traction, the displaced fractures are nearly completely reduced in the oblique view.

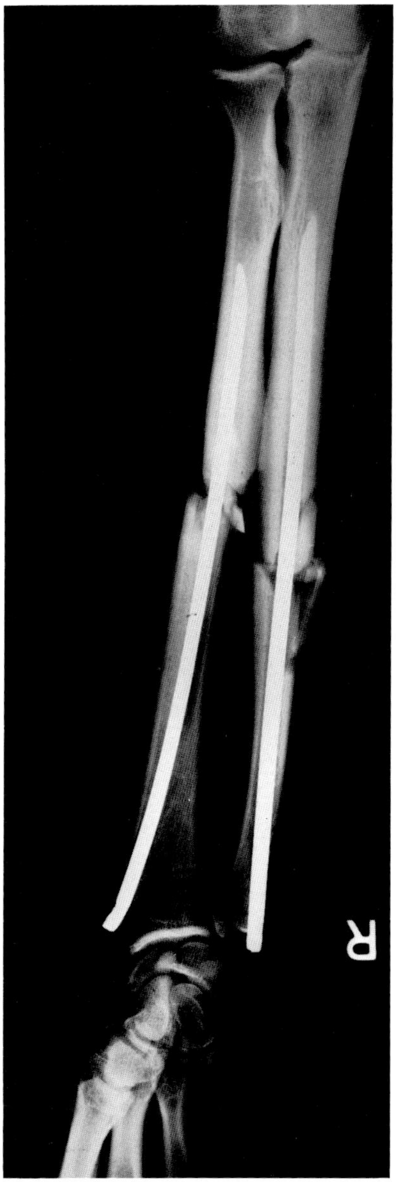

Figure 116 Completed nailing of a fresh fracture of the forearm, AP view. Both bones were nailed from a distal entry.

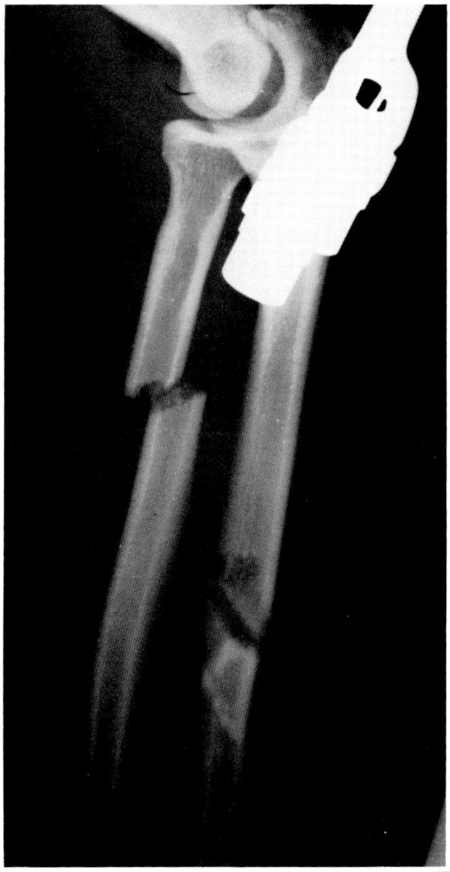

◀ Figure 115 After eight days of traction in the distractor, there is only minimal improvement in the positioning of the radial fracture in comparison with that of the sixth day.

Nailing of Olecranon Fractures with Special Nails

Indications

A transverse fracture of the olecranon, which is not severely comminuted, lends itself to intramedullary nailing with a special olecranon nail. However, the proximal fragment must not be split longitudinally. If these prerequisites are not met, some other type of osteosynthesis must be used.

Positioning and Reduction

The patient is supine on a regular operating table, and the arm is positioned on a radiolucent extension of the table, as described in the chapter concerning the nailing of the forearm. The reduction occurs when the olecranon nail is inserted.

Image Intensification

Preoperative roentgenograms of the elbow joint, comprising two-thirds of the forearm, should be taken in two planes at a 1-m distance. These films will serve as gauges in determining the correct dimensions of the nail. The image intensifier is positioned on the involved side as described for fractures of the forearm (pp. 47-49). Postoperative roentgenograms of the elbow joint comprising two-thirds of the forearm must be taken in two planes.

Operative Technique

Only special olecranon nails are used in the intramedullary nailing of the olecranon fracture. The proximal fragment is held in place by the perpendicular lips of the special v-shaped nail. In order to attain sufficient locking, the nail should be driven at least into the distal third of the ulna.

After the longitudinal incision over the olecranon has been made, the proximal medullary canal is opened at the middle of the olecranon tip. One must consider that the olecranon has been proximally displaced when choosing the middle of the tip. The proximal fragment is reduced by inserting the awl. Then, introduce the guide pin through the proximal fragment into the distal medullary canal of the ulna. Successful reduction must be verified by fluoroscopy. If the reduction proves to be unsatisfactory, the position must be corrected by towel clips or bone hooks. Ream the medullary canal in increments of 0.5 mm until the desired width is obtained, as determined by the preoperative roentgenograms. If the medullary canal is reamed over a ball-point guide pin, this guide pin must then be exchanged for a smooth nail driving guide by first inserting the smooth guide and then withdrawing the original ball-point guide pin. Insert the special olecranon nail and do the final setting of the nail after the removal of the smooth guide. The lips of the special olecranon nail should firmly compress the proximal fragment onto the distal fragment. When nailing a narrow olecranon, the lips of the special nail should be bent toward the olecranon to avoid overhanging. Close the incision.

Common Mistakes

If the proper proximal entry point is not used, a step will form at the articular surface of the fracture site. Decreased mobility of the elbow joint may ensue postoperatively.

If the tip of the V-nail is not bent slightly toward the guide pin, the nail cannot be properly guided by the pin. If the ball-point guide pin was not exchanged for a smooth guide pin before the insertion of the V-nail, the ball-point guide pin cannot be withdrawn. Use of an insufficiently long special olecranon nail causes inadequate longitudinal locking and unsatisfactory compression at the fracture site. In this case, flexing the elbow joint may cause a gap at the fracture site.

Aftercare

Active exercises should be initiated after a sufficient decrease in the soft-tissue swelling.

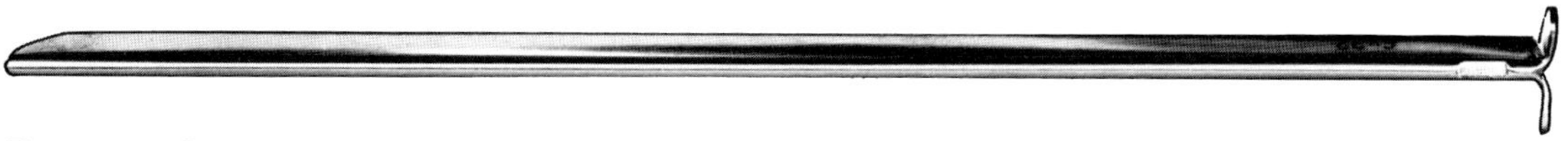

Figure 117 Olecranon nail.

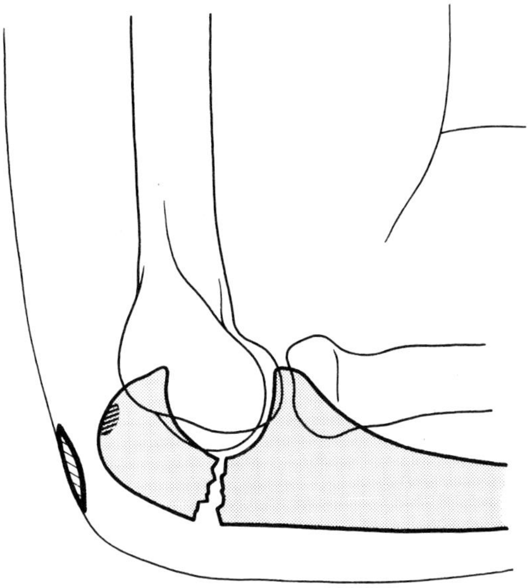

Figure 118 Fracture of the olecranon. Stab incision and the nail entry point at the olecranon.

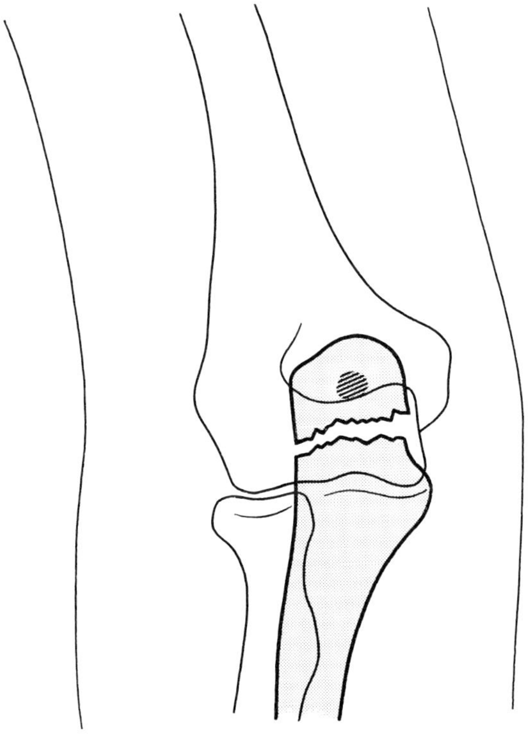

Figure 119 Fracture of the olecranon, AP view, with the nail entry point.

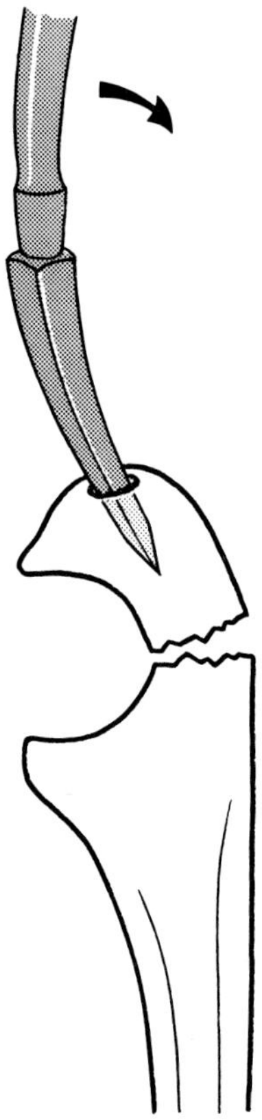

Figure 120 Opening of the medullary canal and reduction of the olecranon fracture with an awl.

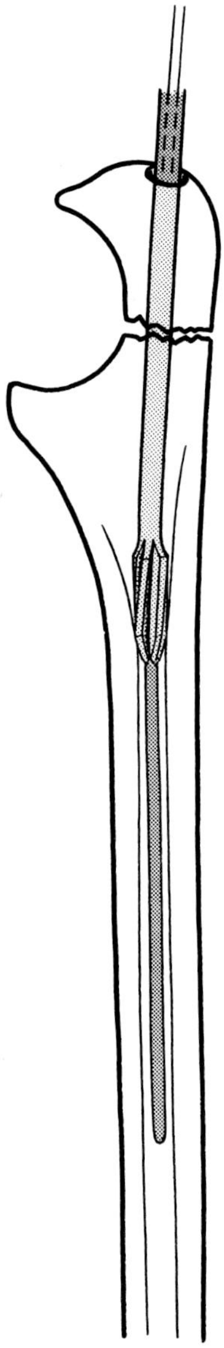

Figure 121 After the reduction of the olecranon fracture, reaming of the medullary canal over the guide pin.

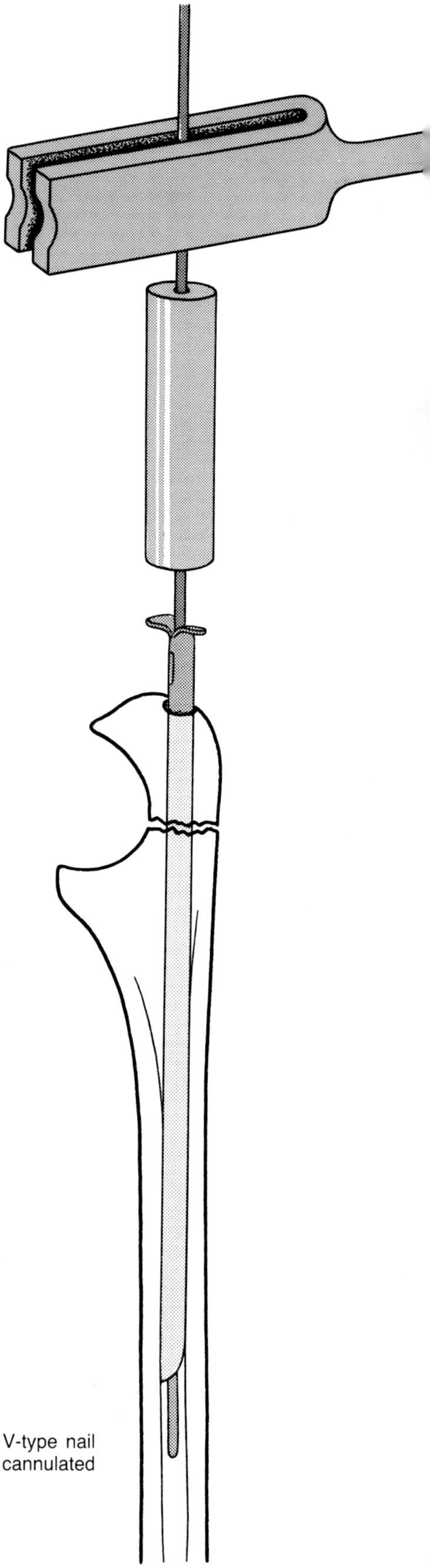

Figure 122 Driving of the olecranon nail (a V-type nail with two lips) over the guide with the aid of a cannulated nail driver.

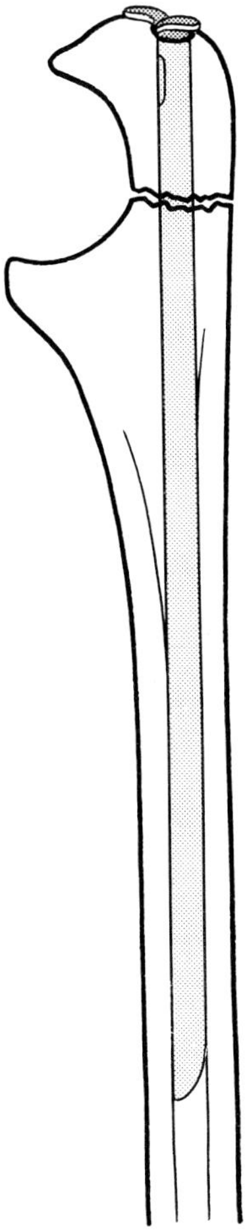

Figure 123 Completed olecranon nailing, lateral view.

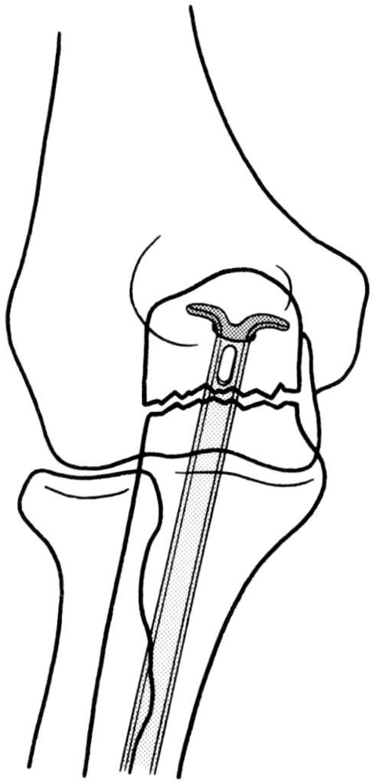

Figure 124 Completed olecranon nailing, AP view.

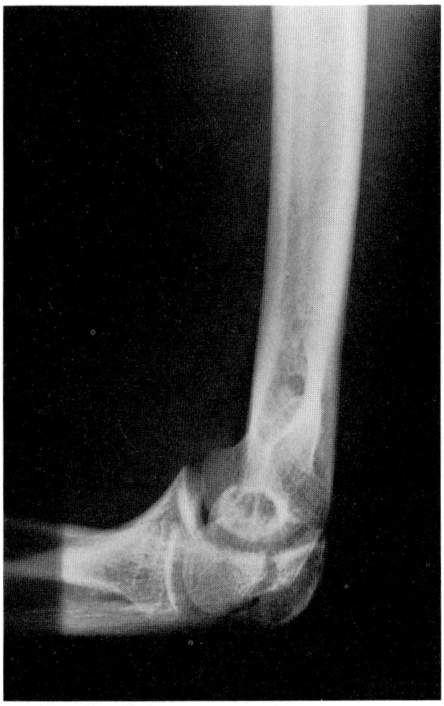

Figure 125 Fresh fracture of the olecranon in a 16-year-old male, lateral view.

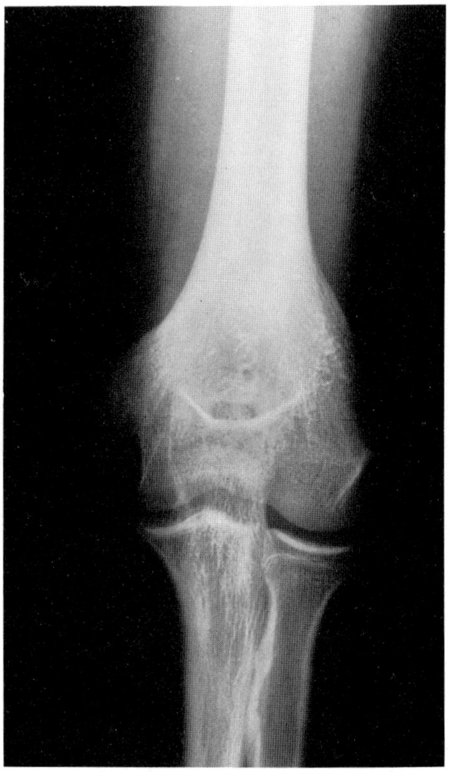

Figure 126 The same olecranon fracture, AP view. Fracture line is visible, proximal to the articular interspace.

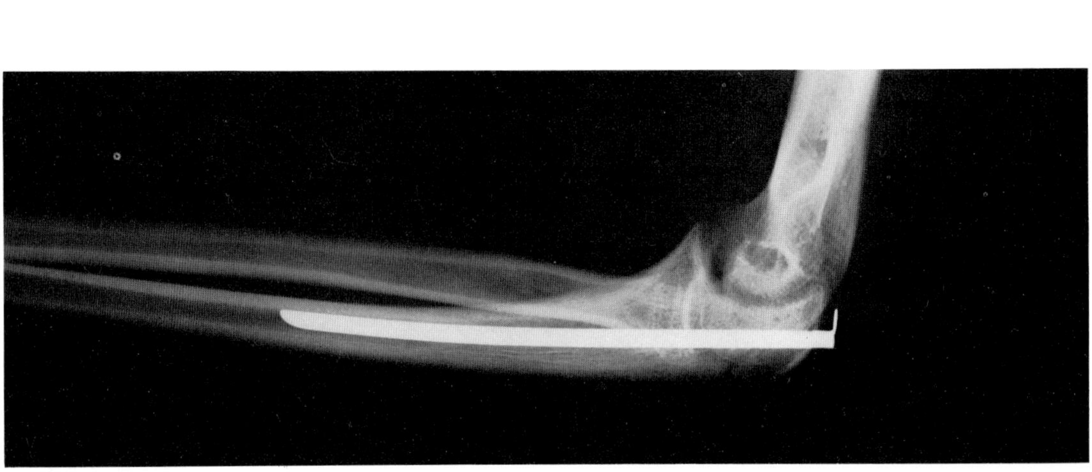

Figure 127 Three weeks after the nailing of the olecranon with a V-type nail, lateral view; the articular surface shows no step.

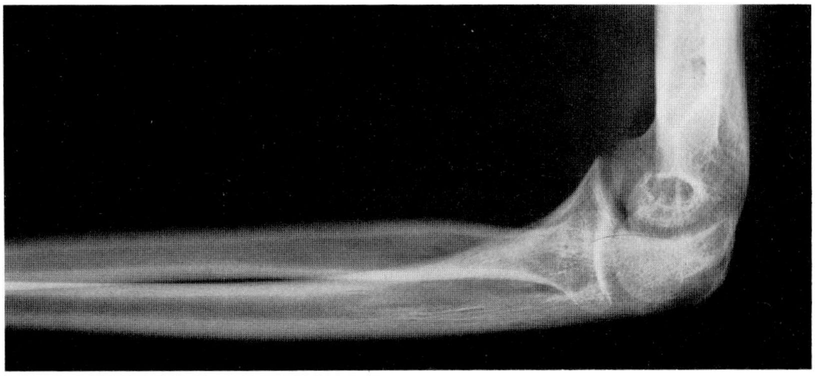

▲ Figure 129 Bony healing of the olecranon fracture after nail removal, 14 months after the accident, lateral view.

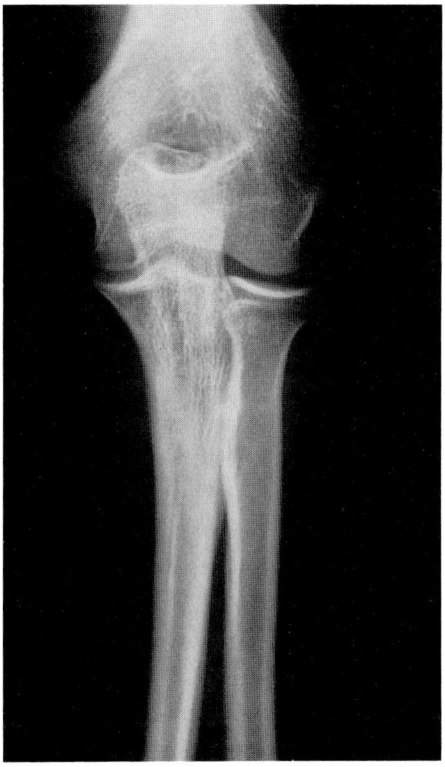

Figure 130 The same in AP view.

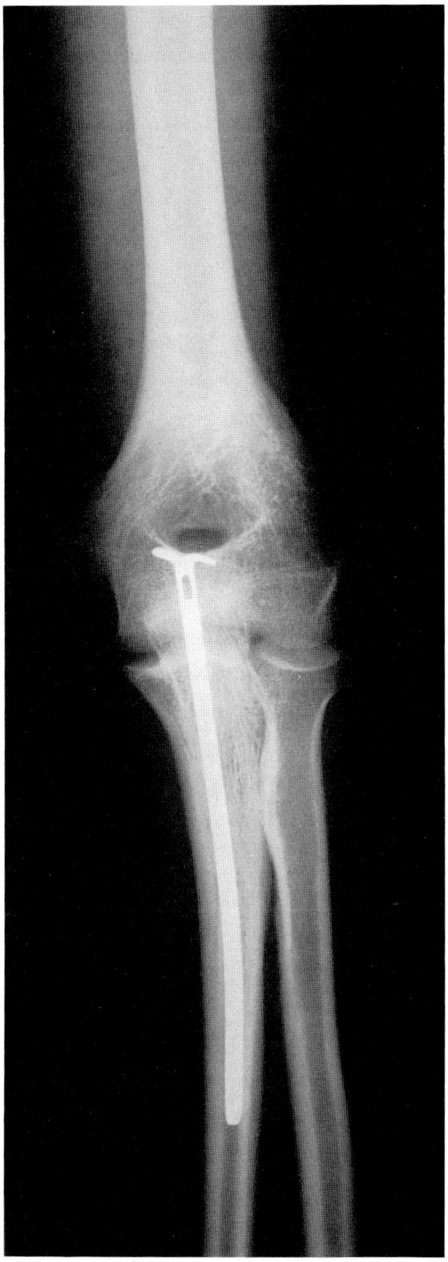

◀ Figure 128 Completed nailing of the olecranon, AP view. One of the lips of the olecranon nail was bent toward the bone to avoid soft tissue damage.

Nailing of Intertrochanteric Fractures

Y-Nailing

The Y-nail is comprised of two parts. A flanged cloverleaf nail is inserted through a femoral neck nail. Both parts interlock in a sliding-brake action when pressure is exerted at the tip of the femoral neck nail. Therefore, the Y-nail requires no bony support within the trochanter.

Indications

Y-nailing is indicated in comminuted fractures of the trochanter and in transverse fractures through the lesser trochanter. Rotational stability is gained by interlocking of the fragments if the patient bears weight directly after the operation.

Instruments

In addition to the standard Küntscher instrument set a Y-nail driver and a Y-nail guide are needed.

Positioning and Reduction

The patient is supine on the fracture table and both legs are abducted. The perineum rests against the radiolucent perineal post. Prepare the foot holder so that the involved leg can be adducted to (or even beyond) the midline of the table. If the fracture table does not allow for this type of adduction, the table is not suitable for Y-nailing. Traction is then applied to both legs. Additional maneuvers, like the interchanging of inward and outward rotation, or the traction-flexion-extension of the hip joint, are seldom necessary for successful reduction. The reduction is simplified. The injured leg is abducted 30 degrees, considerably rotated inward (i.e., the patella should be vertically oriented), attached to the previously prepared foot holder, and then extended.

Image Intensification

Preoperative roentgenograms of the hip joint and the femur are necessary in two planes. The image intensifier is positioned between the abducted legs so that lateral fluoroscopy of the hip joint is possible. If problems arise during the fluoroscopy in the lateral plane, while the injured leg is adducted, the uninvolved leg must be abducted further, or be flexed in the hip joint and supported in a leg holder.

Operative Technique

The localization of the skin incision and the entry point for the femoral neck nail is determined by superimposing the Y-nail on the hip as it is fluoroscoped. Another way of determining the localization of the incision and the entry point is to superimpose the Y-nail on the preoperative roentgenograms and mark its contours. A guide pin is inserted with a hand-chuck through the trochanter into the femoral neck. Comparing the guide pin's fluoroscoped position to the markings on the preoperative roentgenograms yields the exact localization of the incision and the entry point of the femoral neck nail. A skin incision 10 cm long is made over the lateral trochanter, according to the marks. Slit the fascia laterally and expose the trochanter. A longitudinally oval reamer hole is made in the lateral aspect of the trochanter, again using the markings. The opening must be large enough to permit the femoral neck nail to be tilted by several millimeters. The length of the femoral flanged nail is determined by inserting a guide pin and measuring it under fluoroscopy. Y-nails are available in 10- and 12-mm diameters and in varying lengths. One should use the 12-mm nails whenever possible. Remember that the femoral medullary canal is never reamed in Y-nailing. Both nails form an angle of 135 degrees. This angle must be maintained when the Y-nail is homed into the femoral neck and head. The Y-nail should pass over the calcar in the AP projection and should run through the middle of the femoral neck in the lateral projection. The femoral neck nail must be driven deep enough so that its opening for the flanged femoral nail is within the medullary canal. This position must be verified under image intensification. Both parts of the Küntscher Y-nail guide are then inserted, one at a time, through the opening of the femoral neck nail. The portion of the Y-nail guide, acting as a pin, is then tapped through the trochanter tip until it becomes palpable under the skin. Thereafter, the injured leg is adducted and a stab incision is made over the tip of the Y-nail guide. The chosen femoral flanged nail is inserted over the tip of the Y-nail guide pin and advanced while the Y-nail guide pin is simultaneously slowly withdrawn. Withdrawing the Y-nail guide pin slowly ensures that the flanged nail is brought safely into the correct entry point. The flanged nail is then tapped through the cortex of the trochanter, and the Y-nail guide is completely withdrawn. A straight guide pin is advanced through the femoral flanged nail and then through the opening of the femoral neck nail into the distal medullary canal, under fluoroscopy. A periosteal elevator is used to ascertain whether the straight guide pin has passed correctly through the opening of the femoral neck nail or, preferably, the straight guide pin can be directly visualized after the lumen of the femoral neck nail is cleaned with a gauze-tipped hemostat.

If the trochanter is not comminuted, the following operative technique must be used: the reamer awl is guided over the protruding Y-nail guide instead of using the femoral flanged nail, as described. The Y-nail guide is slowly withdrawn, while the reamer awl follows, thus being securely guided through the correct nail entry point at the tip of the trochanter. A hole is created at the trochanter tip by rotating the reamer awl back and forth. The Y-nail guide pin is then completely withdrawn, and a straight guide pin is inserted through the reamer awl and passes through the opening of the femoral neck nail into the distal medullary canal under fluoroscopy. Remove the reamer awl. The correct passage of the straight guide pin through the hole of the femoral neck nail is confirmed either by periosteal elevator or by the direct visualization procedure already described. The chosen femoral flanged nail is driven over the straight guide pin in a way that the nail slit points toward the tip of the femoral neck nail. The passage of the flanged nail through the opening of the femoral neck nail is facilitated by tilting the femoral neck nail in an adductive (or more seldom, an abductive) motion with a Y-nail driver. The flanged nail is homed through the femoral neck nail until the flanged end locks with the femoral neck nail. The position of the Y-nail is visualized by fluoroscopy with the involved leg adducted and then again in the abducted position. If the femoral neck nail traveled laterally when the flanged nail was homed, it may now be tapped in more deeply. The femoral flanged nail should penetrate at least the distal third of the femoral shaft. A drain may be inserted before closure.

Postoperative roentgenograms must be taken in two planes, comprising the hip joint and the femoral shaft.

Common Mistakes

If the inward rotation of the leg is inadequate (i.e., the axis of the patella is not sufficiently pointing vertically), the fracture cannot be satisfactorily reduced, and the correct entry point for the femoral neck nail cannot be chosen. This leads to a postoperative increased outward rotation of the leg. If the entry point for the femoral neck nail is too narrow and is made too far proximally, the femoral flanged nail fails to enter the distal fragment because of the changed angle of the femoral neck nail in reference to the bone. The same can occur if the entry point is made too narrow and too far distally. Both mistakes are easily rectified by enlarging the entry hole longitudinally. The range of tilting of the femoral neck nail is increased through this action, allowing for the correct passage of the femoral flanged nail.

If the straight guide pin cannot pass through the hole in the femoral neck nail into the distal fragment, the guide pin must be exchanged for one with a slightly bent tip. Should this also be unsuccessful, the entry point for the femoral neck nail must be enlarged distally. Following the passage through the femoral neck nail, the guide pin is pulled laterally with a bone hook and guided into the distal medullary canal.

Using too short a femoral neck nail sacrifices the stability of the osteosynthesis under weight-bearing. This allows the femoral neck to tilt, causing a varus deformity.

Using too long a femoral neck nail can cause the nail to perforate the femoral head and cause a painful decrease in joint mobility.

If the femoral flanged nail, with or without the straight guide pin, hits the lateral cranial roof of the femoral neck nail, either the femoral neck nail must be withdrawn a few millimeters, by inserting the tip of the Küntscher nail extractor into the hole of the nail, or the attached Y-nail driver must be tilted toward the foot.

If the femoral flanged nail hits the medial lip of the neck nail's hole, the neck nail must be driven in more deeply and the attached Y-nail driver must be tilted toward the foot.

Aftercare

Because the Y-nail is initially stabilized by weight-bearing, the involved leg should bear full weight as soon as possible.

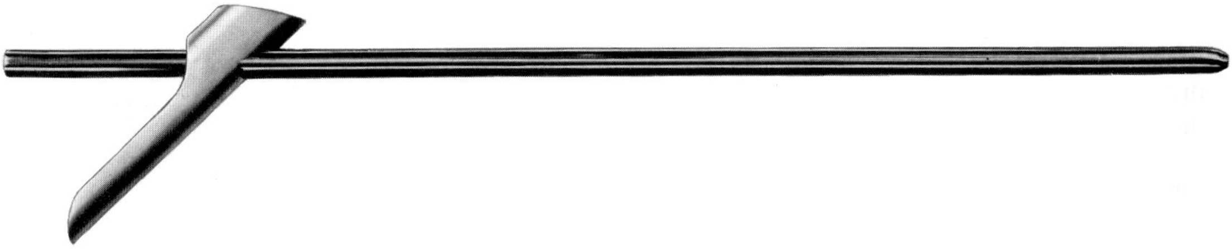

Figure 131 Y-nail.

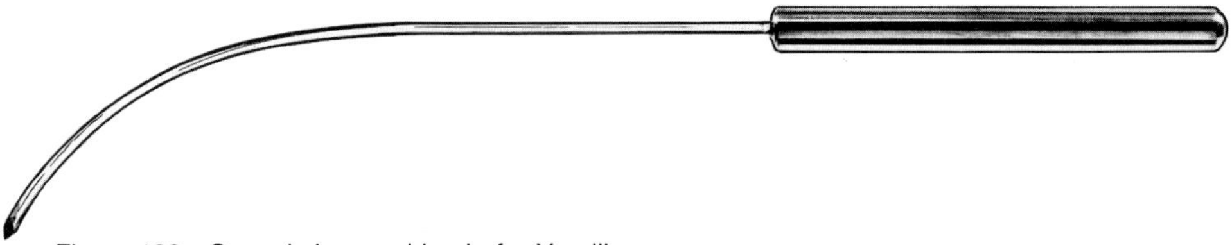

Figure 132 Curved sharp guide pin for Y-nailing.

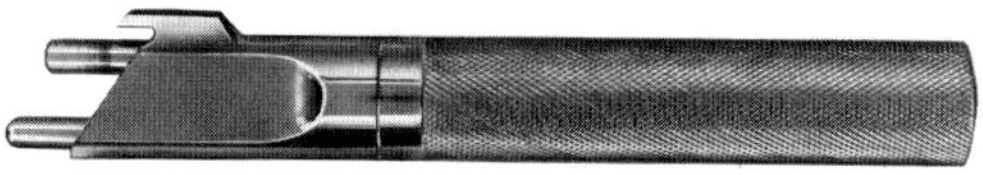

Figure 133 Nail driver for the Y-femoral neck nail.

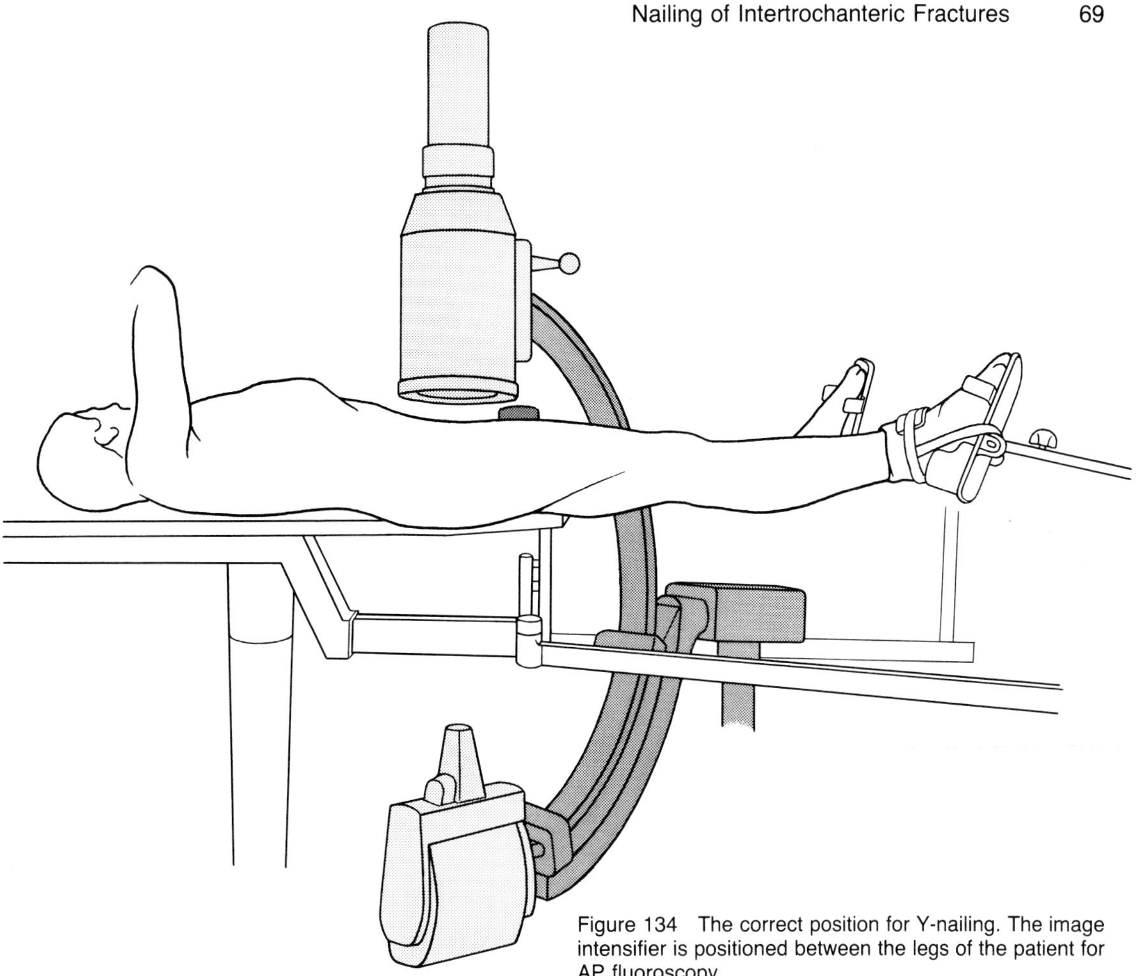

Figure 134 The correct position for Y-nailing. The image intensifier is positioned between the legs of the patient for AP fluoroscopy.

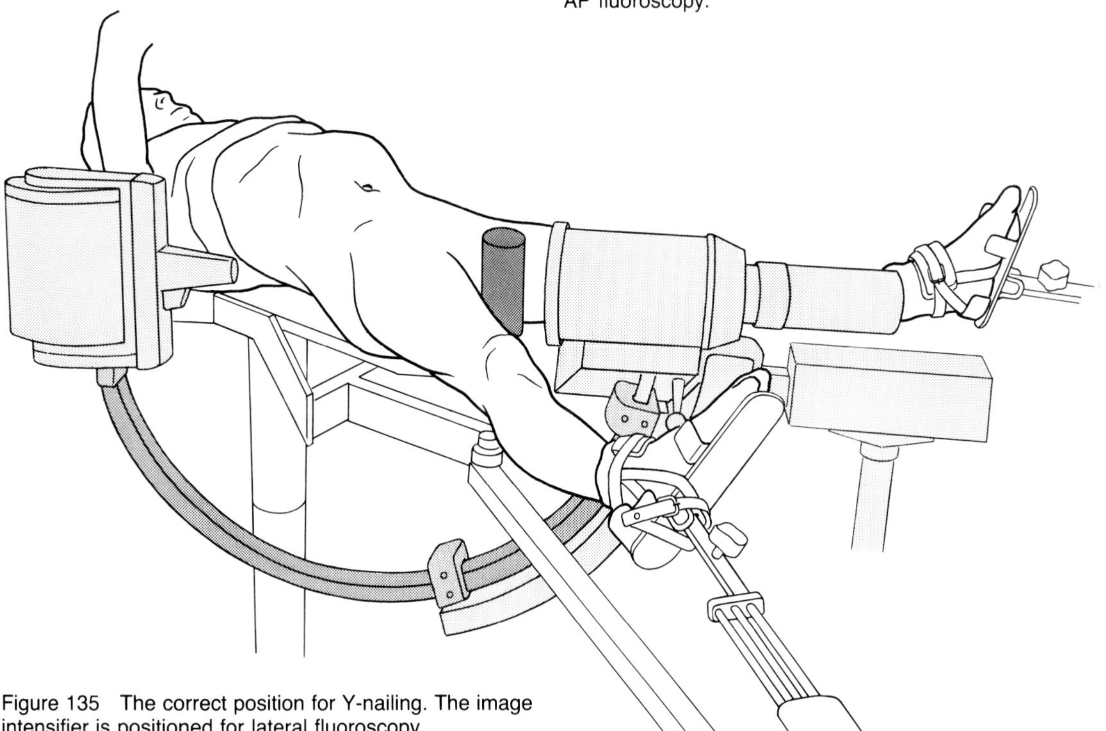

Figure 135 The correct position for Y-nailing. The image intensifier is positioned for lateral fluoroscopy.

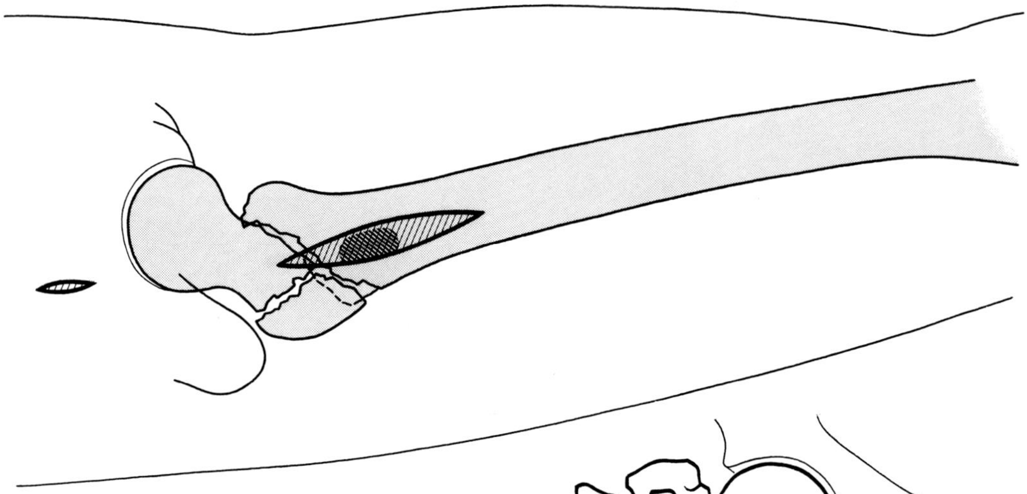

Figure 136 The correct position of the skin incision for the Y-nailing and the entry point for the femoral neck nail in the trochanter area.

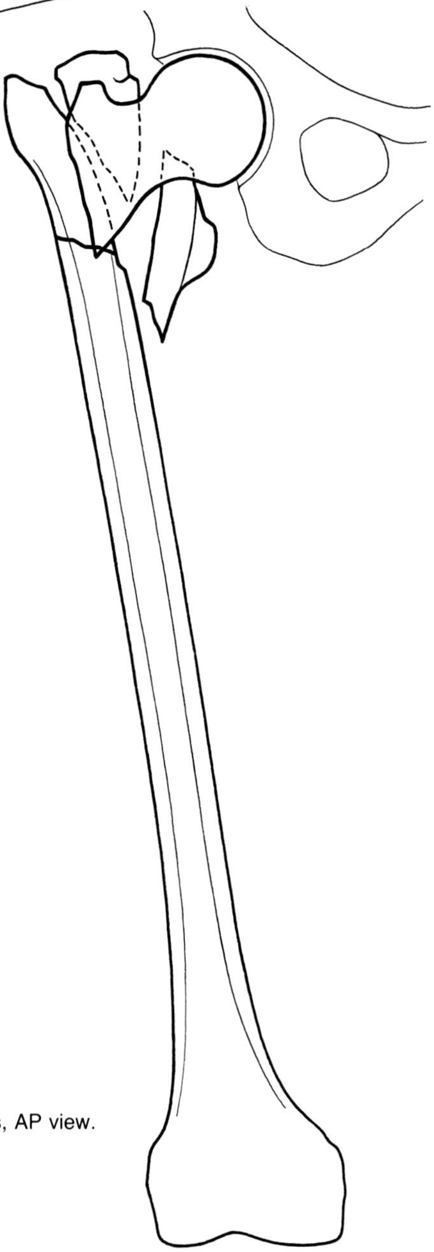

Figure 137 Comminuted intertrochanteric fractures, AP view.

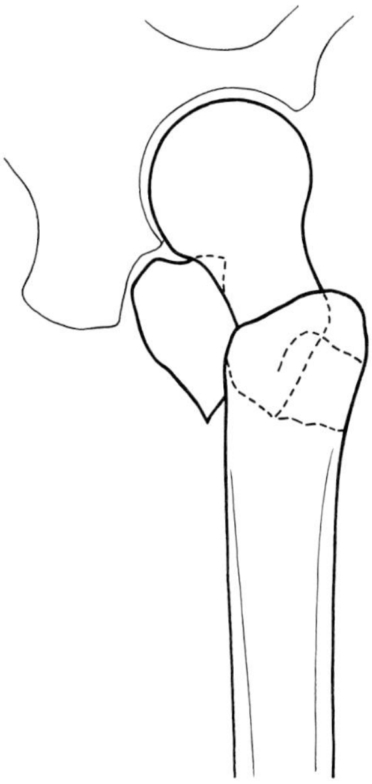

Figure 138 Comminuted intertrochanteric fractures, lateral view.

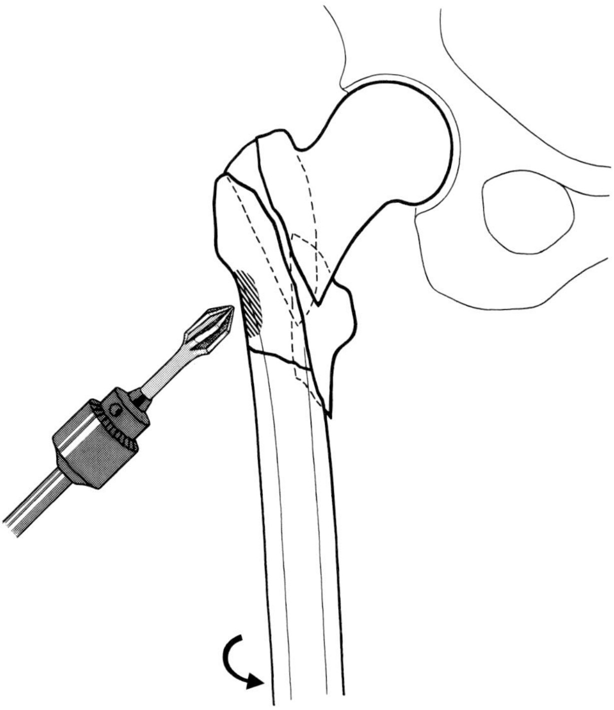

Figure 139 After the reduction of the comminuted intertrochanteric fracture, preparation for the entry port for the femoral neck nail.

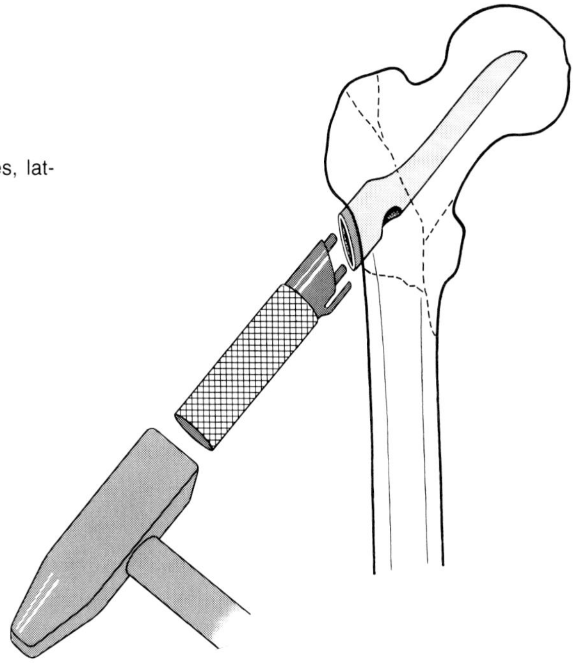

Figure 140 Driving of the Y-femoral neck nail.

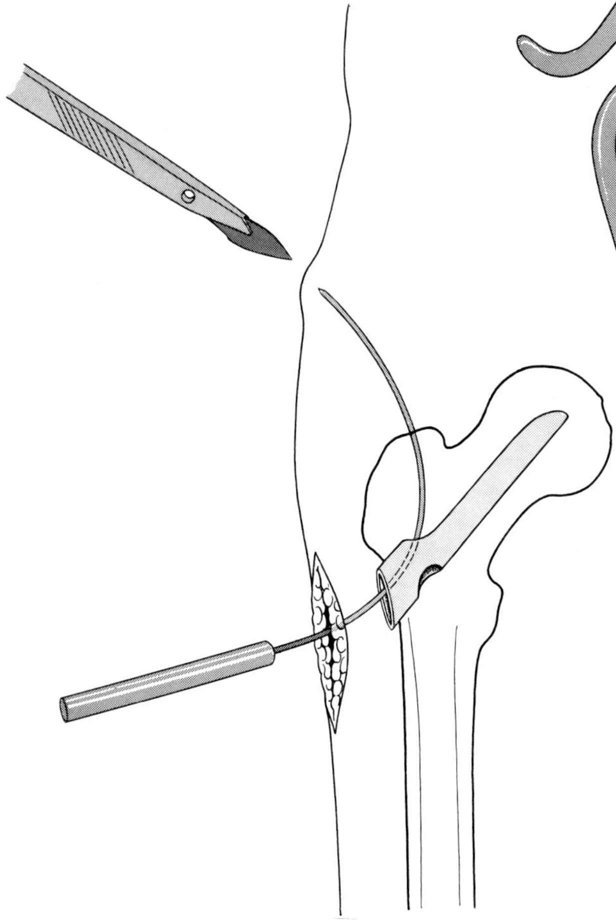

Figure 141 Inserting the curved sharp guide pin through the Y-femoral neck nail and through the trochanter tip until reaching the skin. Stab incision.

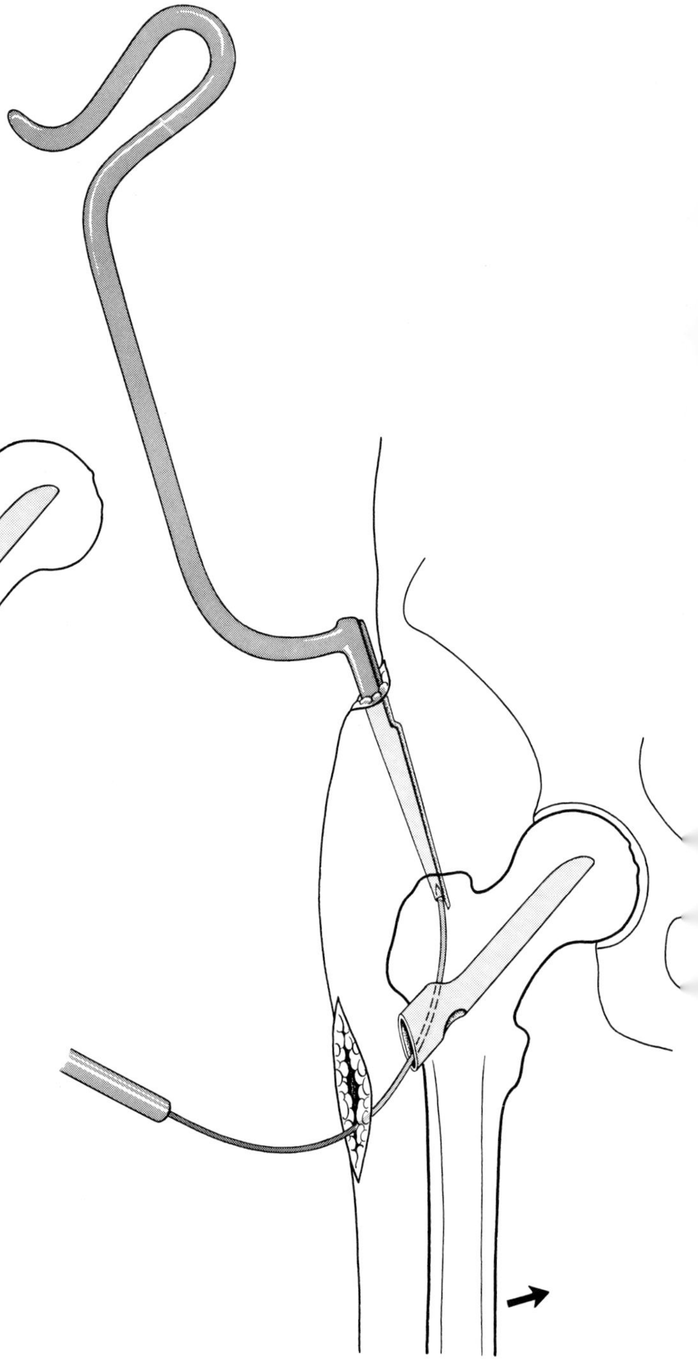

Figure 142 Leading of the reamer awl to the trochanter tip by the curved sharp guide pin. Reaming of the entry point of the flanged femoral nail.

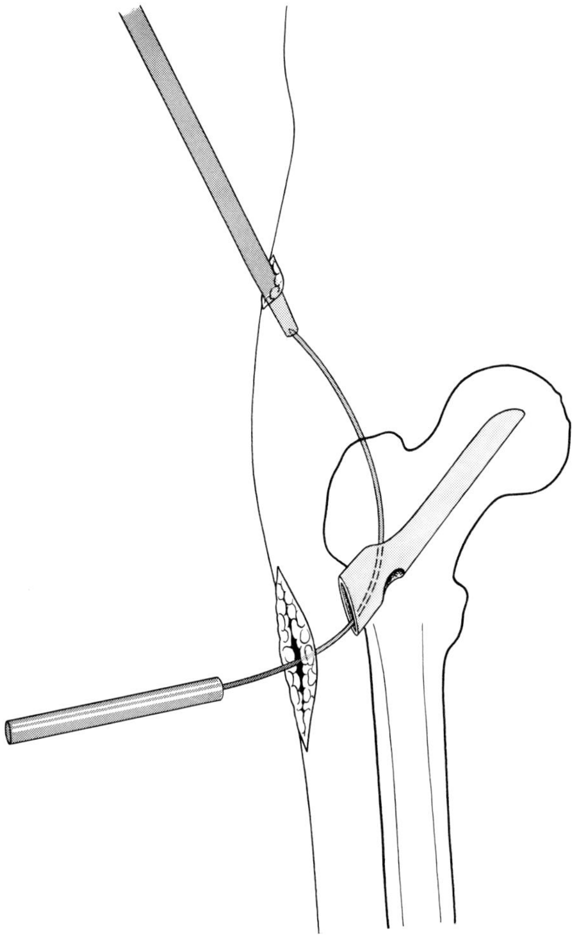

Figure 143 Leading of the flanged femoral nail to the trochanter tip by the curved sharp guide pin.

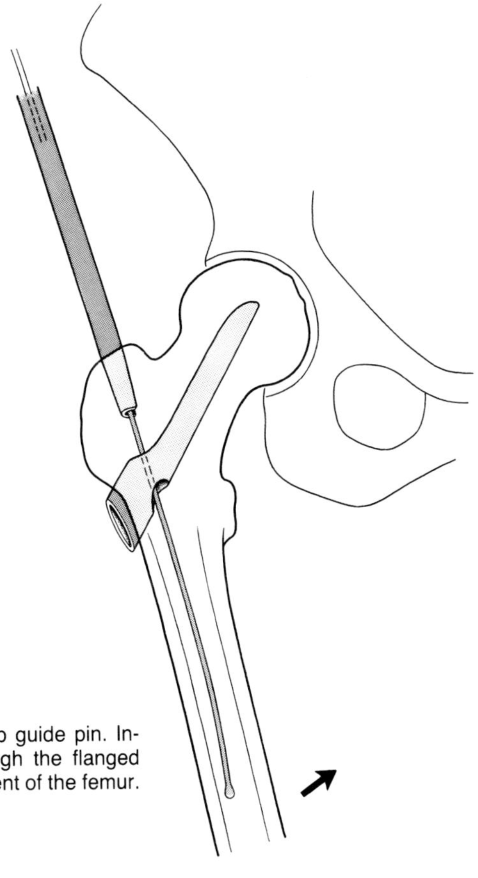

Figure 144 Removal of the curved sharp guide pin. Introduction of the straight guide pin through the flanged femoral nail until reaching the distal fragment of the femur. Adduction of the leg.

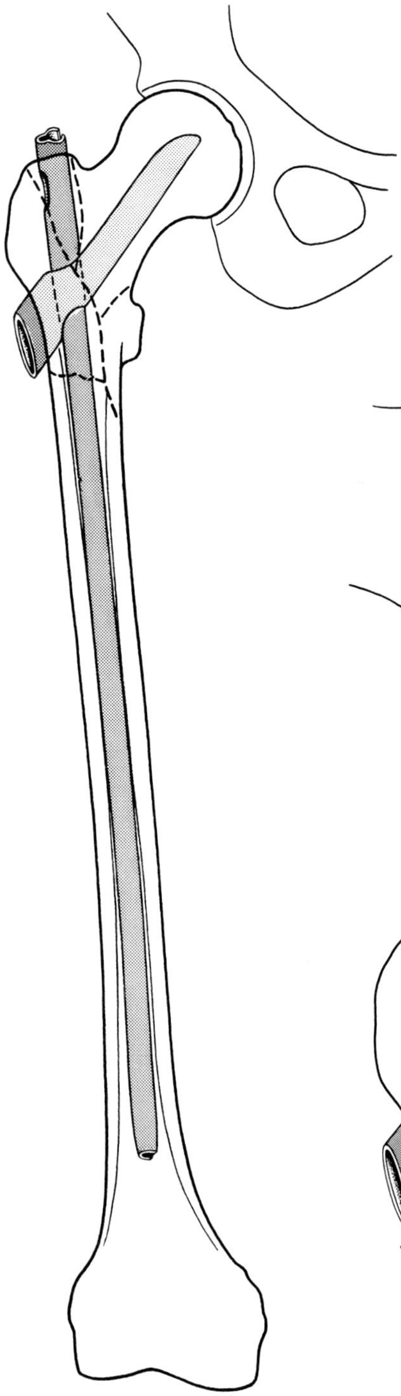

Figure 145
Completed Y-nailing, AP view.

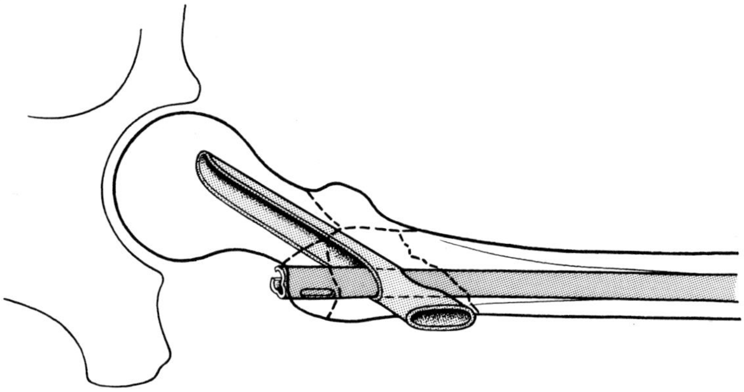

Figure 146 Completed Y-nailing, lateral view.

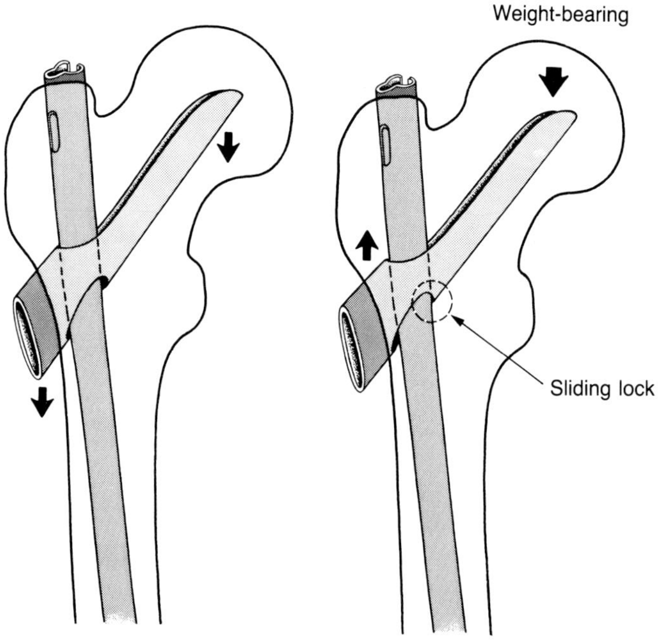

Figure 147 The principle of the Y-nail. Weight-bearing exerts pressure on the Y-femoral neck rail, thereby locking the Y-femoral neck nail onto the flanged femoral nail.

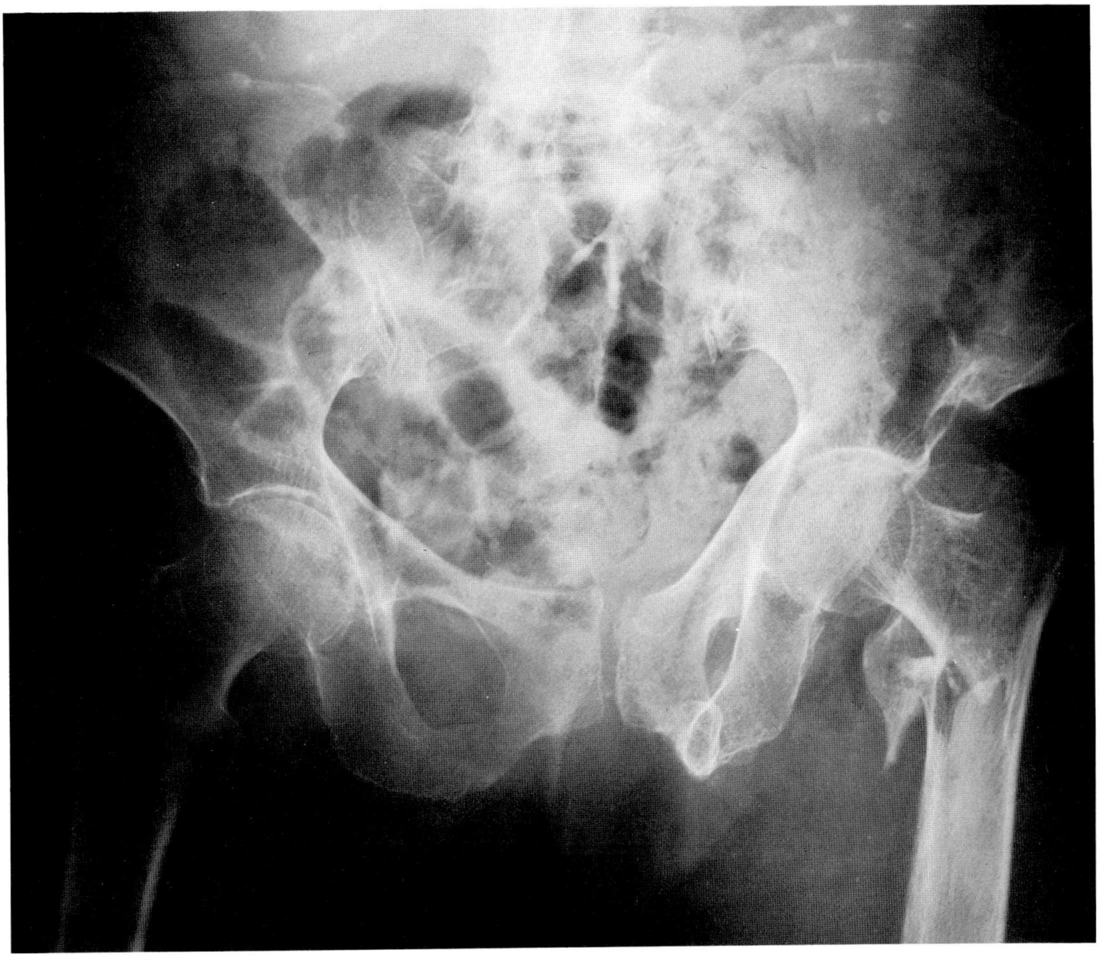

Figure 148 Severely comminuted fracture of the left trochanter with evulsion of the lesser trochanter, AP view.

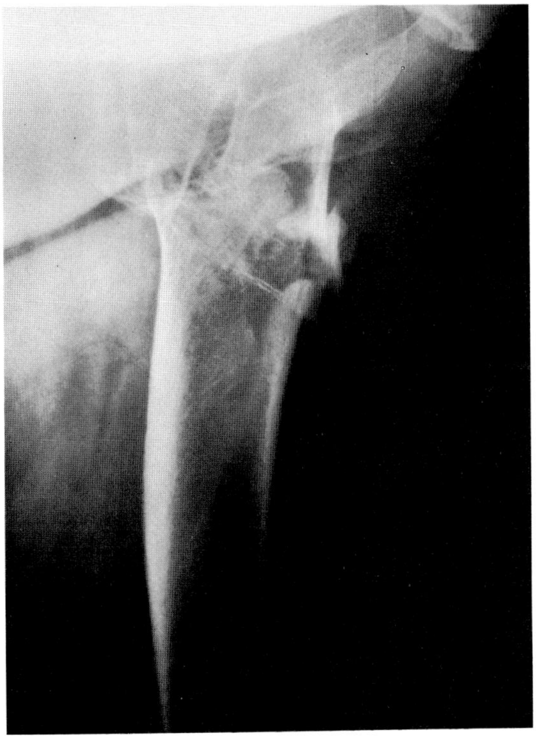

Figure 149 Lateral view of the left comminuted trochanter fracture.

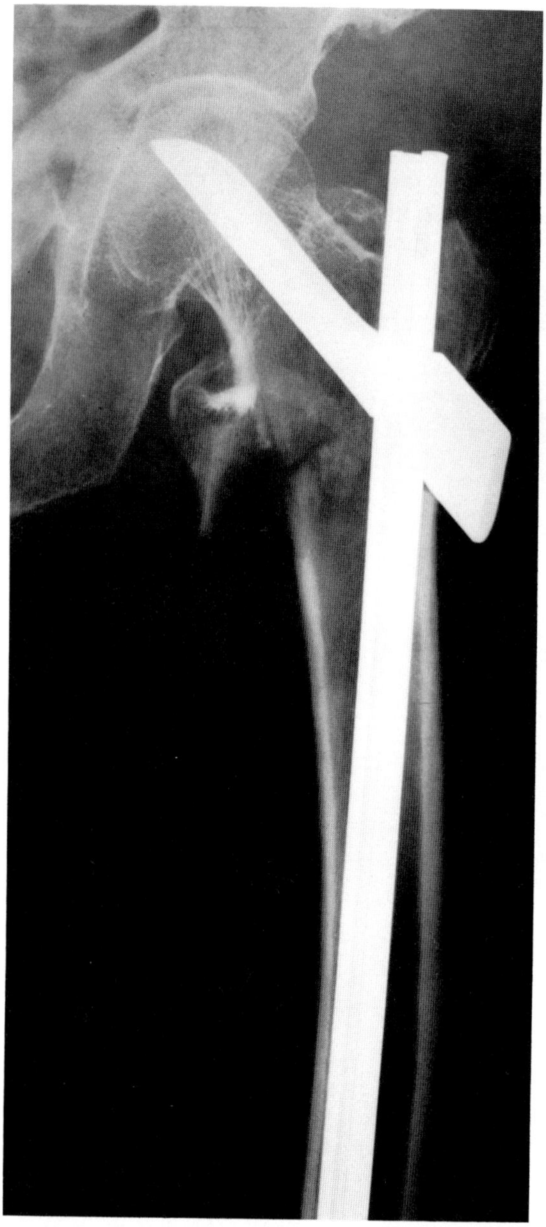

Figure 150 The same fracture after Y-nailing, AP view. The displacement of the lesser trochanter is of no significance. The proper femoral neckshaft angle is restored. The elastic longitudinal locking of the flanged femoral nail is obvious in this varus-deformed femur.

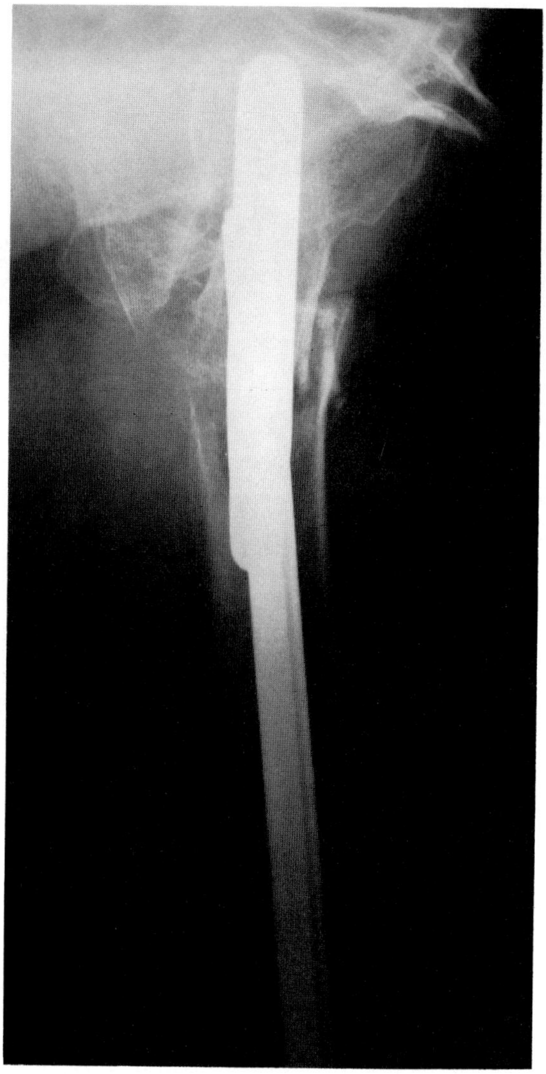

Figure 151 Lateral view after Y-nailing. The anteversion of the femoral neck is restored.

Trochanter Nailing

Indications

All noncomminuted intertrochanteric fractures, either with or without fractures of the lesser trochanter, excluding subtrochanteric fractures, are indications for trochanter nailing. Fragmented fractures of the trochanter mass can be nailed if the calcar has satisfactory cortical support. These indications can be widened for bedridden patients to include trochanteric, intertrochanteric, and subtrochanteric fractures. This osteosynthesis, which causes only little stress to the patient, allows for more comfortable and efficient nursing.

Instruments

The standard Küntscher intramedullary nail set is used for trochanter nailing. A bendable smooth (i.e., without a ball-point tip) long guide pin, a special pin handgrip, a curved nail driver, and a nail bender are additionally used. The trochanter nails have either 9- or 10-mm diameters and come in varying lengths. Each nail comes with a condylar fixation pin.

Positioning and Reduction

The patient is supine on the fracture table with both legs abducted. The perineum rests against the radiolucent perineal post. Both feet are usually attached to the traction device. The reduction necessitates a strong inward rotation and traction of the involved leg. If the fragments are interlocked, they must be mobilized by interchanging inward and outward rotation with traction and longitudinal compression. Occasionally the leg must be raised or lowered in order to obtain the phsysiologic angle of the femoral shaft.

Image Intensification

Preoperative roentgenograms in two planes of the entire femur, comprising the hip and knee joint, are necessary. The femoral neck and the knee joint must be fluoroscoped in two planes. For this reason, the image intensifier must be obliquely positioned on the injured side. Postoperative roentgenograms of the hip joint are to be taken in two planes.

Operative Technique

The surgeon stands between the abducted legs. A 2- to 3-cm long skin incision is made just proximal to the interarticular space over the epicondyle, longitudinal to the femoral axis. The entry point into the femoral condyle is then opened by the awl. After the awl pierces the cortex, its handle is tilted toward the lower leg, so that the tip of the awl points into the medullary canal. Insert the smooth (i.e., without ball-point) guide pin until the proximal lateral quadrant of the femoral head is reached under image intensification. The guide pin should pass the fracture eccentrically close to the calcar. Occasionally the pin's tip must be bent in order to reach the proximal lateral quadrant more easily. Trochanter nails are driven into the medullary canal without reaming. The guide pin should be 3mm thick so that it can emerge from the slit of the nail, thus guiding the nail at its narrow tip only. If the guide pin is too thick it cannot be adjusted to the shape of the medullary canal by subsequent bending without the nail getting wedged to the pin as it is driven in, thus advancing the pin further into the hip joint or pelvic bone as the nail proceeds. The length of the nail is calculated by subtracting the protruding part of the guide pin from the known length of the guide pin. One should bend the selected nail into the shape of the bone with the nail bender. One can check to see if the altered shape of the nail matches the bone by laying the nail on top of the leg and fluoroscoping. The trochanter nail is then driven over the guide pin and an elevator is placed through the nail slot. Occasionally minor corrections of the nail's position can be made while driving the nail by rotating it with the elevator. Once the nail reaches the desired position, withdraw the guide pin. The curved driver is used to drive the nail under the soft tissue. The fixation pin is driven into the nail to prevent any movement of the nail. One should bend the overhanging lips of the fixation pin, which lie in the soft tissue, with a pair of pliers. Incision is then closed.

Common Mistakes

If the entry point is made too far proximally into the medial femoral condyle, the nail meets the contralateral cortex of the femoral shaft at too steep an angle. This causes a bony lamella to crack off from the transition of the medial femoral condyle into the shaft. An entry point that is too far distal opens the knee joint, often resulting in joint effusion. An entry point that is too far ventral can also lead to opening of the knee joint and to joint effusion. An entry point that is too far dorsal can cause the nail to exit the fracture site dorsally and impose torsional strain on the nail. A trochanter nail that is insufficiently bent at the tip can fracture the lateral femoral cortex. Another result of this mistake can be the exiting of the nail at the proximal lateral quadrant.

Bending the trochanter nail excessively can split the femoral shaft.

Insufficient bending of the trochanter nail can lead to the nail's distal end breaking into the convexity of the medial femoral condyle. Using too short a nail allows a varus deformity under weight-bearing. The fracture site is thereby gapping in the area closest to the trochanter tip.

If the trochanter nail is too long, it will penetrate the femoral head when the fracture impacts. This causes a painful decrease in hip mobility. A long trochanter nail may, on rare occasions, even push out distally and restrain motion of the knee joint. The combination of nailing with too long a nail into the incorrect entry point can lead to the fixation pin's penetration into the knee joint.

Aftercare

Because the trochanter nailing is designed for immediate weight-bearing, physiotherapy is initiated as soon as soft-tissue healing will allow. No special aftercare is necessary, except for active exercises and supervised ambulation.

Figure 152A Trochanter nail with stop pin.

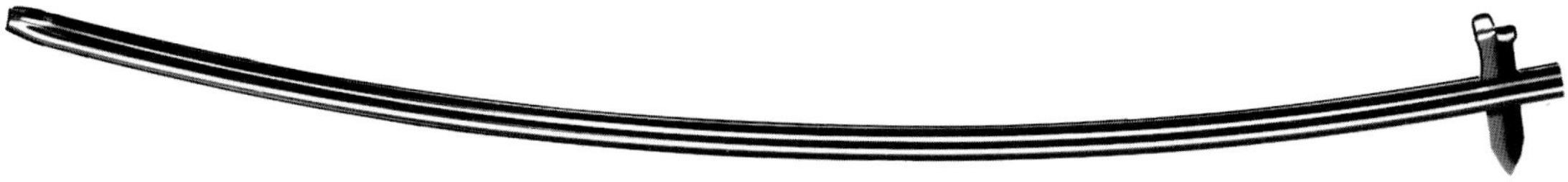

Figure 152B Trochanter nail with stop pin through the slot.

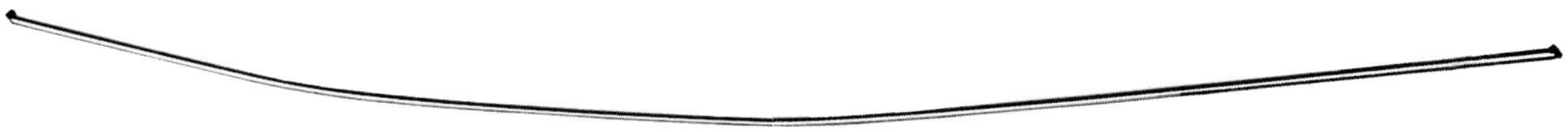

Figure 153 Bendable smooth guide pin.

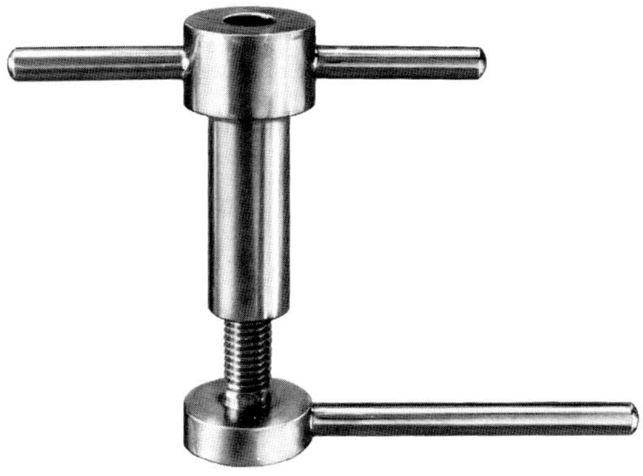

◀ Figure 154 Guide pin extractor for trochanter nailing.

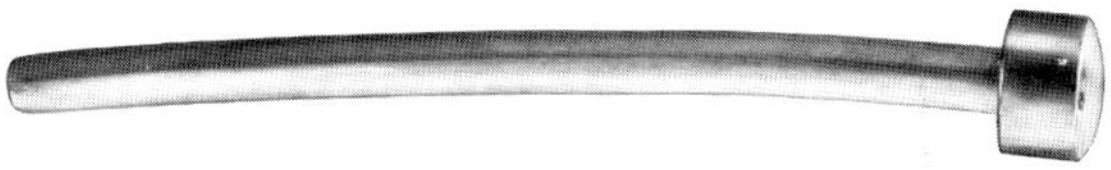

Figure 155 Curved nail driver.

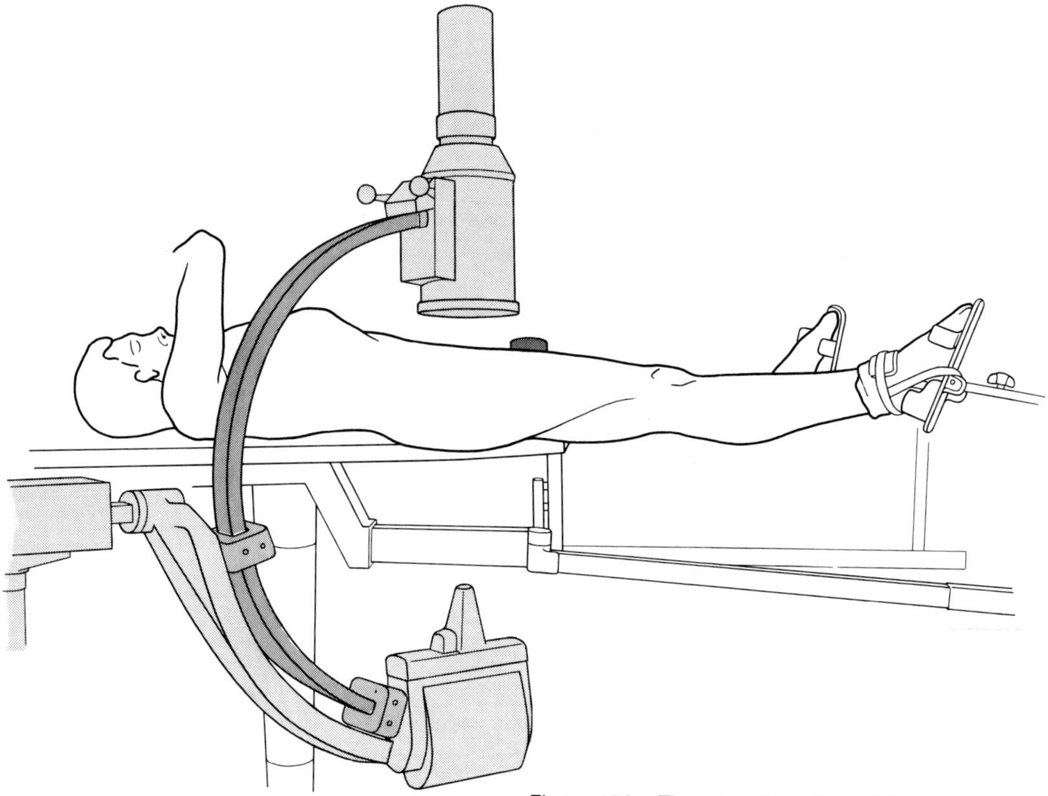

Figure 156 The correct position of the patient on the fracture table for trochanter nailing. The correct position of the image intensifier for AP fluoroscopy.

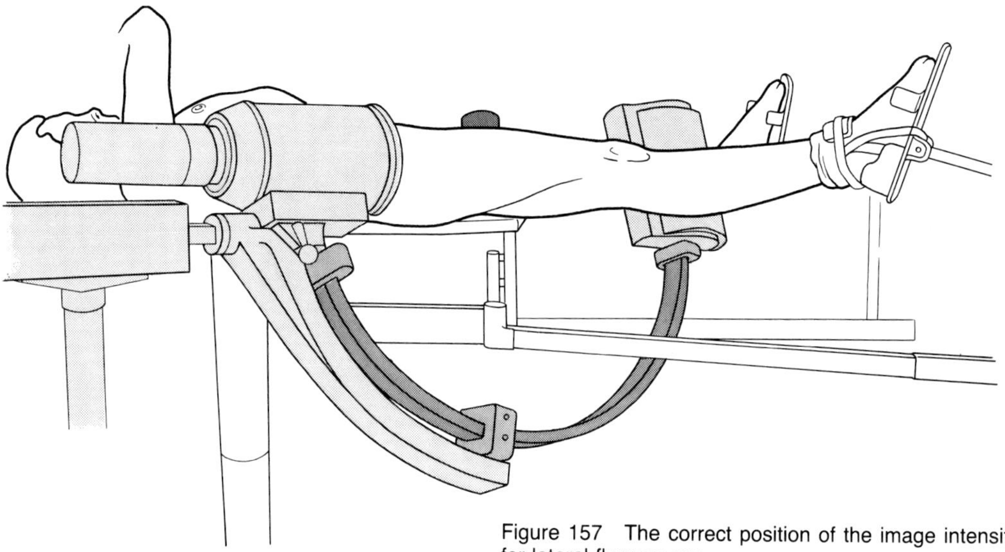

Figure 157 The correct position of the image intensifier for lateral fluoroscopy.

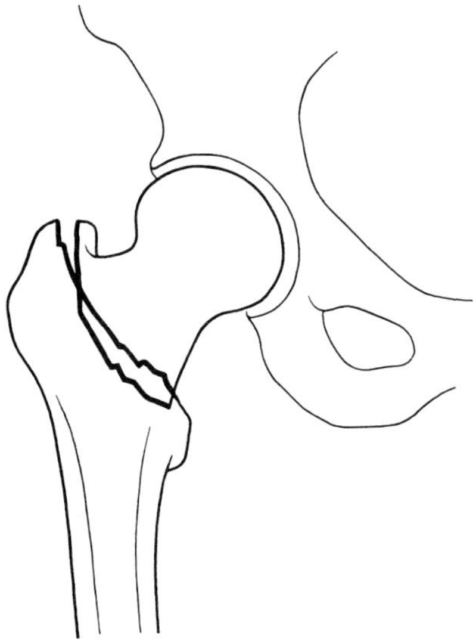

Figure 158 Intertrochanteric fractures of the femur.

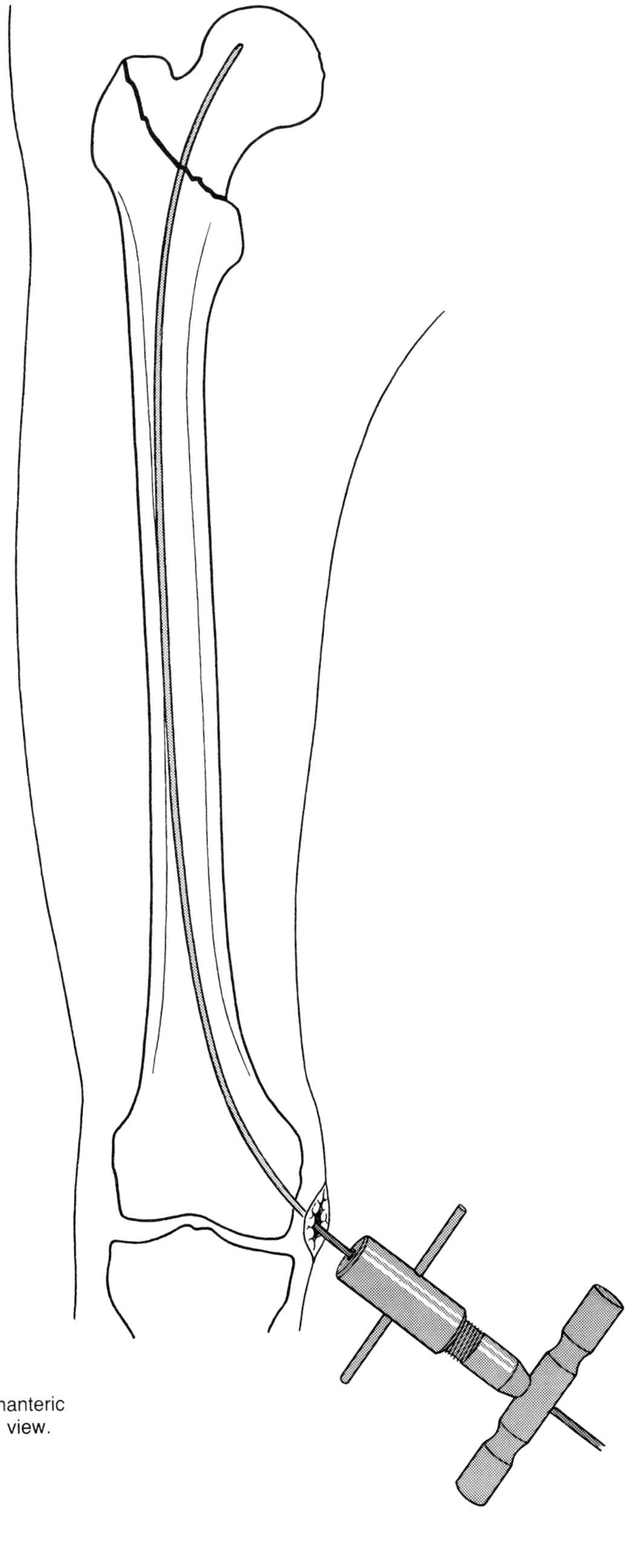

Figure 159 After the reduction of the intertrochanteric fractures, stab incision and inserted guide pin, AP view.

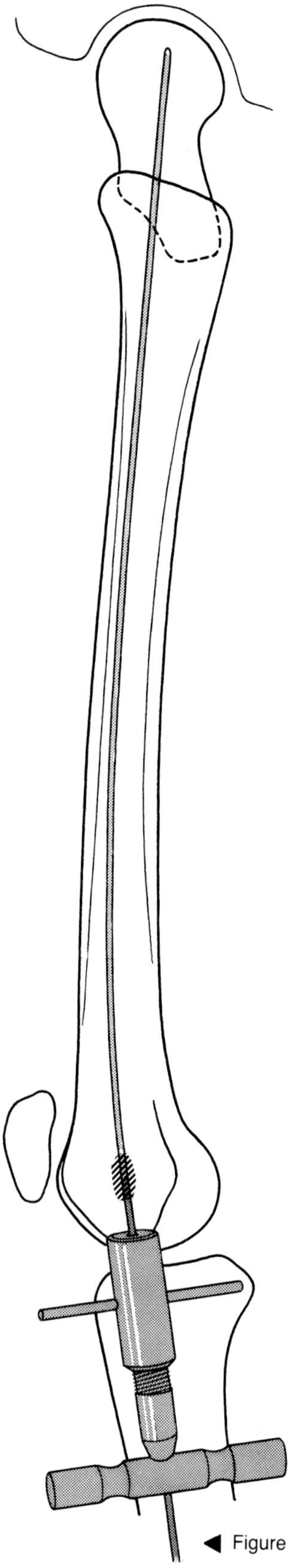

◀ Figure 160 The same case in lateral view.

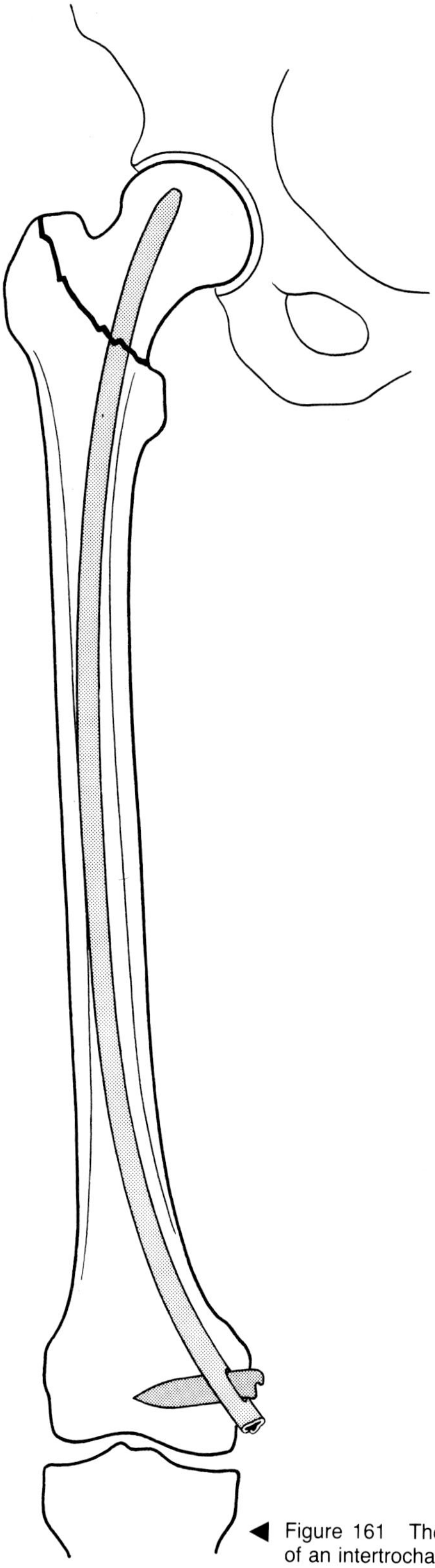

◀ Figure 161 The completed trochanter nailing of an intertrochanteric fracture, AP view.

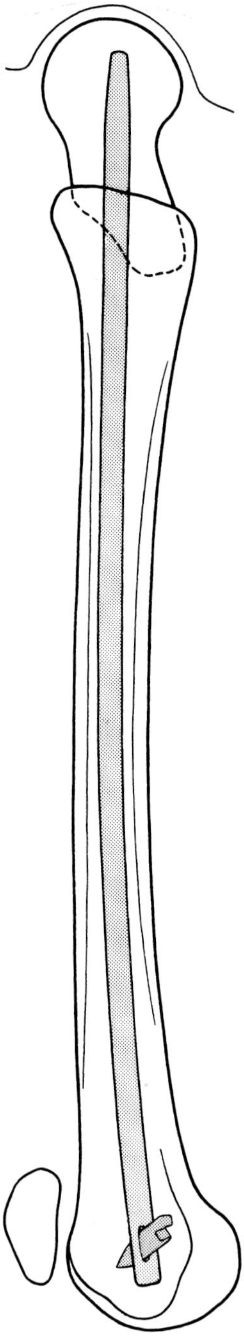

Figure 162 Condition after trochanter nailing, lateral view.

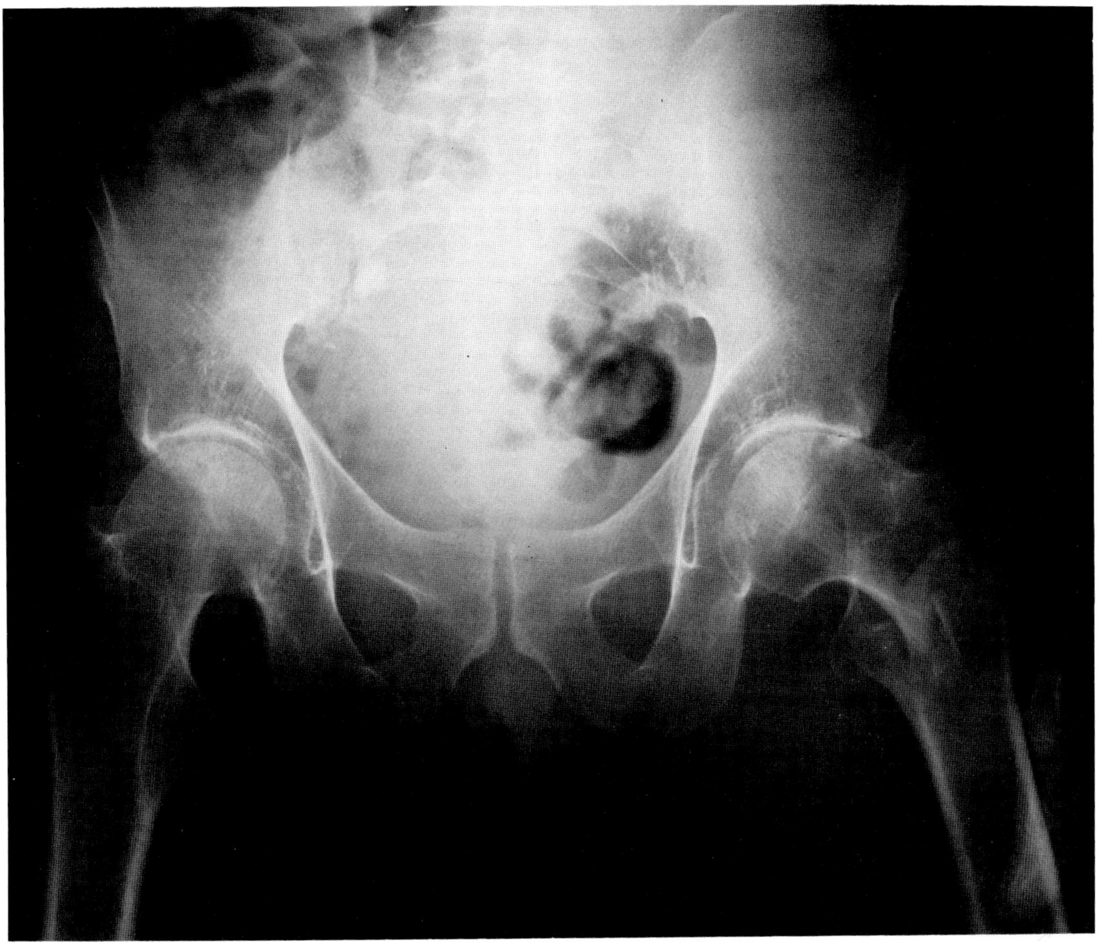

Figure 163 Left intertrochanteric fracture with varus deformity and outward rotation of the leg.

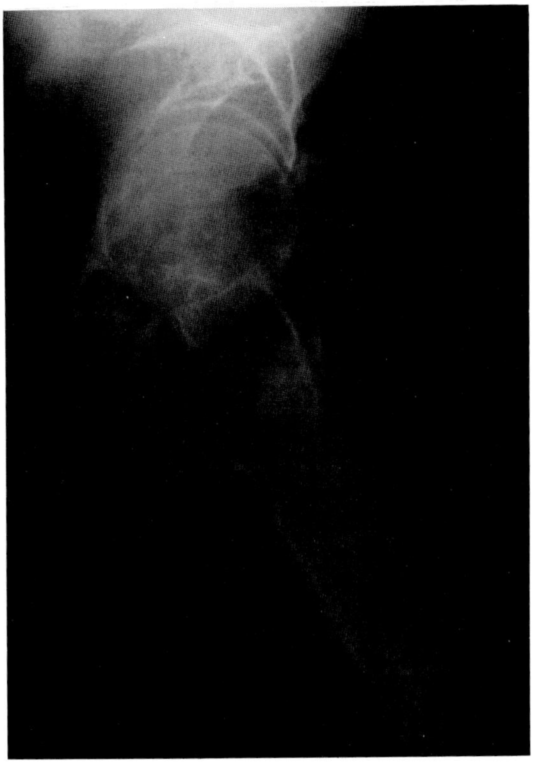

Figure 164 Lateral view of the same intertrochanteric fracture.

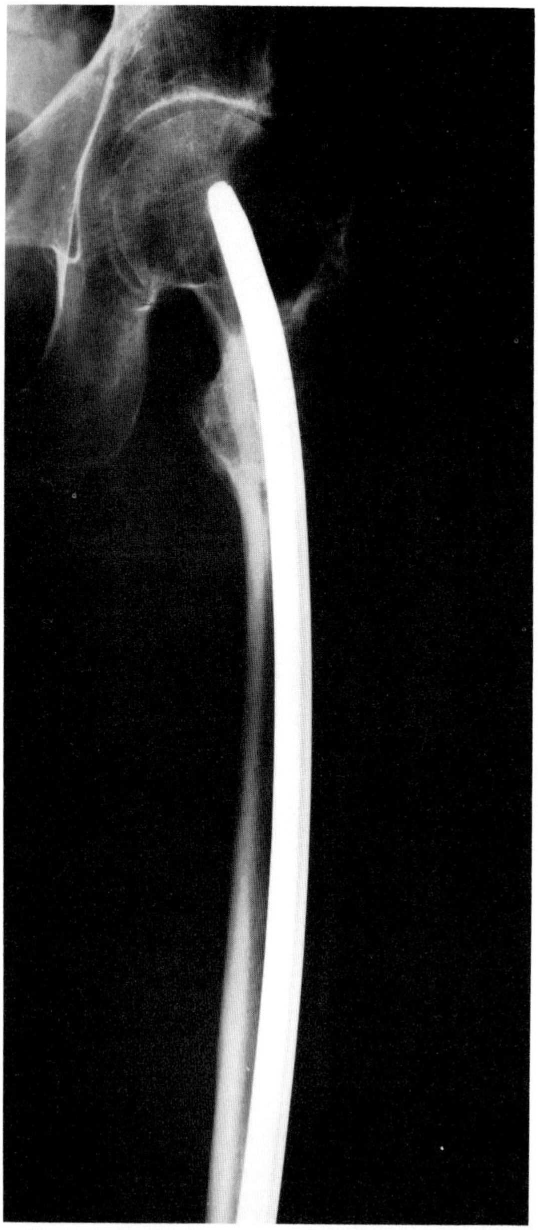

Figure 165 The same fracture after trochanter nailing, 12 months after the accident, AP view.

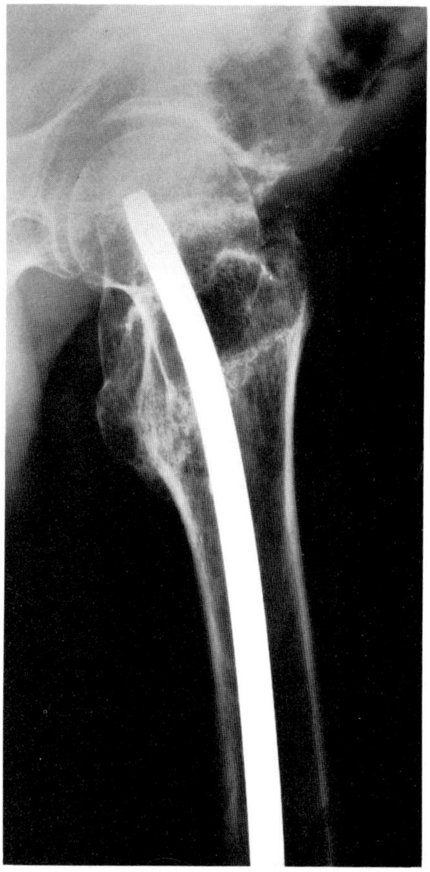

Figure 166 Lateral view after trochanter nailing and bony healing.

Figure 169 The same intertrochanteric fracture after bony healing and nail removal, AP view. ▶

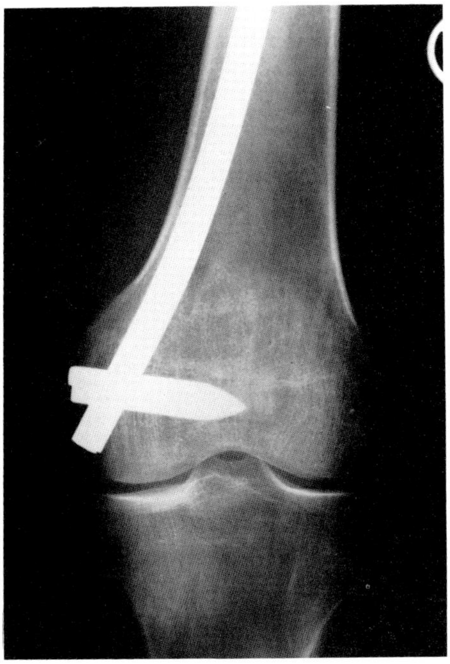

Fig. 167

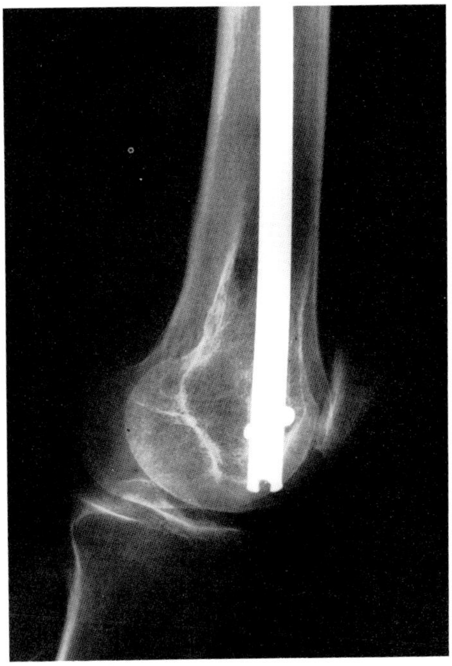

Fig. 168

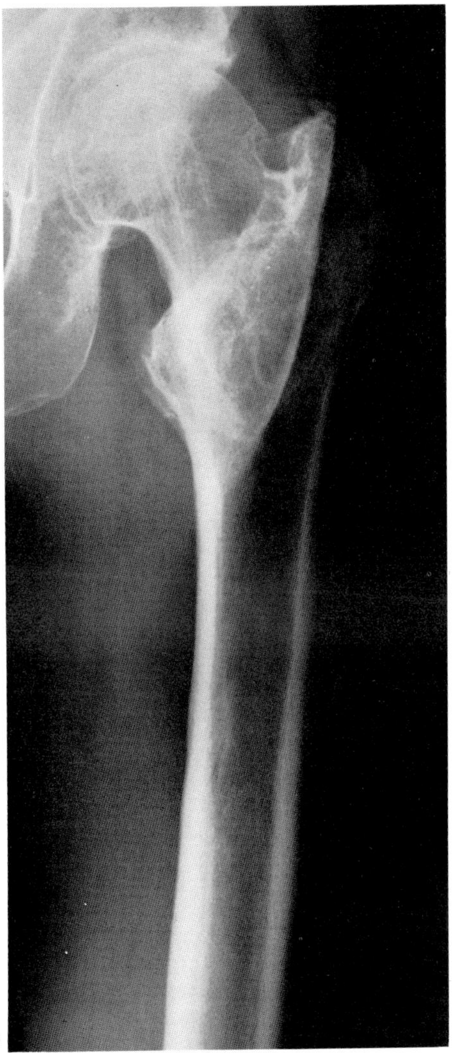

Fig. 169

Figure 167 Nail entry point at the medial femoral condyle, showing the nail's end, with the stop pin inserted through the slot, AP view.

Figure 168 Lateral view of the nail's end with stop pin through the slot.

Figure 170 Lateral view of the intertrochanteric fracture after bony healing and nail removal, 12½ months after the accident.

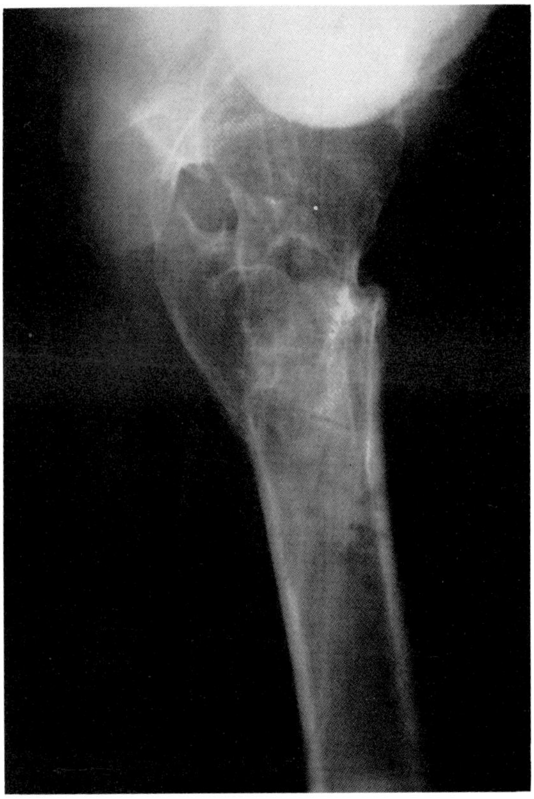

Nailing of the Clavicle

Indications

There are only a few indications for clavicle nailing. Nailing is warranted only in cases when the fracture occurs in the middle portion of the clavicle and is accompanied by either nerve or vascular damage, or is completely offset with or without considerable shortening. Another candidate for nailing, however, is the painful pseudarthrosis occurring in the middle third portion of the clavicle.

Instruments

A handchuck and twist drill, along with clavicle nails, are needed in addition to the standard intramedullary nailing instruments. The clavicle nails have a V-shaped profile with two narrowed, easily bendable ends. These nails are available in varying lengths and diameters.

Positioning and Reduction

The patient should be in a supine position on a regular operating table. The injured shoulder should be positioned as far over the edge of the regular table as needed, to make clavicle x-ray exposures possible. The clavicle may also be positioned on an accessory radiolucent head end for the table. The fracture will be reduced after its surgical exposure.

Image Intensification

Preoperative roentgenograms of the clavicle, including the shoulder joint, are necessary. Because the fracture is reduced while the wound is opened, the image intensifier need only be pushed under the clavicle from the involved side if necessary. However, postoperative films of the clavicle should be taken in two planes.

Operative Technique

A skin incision 3 cm long is made over the fracture. Visualize the fragments and expose the distal fragment outside of the incision with a bone hook. Ream the medullary canal of the distal fragment with the handchuck and drill bits in increasing diameters. Because of the S shape of the clavicle, the drill exits dorsally. A stab incision is made over the protruding tip of the drill bit. Withdraw the drill bit. The proximal clavicle fragment is drilled in the same fashion, until the tip of the twist drill is noticed under the skin before the sternoclavicular joint. Make another stab incision over the protruding tip of the drill. Remove the twist drill. Hammer the chosen clavicle nail, slotted end first, from the site of the fracture distally until the slot of the nail protrudes out of the stab incision. Insert the hook of a nail extractor into the slot and use a slotted driver to pull the clavicle nail out until its medial end is flush with the distal fracture site. Reduce the fracture and drive the clavicle nail retrograde into the proximal fragment until the narrowed nail end exits the clavicle drill hole near the sternoclavicular joint. The nail is then bent at the proximal end and shortened as necessary. Thereafter, insert the hook of the nail extractor and compress the fracture by driving the nail distally, using a slotted driver. Bend the distal narrowed nail end at the exit site to maintain the compression and shorten as necessary. Close the incisions.

Common Mistakes

If both nail ends are not bent, the possibility of nail migration exists. Nail ends that are not sufficiently bent may lead to soft-tissue irritation and even necrosis.

Aftercare

No special aftercare is necessary. The beginning of active exercises depends on the condition of the soft tissue.

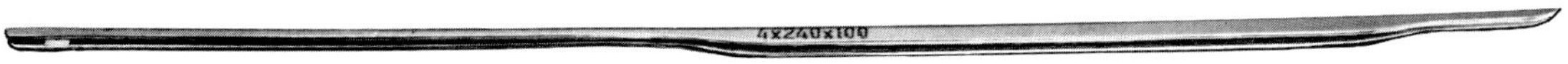

Figure 171 Clavicle nail.

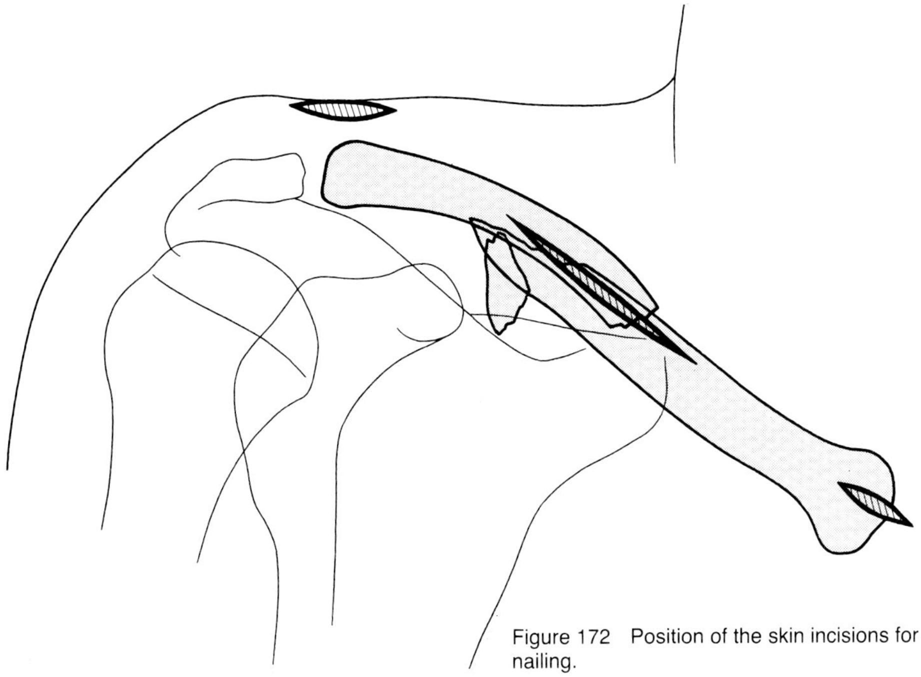

Figure 172 Position of the skin incisions for clavicular nailing.

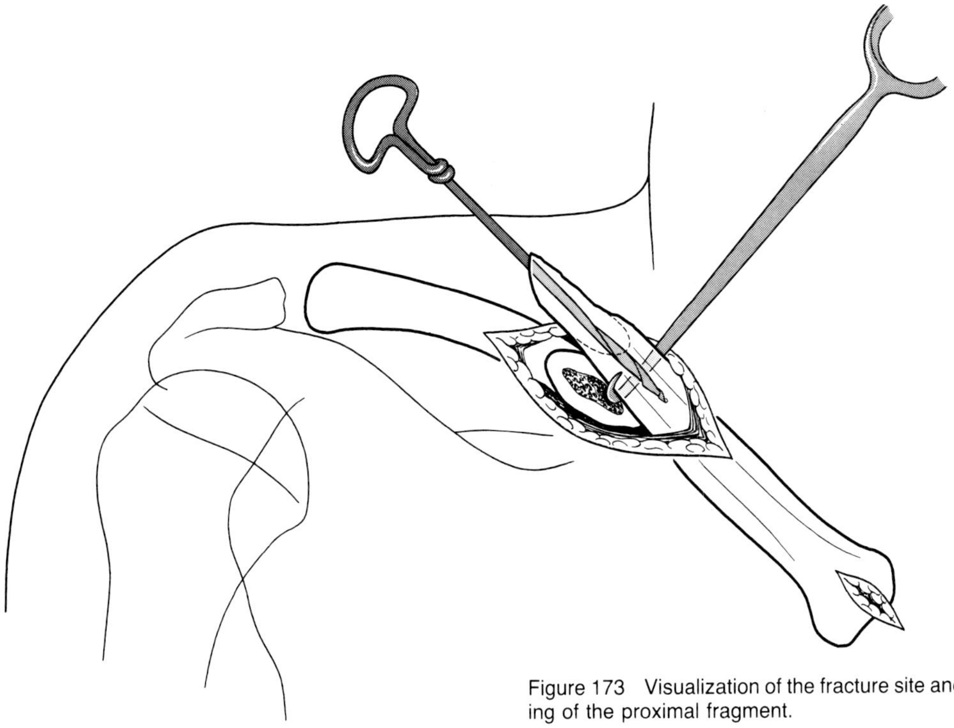

Figure 173 Visualization of the fracture site and reaming of the proximal fragment.

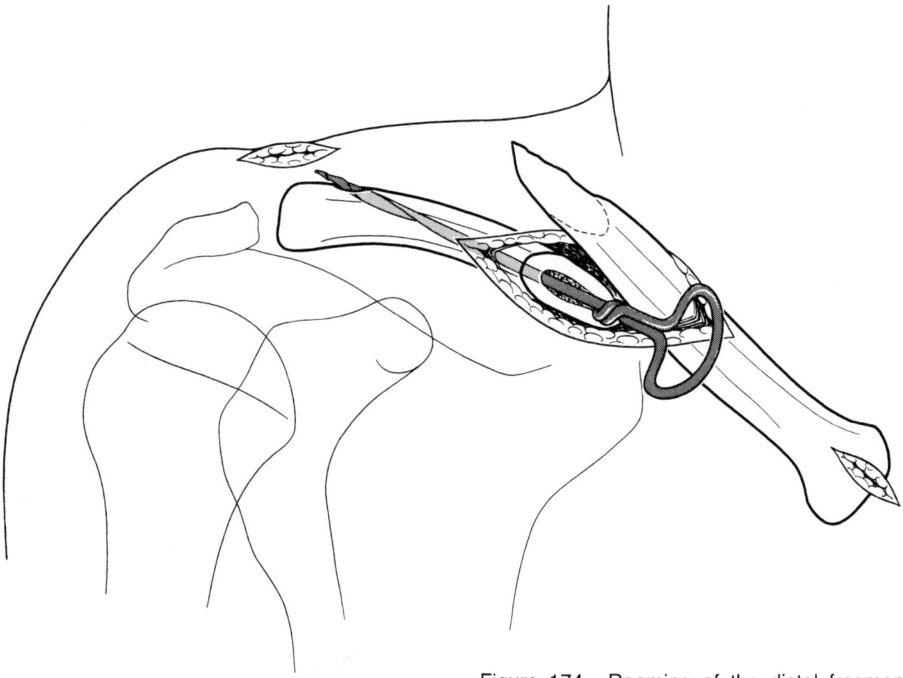

Figure 174 Reaming of the distal fragment with the hand reamer.

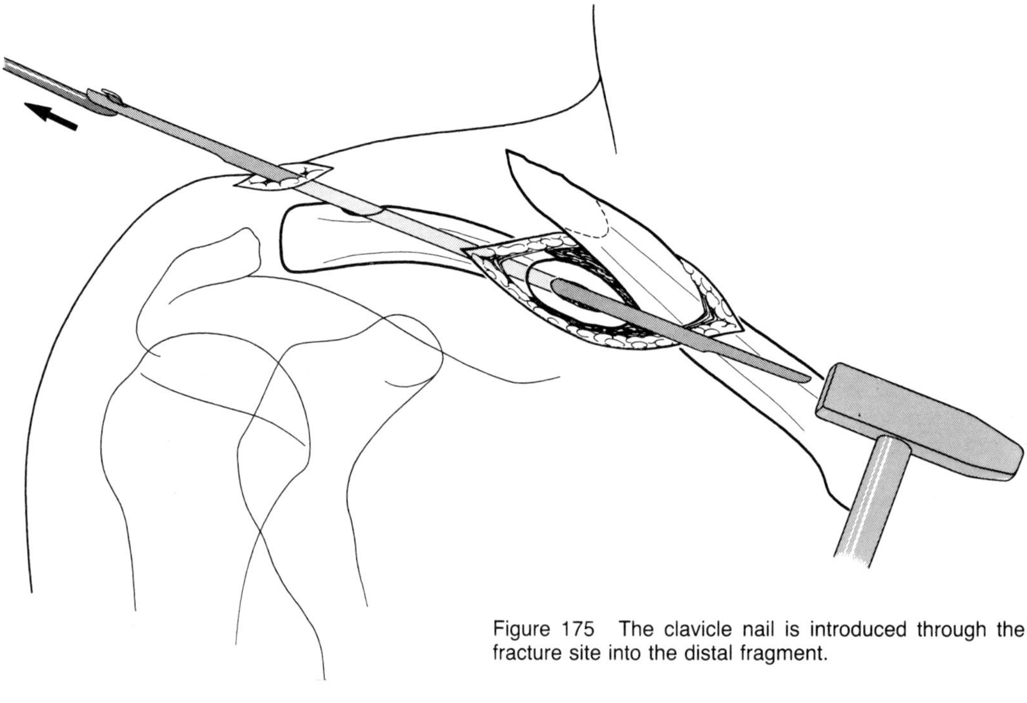

Figure 175 The clavicle nail is introduced through the fracture site into the distal fragment.

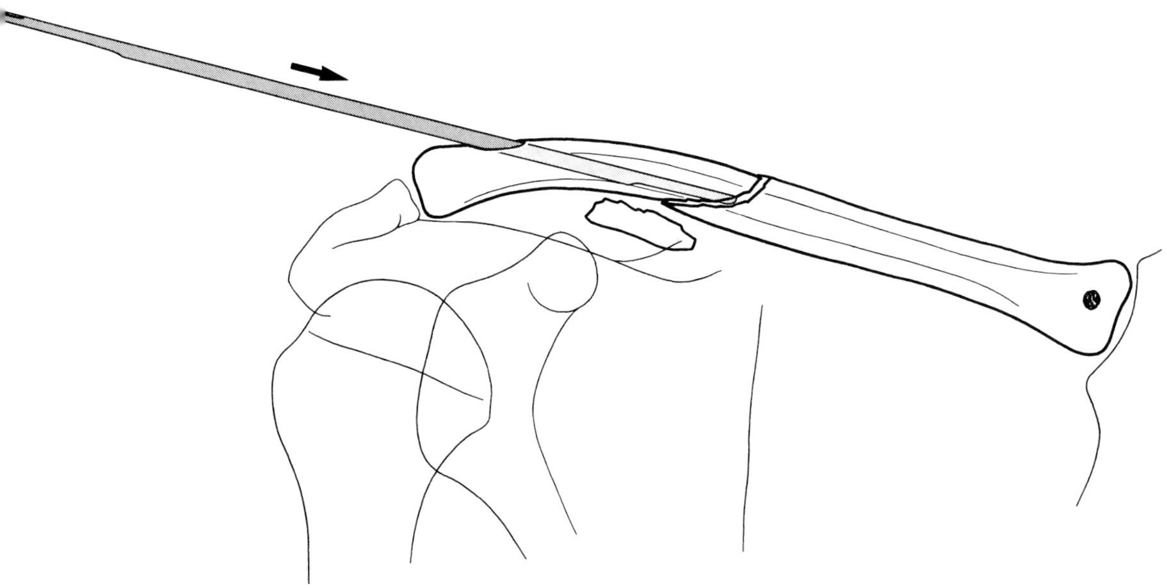

Figure 176 After reduction of the fracture, driving the clavicle nail from the distal into the proximal fragment.

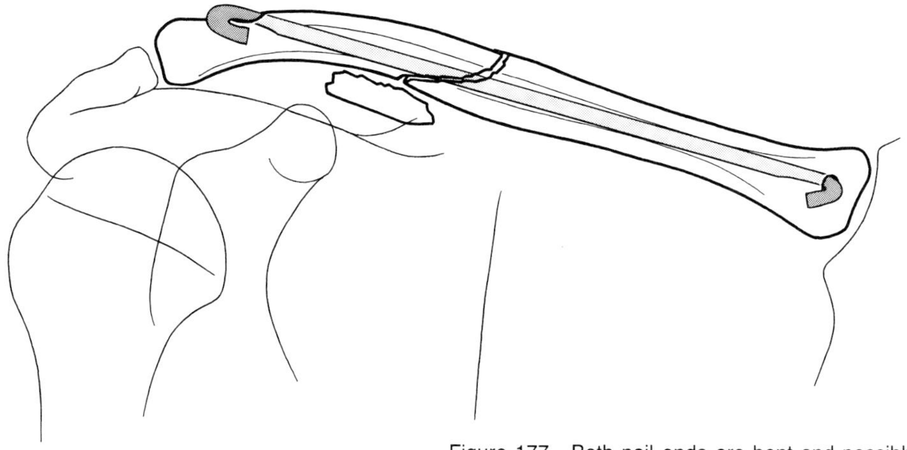

Figure 177 Both nail ends are bent and possibly shortened to avoid any migrating of the nail.

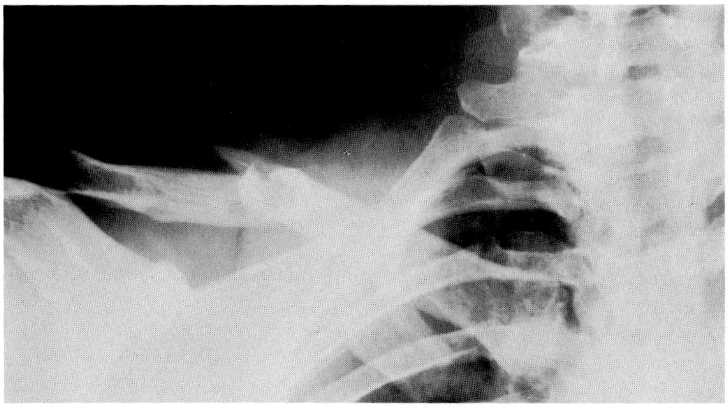

Figure 178 Fresh fracture of the clavicle, middle third.

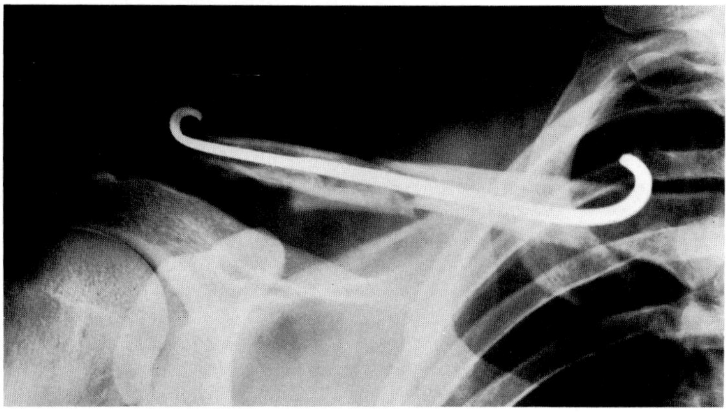

Figure 179 The same fracture after nailing. Both nail ends were bent.

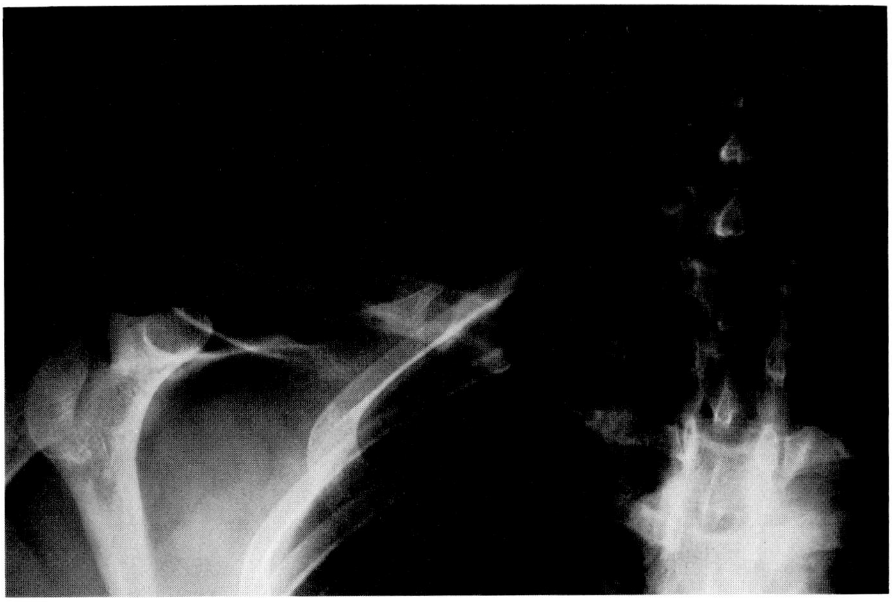

Figure 180 The same fracture of the clavicle after bony healing and nail removal, AP view, after 21 months.

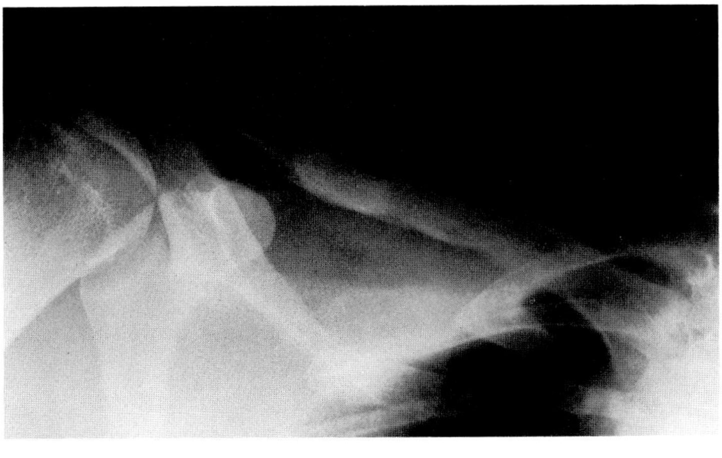

Figure 181 Oblique view after the removal of the clavicle nail.

Interlocking Nail Osteosynthesis

Interlocking Nail Osteosynthesis of the Femur

The interlocking nail is a Küntscher nail with two to four transverse holes, through which transverse screws can be inserted, providing the interlocking features.

Indications

The indications for the femoral intramedullary nailing are significantly widened by using the interlocking nail. Spiral fractures, fragmented fractures, severely comminuted fractures, and transverse fractures in bone segments with wide medullary canals can all be stabilized satisfactorily with interlocking nails. Furthermore, all fractures with unsatisfactory longitudinal stabilization, in which the danger of postoperative shortening exists, lend themselves to interlocking nail osteosynthesis. The location of indicated fractures ranges from the supracondylar to the subtrochanteric area of the femur.

Instruments

The standard femoral Küntscher nail set is used. In addition, a triangular awl with an aluminum handgrip is used to ream the holes needed for the transverse screws. A 4-mm twist drill bit and a matching hexagonal screwdriver are also necessary. For some cases the femoral interlocking nail must be specially manufactured and tailored to the shape of the fracture in question on the preoperative roentgenograms taken at a 1-m distance. For the more common fractures, standardized interlocking nails and instruments are available (developed by K. Klemm, J. Kempf, et al.).

Positioning and Reduction

The patient is positioned on the fracture table with his fractured side up, as described for femoral nailing, and the fracture is reduced (p. 13).

However, the patient may also be supine on the fracture table as described for the Y-nailing (p. 66).

Image Intensification

Preoperative roentgenograms of the femur and both adjacent joints are necessary in two planes. These films must be taken at a 1-m distance in order to serve as gauges for determining the dimensions of the interlocking nail. The image intensifier must be positioned in such a way that the femur can be fluoroscoped in two perpendicular planes. Postoperative roentgenograms of the entire femur are to be taken in two planes.

Operative Technique

The operative technique is initially identical with that described for femoral nailing (p. 13). The medullary canal should be reamed, if possible. The reaming must be done very carefully in comminuted and fragmented fractures. The reamer can cause spinning of larger fragments and this must be avoided by fixating the fragment with a bone holder. Ream in 0.5-mm increments until the predetermined diameter is reached. The intramedullary nail must be driven in such a way that the longitudinal slot points posteriorly and that the transverse holes point laterally. The reduction of the fracture should be verified by fluoroscopy before any attempt is made to drill the transverse holes for the transverse screws. The location for the initial transverse screw is marked with the aid of fluoroscopy. A stab incision is then made at the indicated mark. A tissue protector must be used at all times to prevent any soft-tissue damage, while preparing the hole for the transverse screw with the triangular awl. The canal is prepared by using the awl through the cortex, the transverse holes of the nail, and the contralateral cortex. The holes are prepared, one at a time, from distal to proximal, in this fashion. The selected self-tapping transverse screw is inserted and must firmly penetrate the contralateral cortex. If an interlocking nail with obliquely inserted proximal transverse screws, as designed by Klemm and Schellmann, is used, a drill jig is needed to prepare the canal for the long transverse screws. The incision is then closed.

Common Mistakes

The same mistakes as described in the femoral nailing section can occur (p. 14). Difficulties arise when inserting the transverse screws if the interlocking nail is driven in with its longitudinal slot not exactly pointing posteriorly. Imprecise preparation of the canal can lead to the transverse screws either deadlocking or missing the transverse holes of the nail. If the screw is forced through an imprecise canal, the cortex may split.

If the length of the interlocking nail is not exact, or the correct nail is not driven deeply enough, the transverse holes of the nail may be within the fracture area. Thus, the transverse screws cannot stabilize the fracture firmly.

Aftercare

The interlocking nail osteosynthesis always permits postoperative exercises. Active exercises should be initiated as soon as possible, depending on the severity of the soft-tissue damage. The bony stability and the progress of the fracture healing determine the time for full weight-bearing. The interlocking nail osteosynthesis of transverse fractures allows for immediate postoperative full weight-bearing.

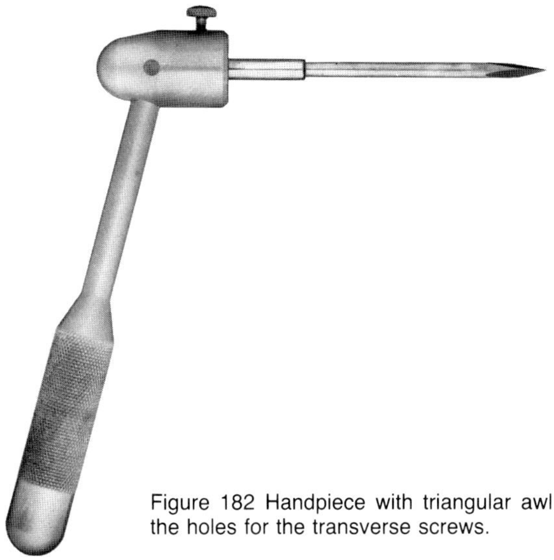

Figure 182 Handpiece with triangular awl to start the holes for the transverse screws.

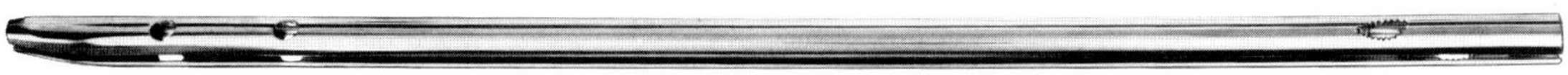

Figure 183 Standard interlocking femoral nail by Klemm.

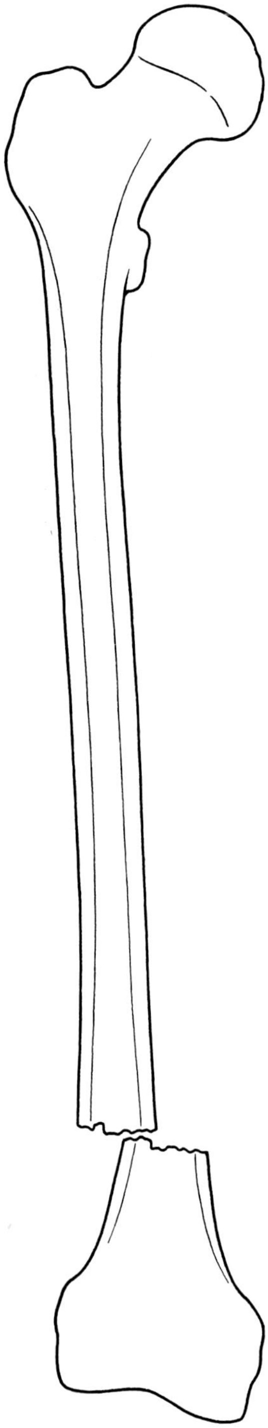

Figure 184 Femur fracture, distal third, within the widening medullary canal zone.

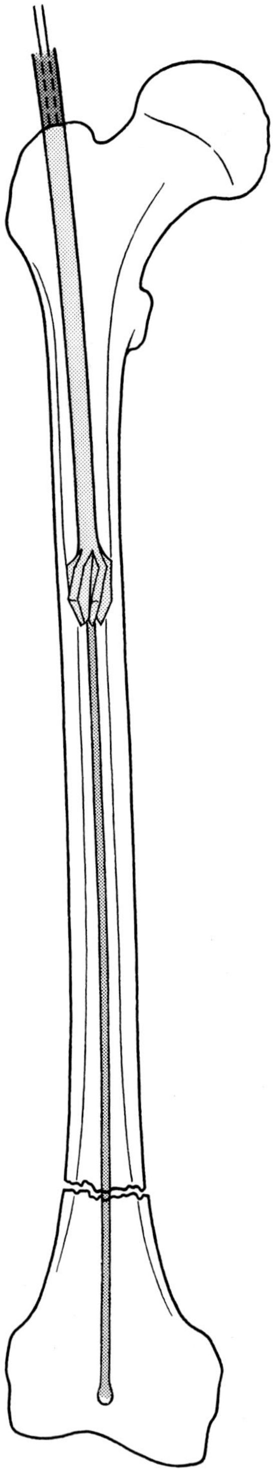

Figure 185 Reaming of the proximal narrow medullary canal after the reduction of the fracture.

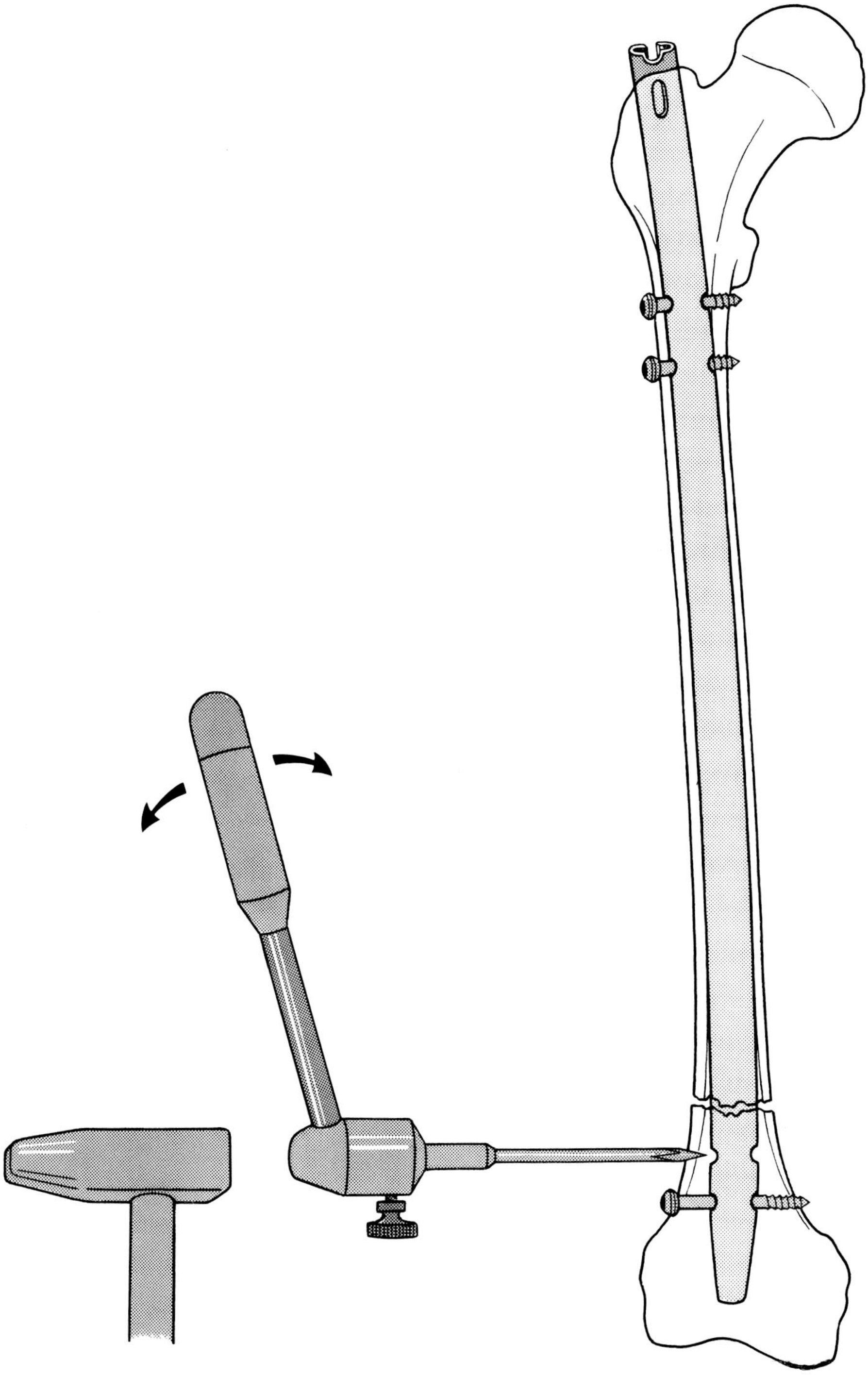

Figure 186 After driving the interlocking nail, preparation of the holes for the transverse screws.

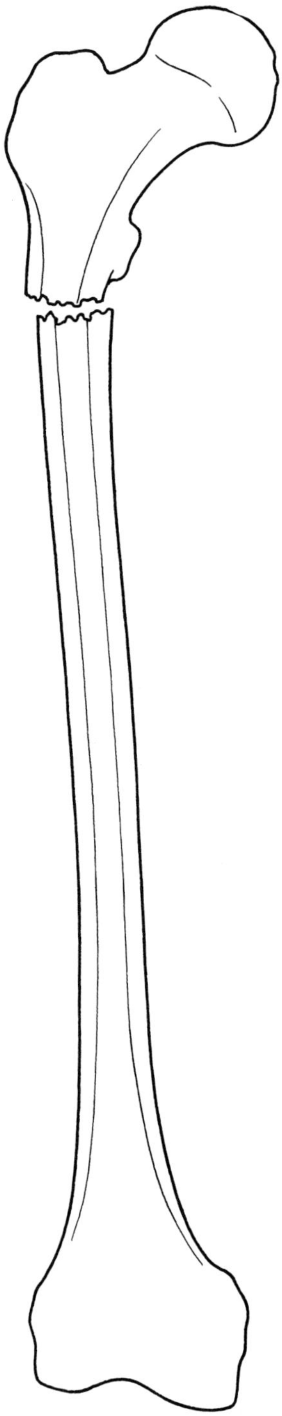

Figure 187 Fracture of the femur, proximal third, in the area of the widening medullary canal.

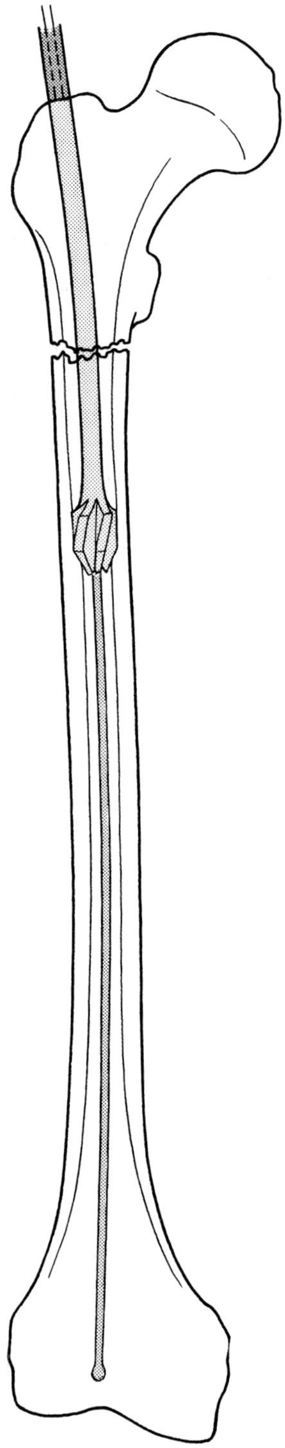

Figure 188 After reduction of the fracture, reaming of the narrow distal medullary canal.

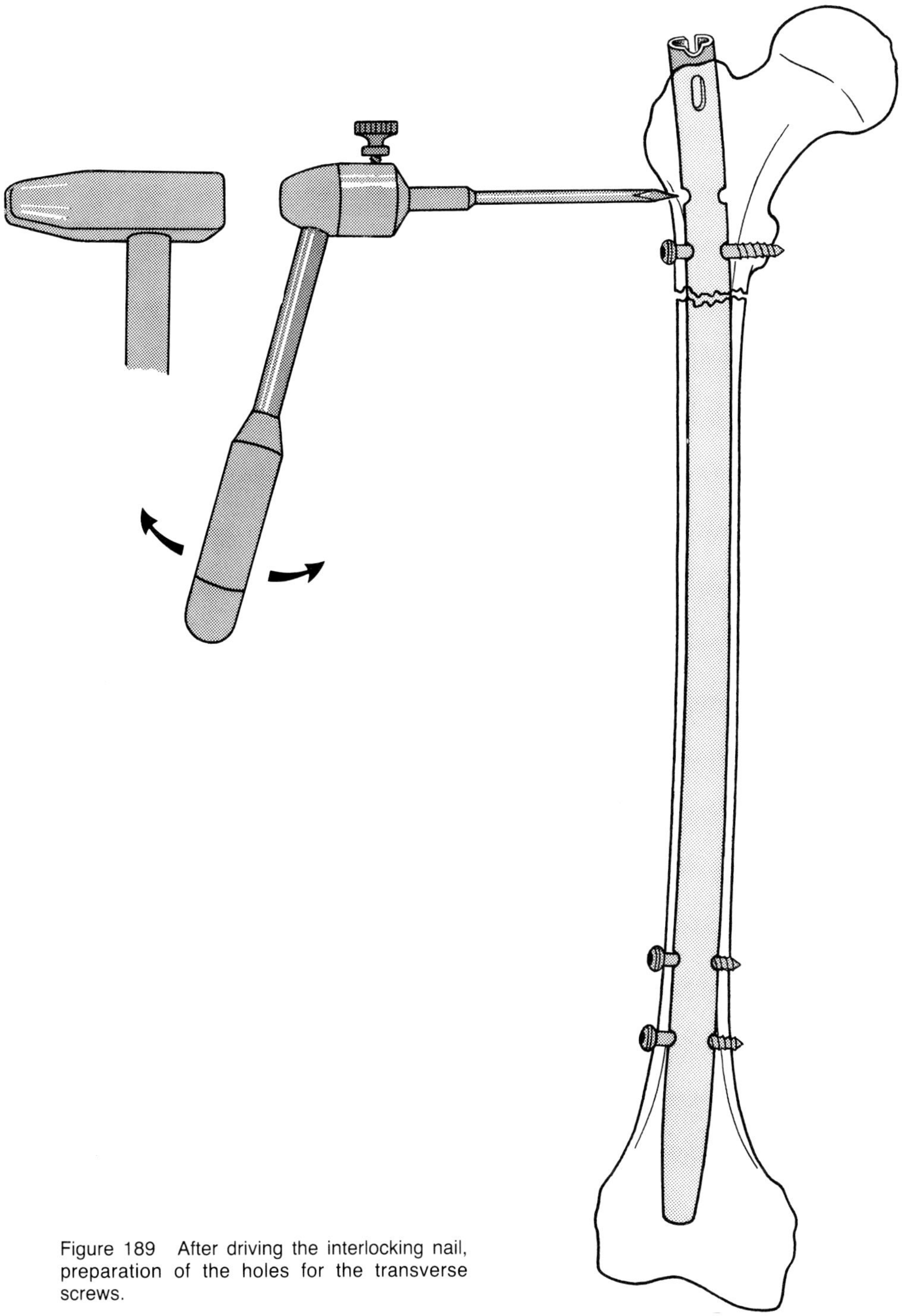

Figure 189 After driving the interlocking nail, preparation of the holes for the transverse screws.

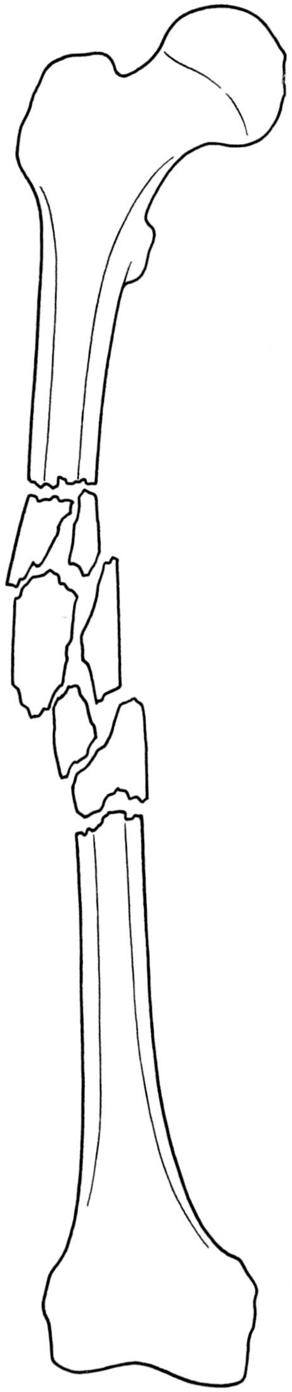

Figure 190 Severely comminuted fracture of the femur, middle third.

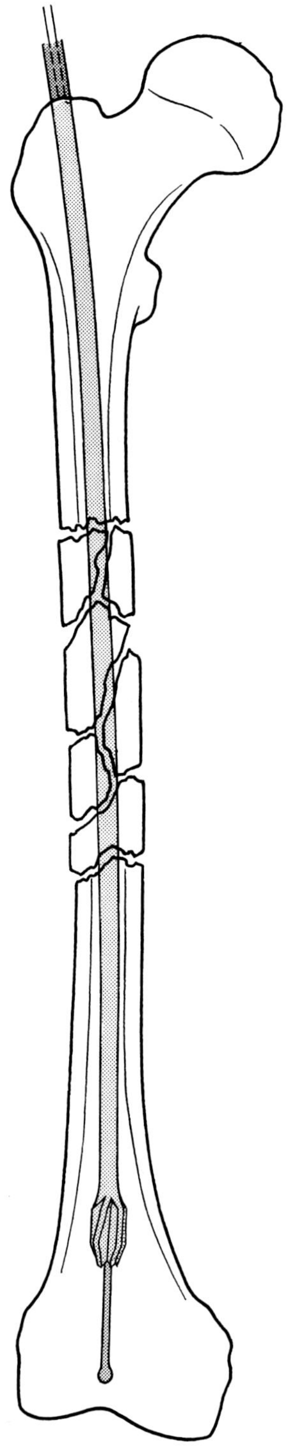

Figure 191 Careful reaming of the medullary canal, after reduction of the fracture by strong traction and stringing of the fragments by the guide pin.

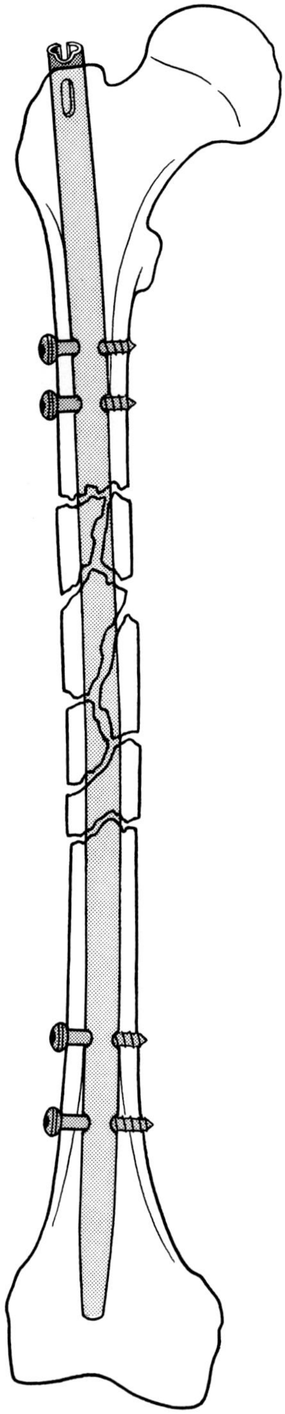

Figure 192 Completed interlocking nailing of the severely comminuted femoral shaft fracture.

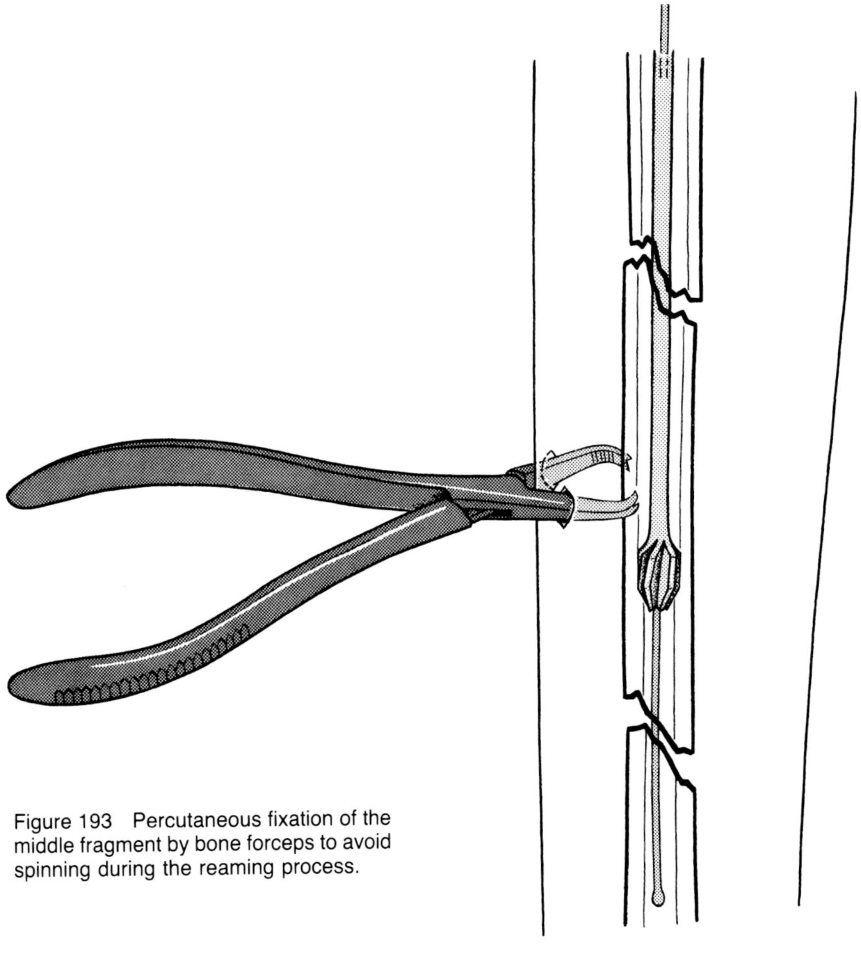

Figure 193 Percutaneous fixation of the middle fragment by bone forceps to avoid spinning during the reaming process.

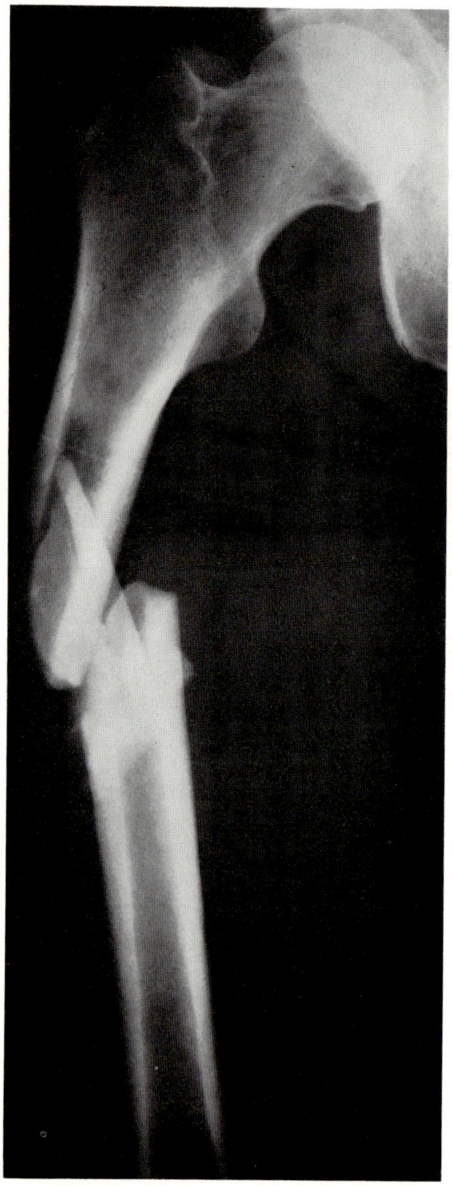

Figure 194 Fracture of the femoral shaft, proximal third, with comminution, AP view.

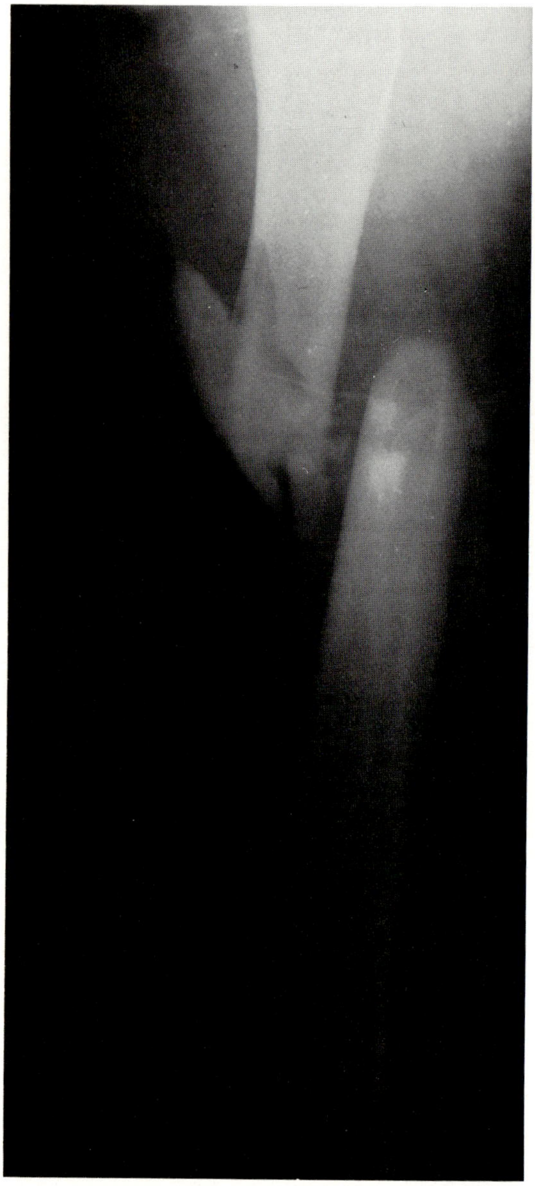

Figure 195 Lateral view of the same fresh femoral fracture.

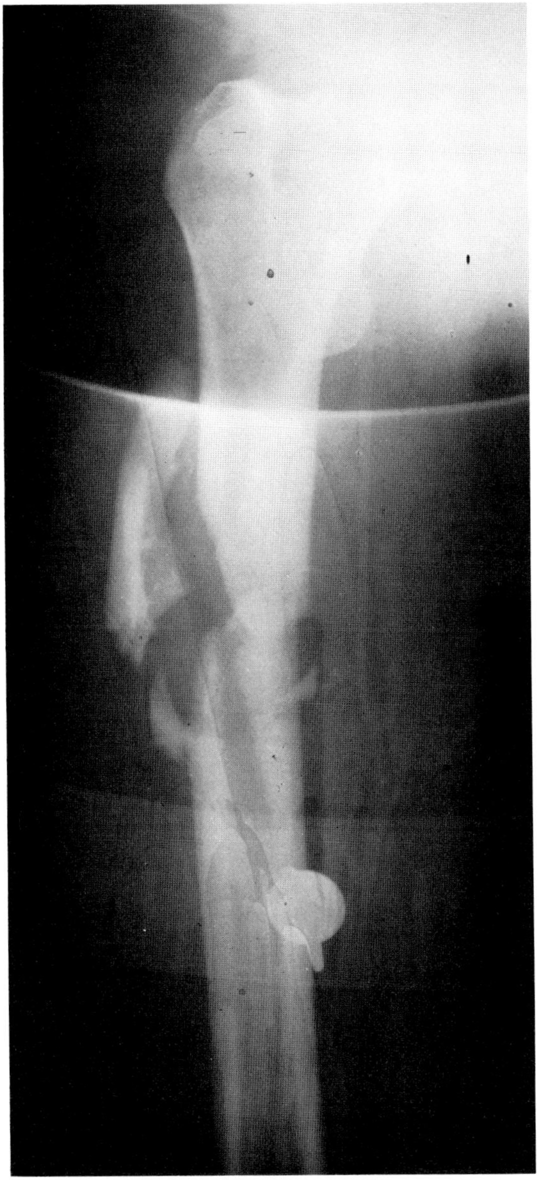

Figure 196 The same fracture after reduction in the distractor seven days later. A special interlocking nail was manufactured during this period.

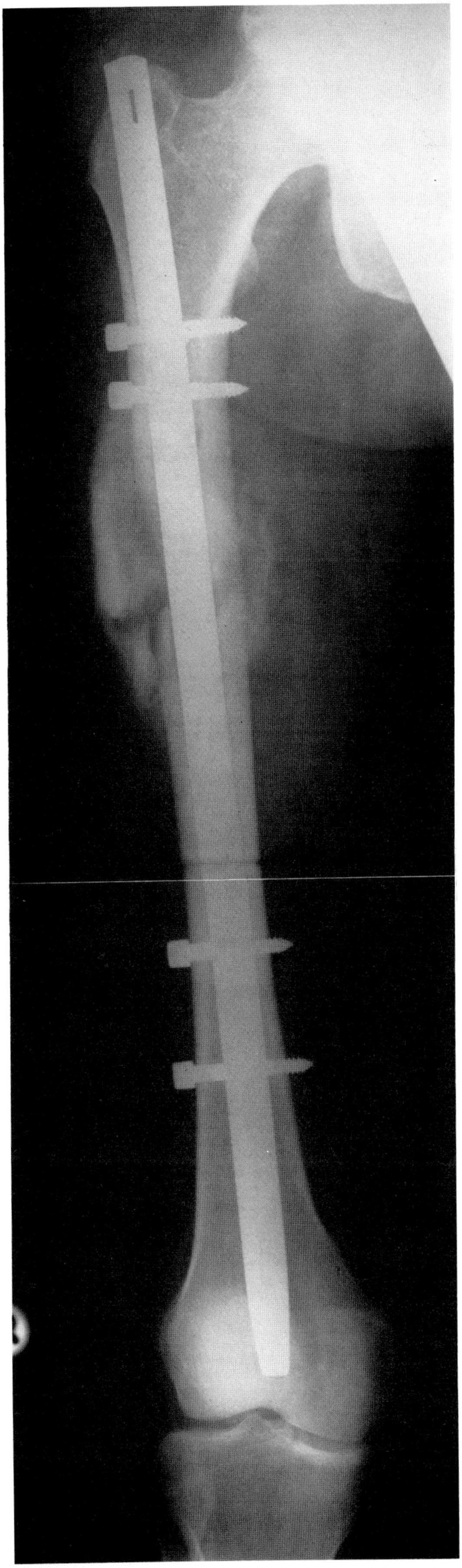

Figure 197 Beginning callus formation three months after the nailing, using the custom-made interlocking nail with full weight-bearing, AP view.

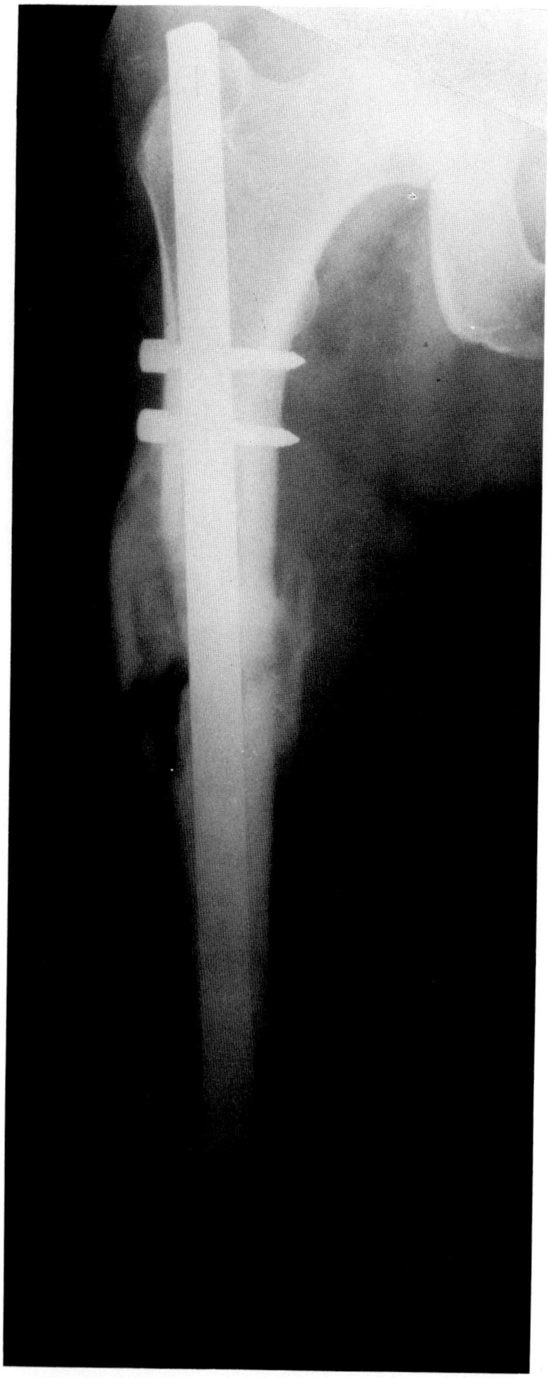

Figure 198 The same fracture after five months, showing beginning bone healing, AP view.

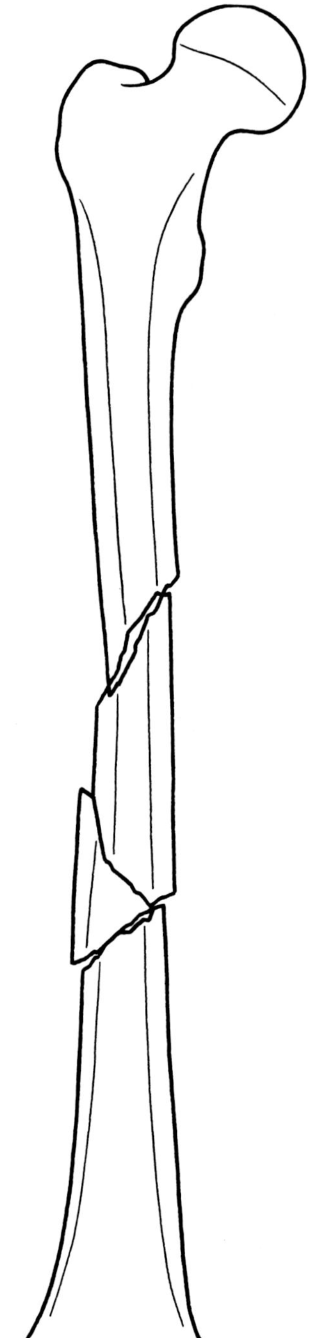

Figure 199 Fragmented femoral shaft fracture.

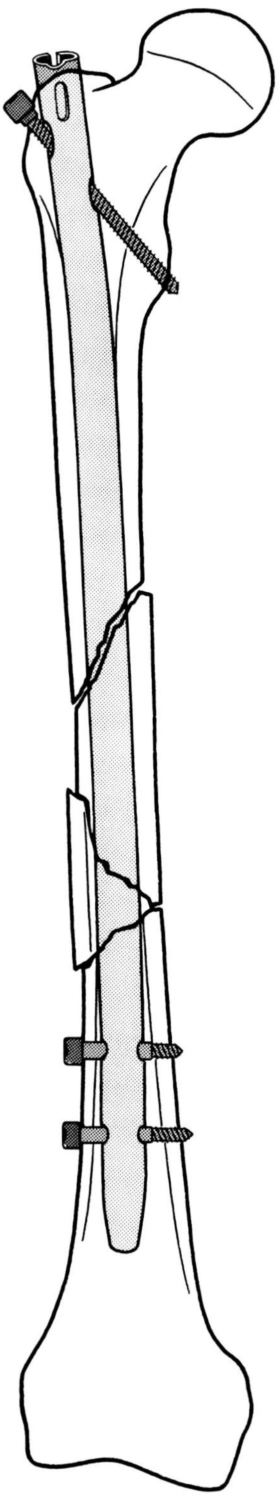

Figure 200 Nailing of the fragmented femoral shaft fracture with an interlocking nail by Klemm.

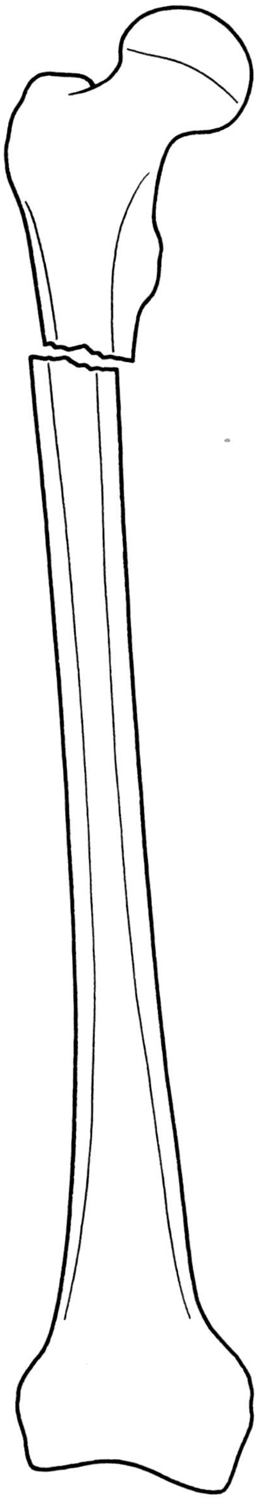

Figure 201 Fragmented femur fracture, proximal third, in the widening medullary canal zone.

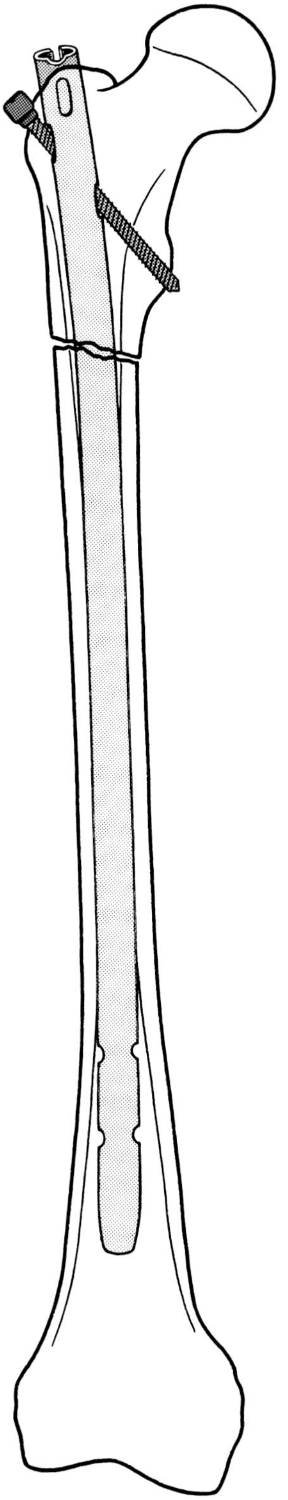

Figure 202 Nailing of the femoral shaft fracture, proximal third, with an interlocking nail by Klemm. Distal transverse screws are unnecessary—dynamic interlocking.

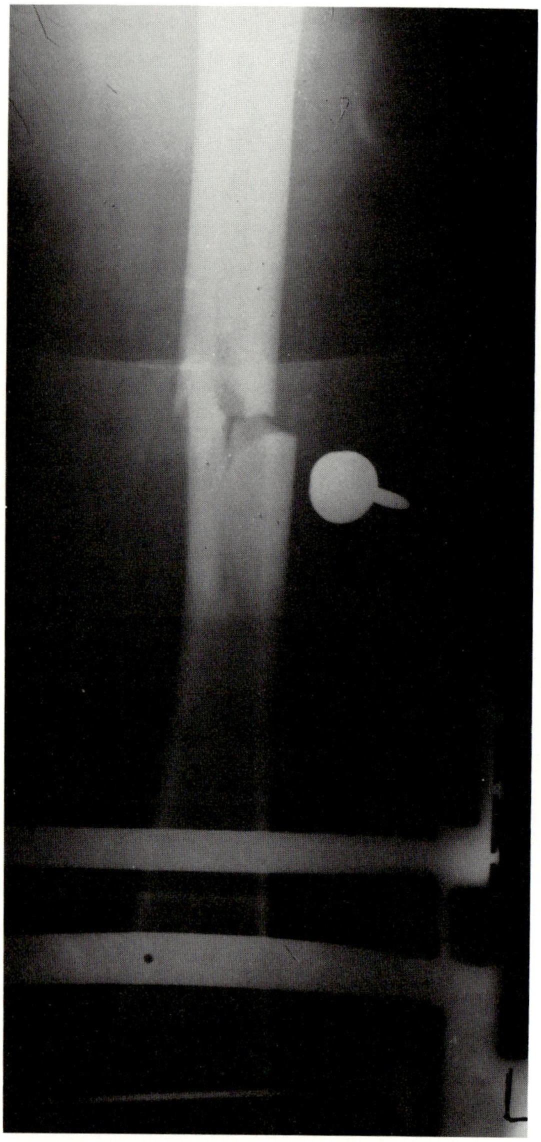

Figure 203 Fracture of the femoral shaft at the border of the narrow medullary canal with longitudinal fractures proximally and distally in supracondylar skeletal traction.

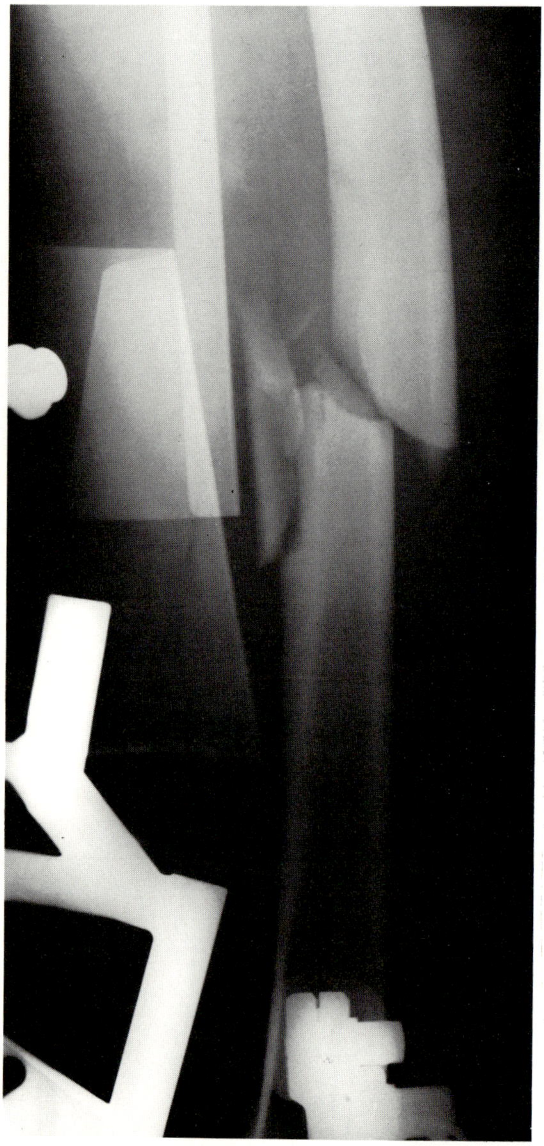

Figure 204 Lateral view of the same fracture. A large wedge-shaped fragment is visible.

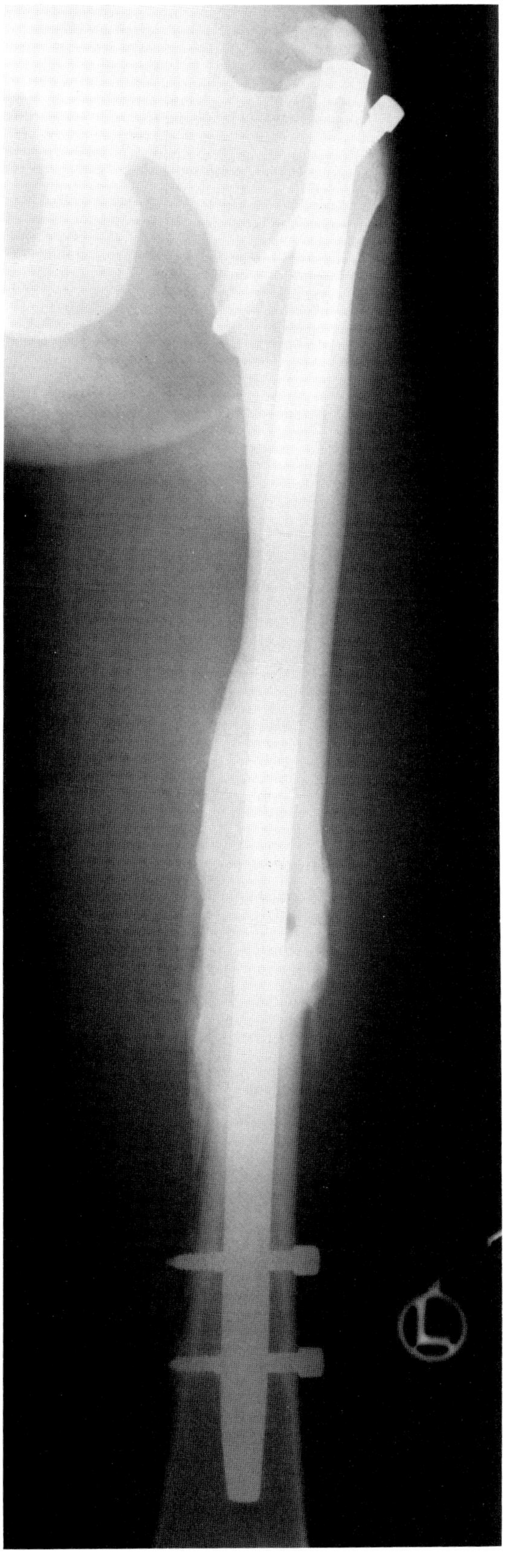

Figure 205 The same fracture, nine months after the nailing with a standard interlocking nail by Klemm. The bone healing is completed, AP view.

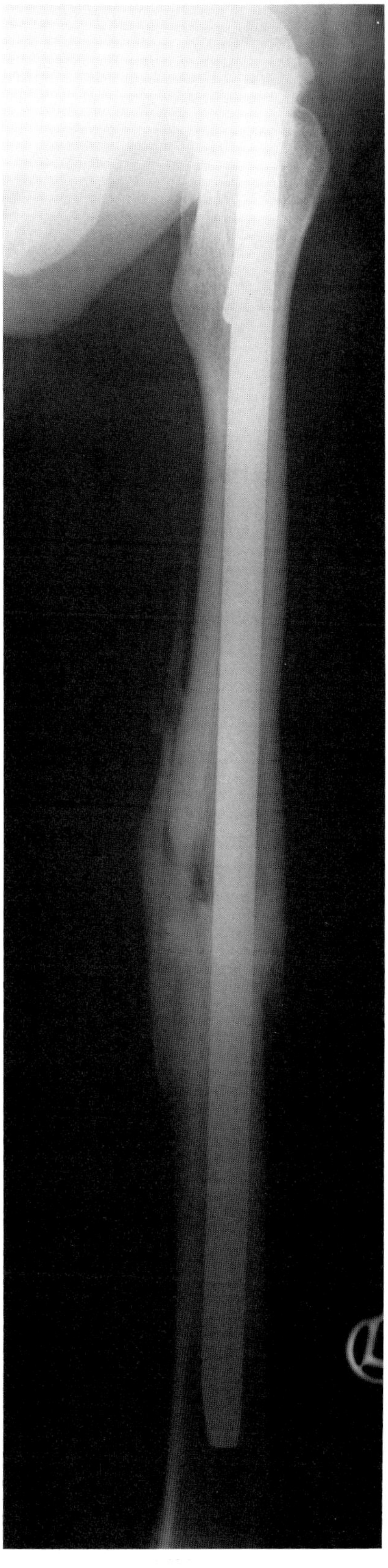

Figure 206 Lateral view after bone healing of the same fracture. The wedge-shaped fragment is fused within the callus mass.

Interlocking Nail Osteosynthesis of the Tibia

Indications

Interlocking nail osteosynthesis of the tibia is indicated in fractures that are beyond the indications for the regular intramedullary nail: severely comminuted fractures, fragmented fractures, spiral fractures, and large oblique fractures. The type and localization of the fibular fractures play no role in the indications for the interlocking nail osteosynthesis of the tibia.

Instruments

The standard Küntscher nail set for the tibia nailing is used in conjunction with the special instruments listed in the preceding chapter. Standardized interlocking nails can be used if the type of fracture does not demand a specially manufactured interlocking nail with distal or proximal transverse holes.

Positioning and Reduction

The patient is positioned as illustrated in the tibia nailing chapter (p. 25). The extension attachment of the foot must allow access to the distal tibia, so that the most distal transverse screw can be inserted. Occasionally, the skeletal traction through the os calcis must be done; the Kirschner wire tractor is attached to the traction device of the fracture table. The fracture is reduced as described on page 23.

Image Intensification

Preoperative roentgenograms of the entire tibia comprising both adjacent joints must be taken in two planes at a 1-m distance. The image intensifier is positioned as illustrated on pages 25 and 26. Postoperative roentgenograms of the entire tibia in two planes are necessary.

Operative Technique

The operative technique of the tibia interlocking nail osteosynthesis is initially identical with that of the Küntscher nailing of the tibia (p. 23). The medullary canal must always be reamed. Fragmented fractures must be carefully reamed to avoid spinning of the middle fragment. This fragment must occasionally be held percutaneously with a bone holder. The selected nail must be driven in such a way that the transverse holes are exactly in the transverse plane. The transverse screws are laterally inserted so that a soft-tissue cover over the heads of the screws can be provided. The preparation and insertion of the screws are done as described on page 92. The lengths of the screws are determined either by the preoperative roentgenograms or by direct measurements. The fixation of a nail in the short fragment necessitates the use of two screws.

Common Mistakes

If the interlocking nail is too short in a fracture of the distal tibia, only one fixation screw can be inserted into the distal fragment, which may tilt under weight-bearing. If imprecise holes are prepared, the same complications may arise as those described on page 92.

Aftercare

The interlocking nail osteosynthesis of the transverse fractures allows for immediate postoperative weight-bearing. All other interlocking nail osteosyntheses enable immediate postoperative exercises. Weight-bearing in these fractures is dependent on the strength and healing of the bone. Only partial weight-bearing should be undertaken when insufficient bone strength exists.

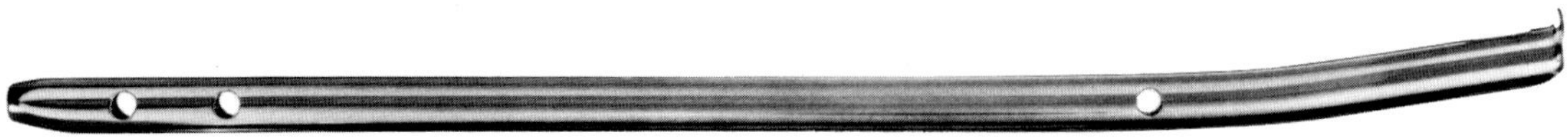

Figure 207 Standard tibial interlocking nail.

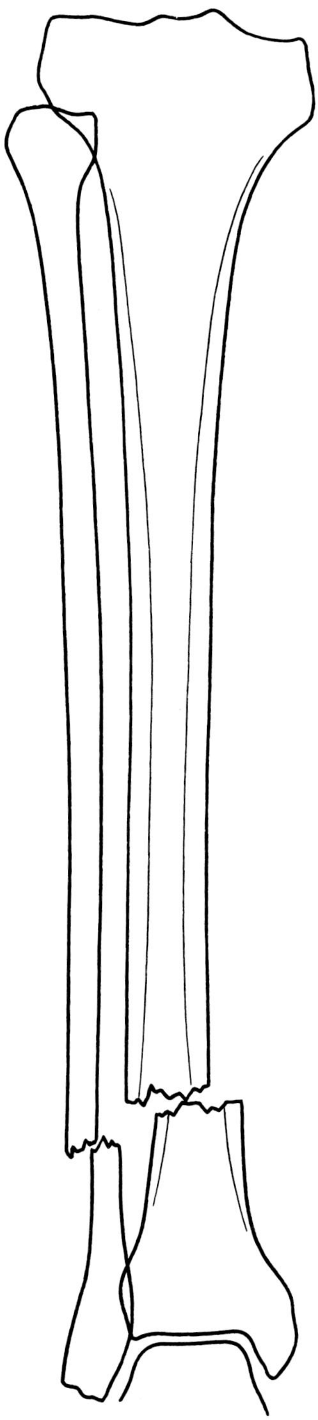

Figure 208 Tibial fracture, distal third, in the area of the widening medullary canal, AP view.

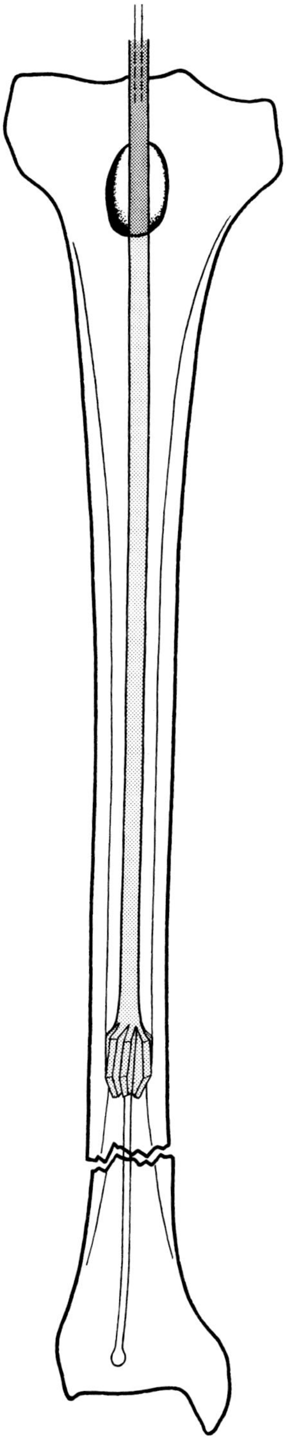

Figure 209 Reaming of the proximal medullary canal over the guide pin in distal fracture of the tibia.

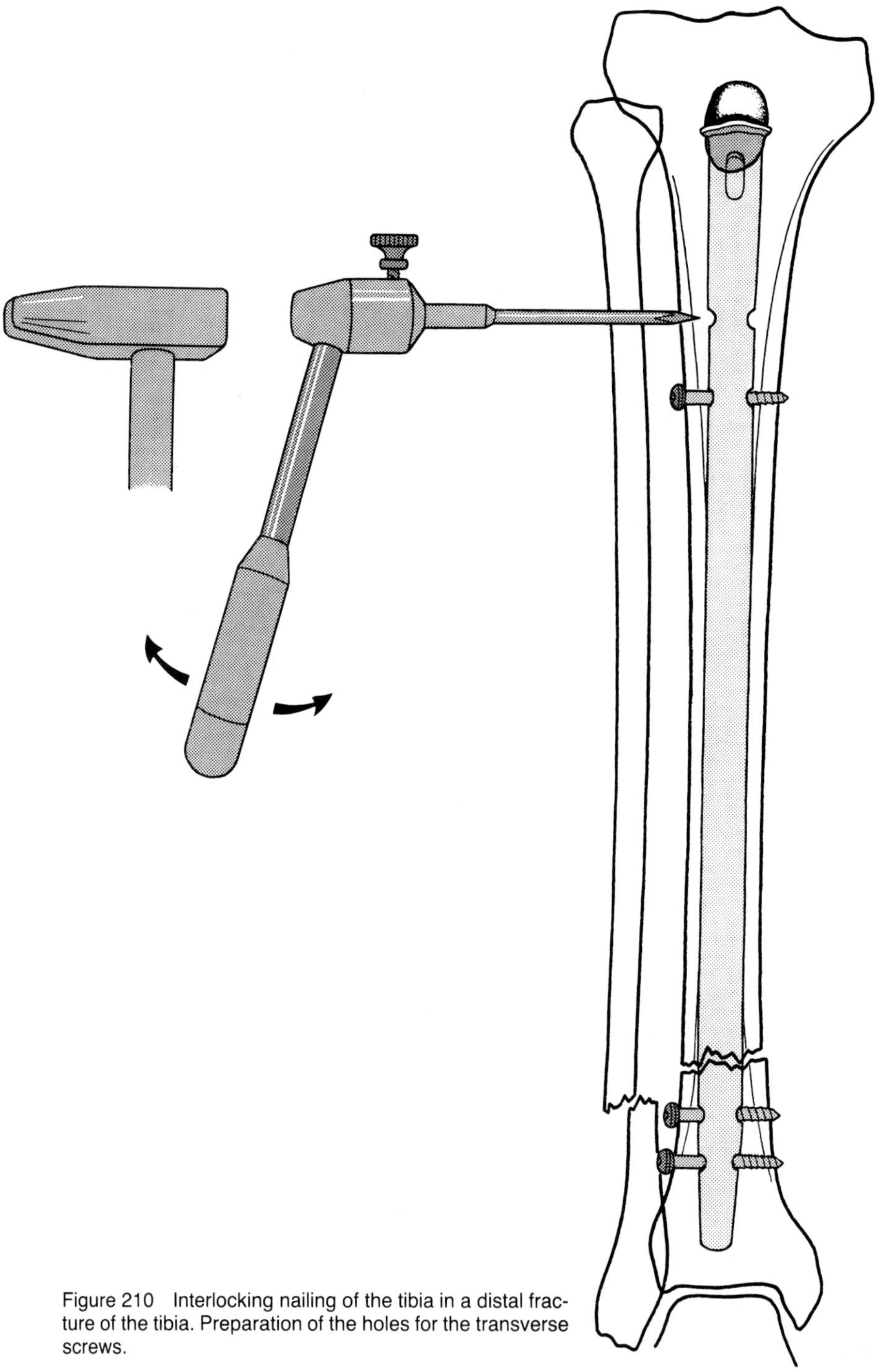

Figure 210 Interlocking nailing of the tibia in a distal fracture of the tibia. Preparation of the holes for the transverse screws.

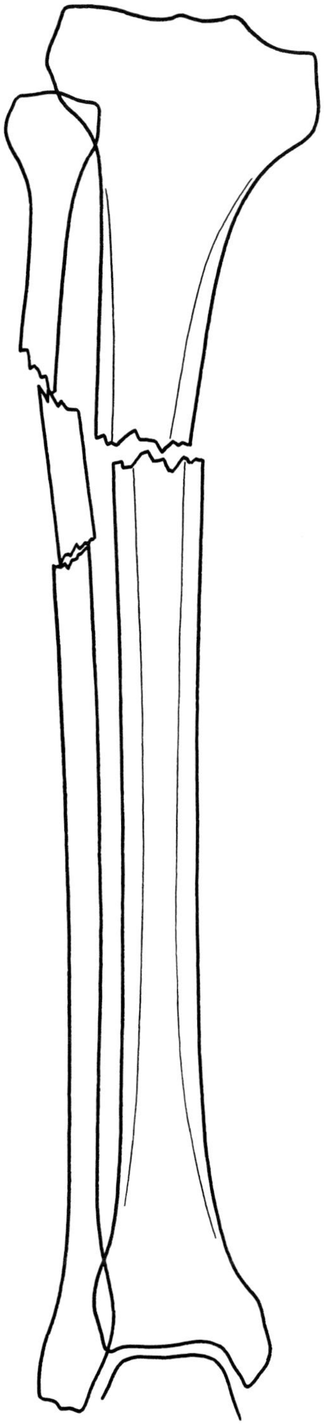

Figure 211 Tibial fracture, proximal third, in the area of the widening medullary canal.

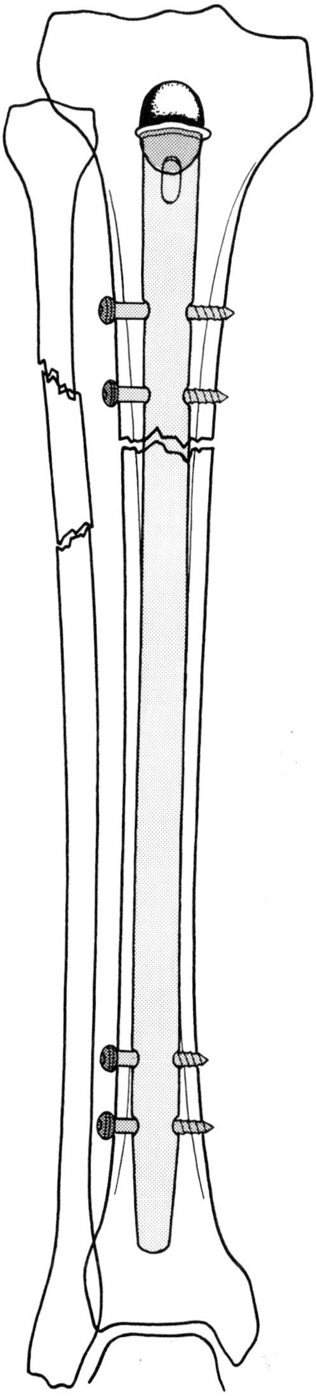

Figure 212 Completed interlocking nailing of a tibial fracture in the proximal third, in the area of the widening medullary canal.

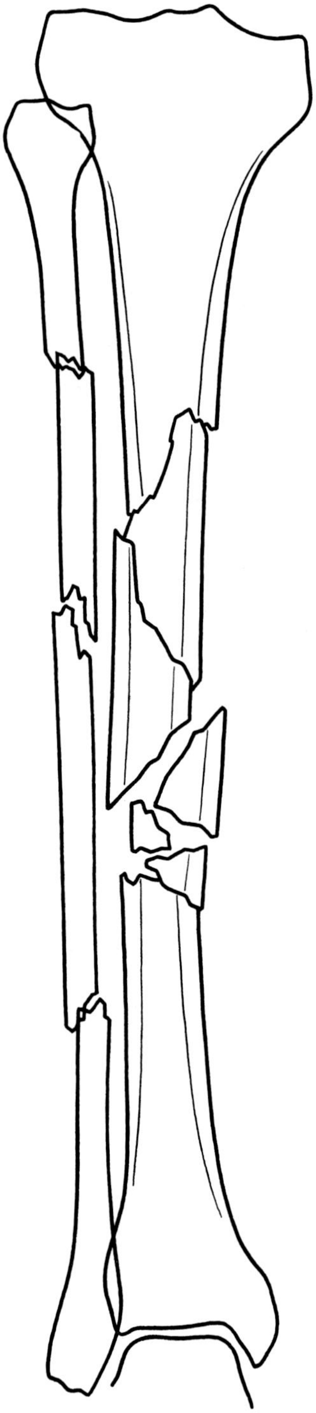

Figure 213 Severely comminuted fracture of the tibial and fibular shafts.

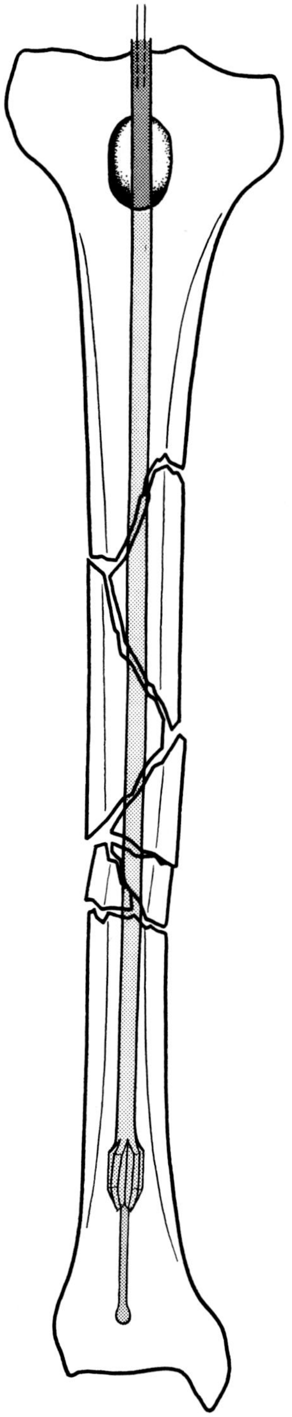

Figure 214 Reaming of the medullary canal of the tibia over the guide pin after closed reduction with strong traction.

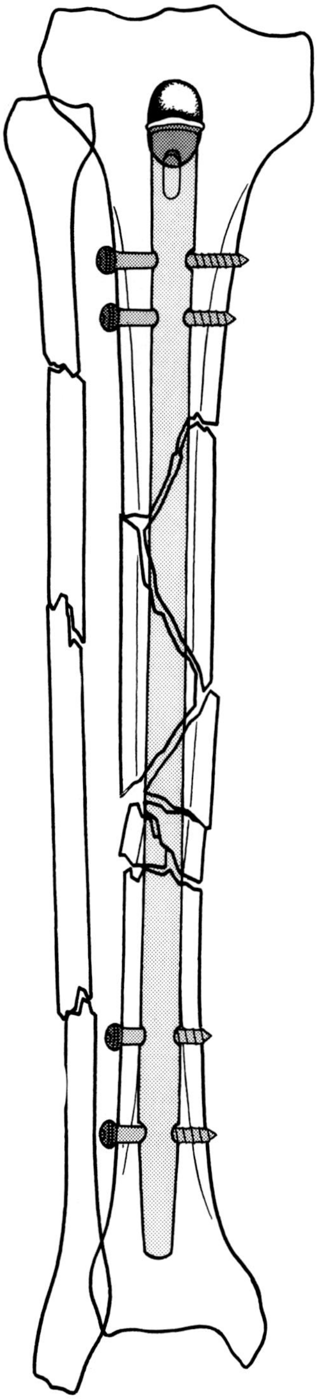

Figure 215 Completed interlocking nailing of the tibia in severely comminuted tibial and fibular fractures.

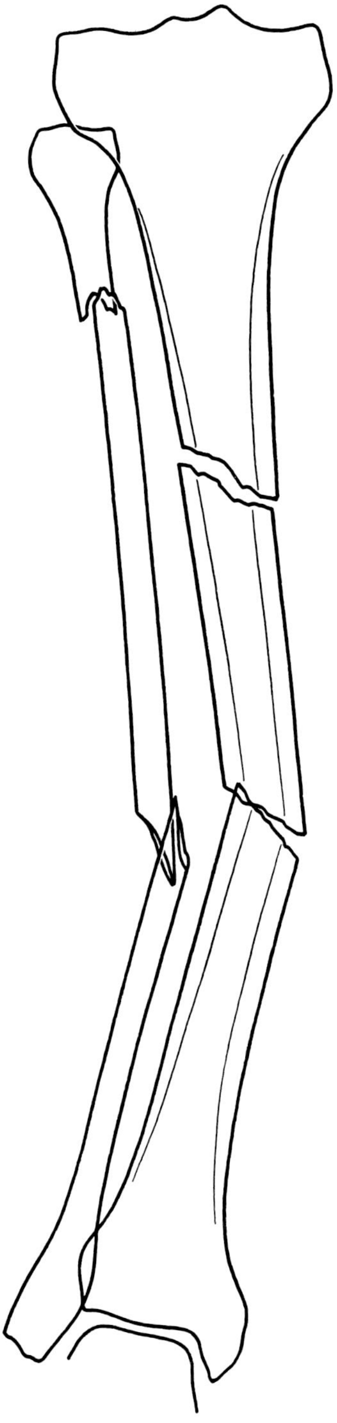

Figure 216 Fragmented tibial and fibular fractures, AP view.

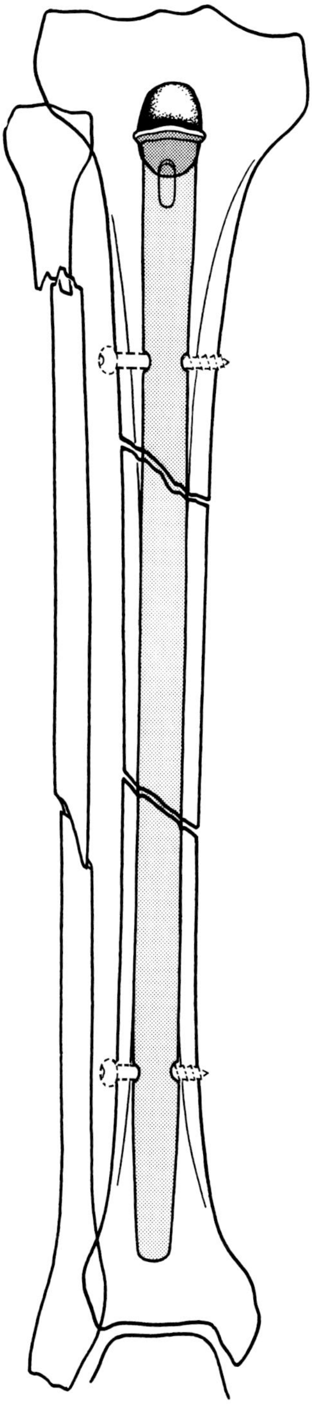

Figure 217 Completed nailing of a fragmented tibial fracture. Cases of instability necessitate interlocking nails.

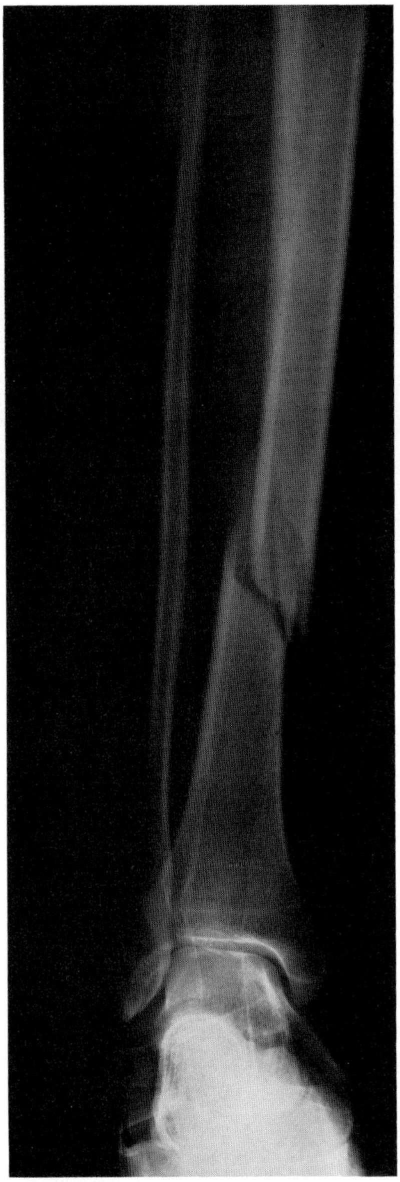

Figure 218

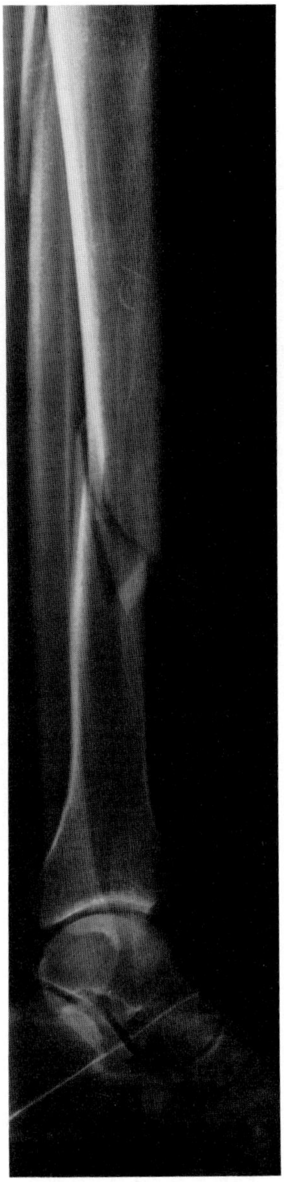

Figure 219

Figure 218 Fresh fracture of the tibia, AP view. The fracture site is in the area of the widening medullary canal.

Figure 219 The same tibial fracture, lateral view, showing the medullary canal to be already wider at the fracture site.

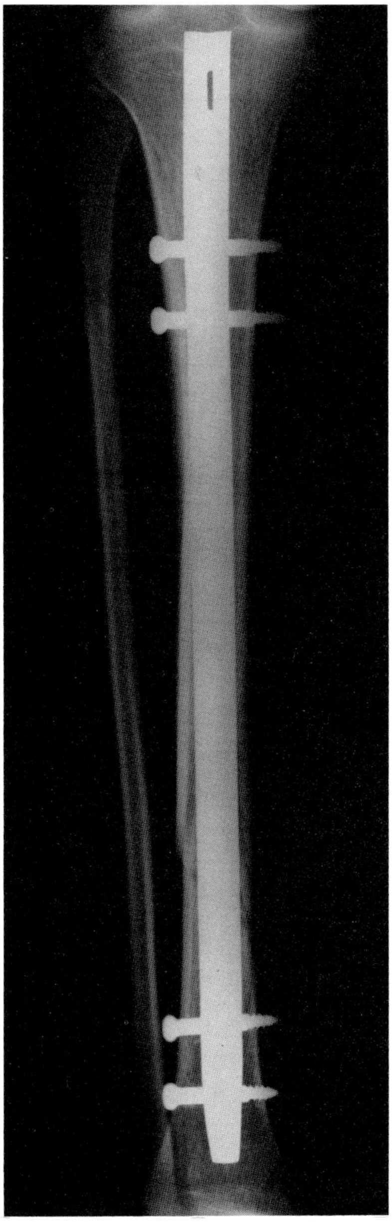

Figure 220

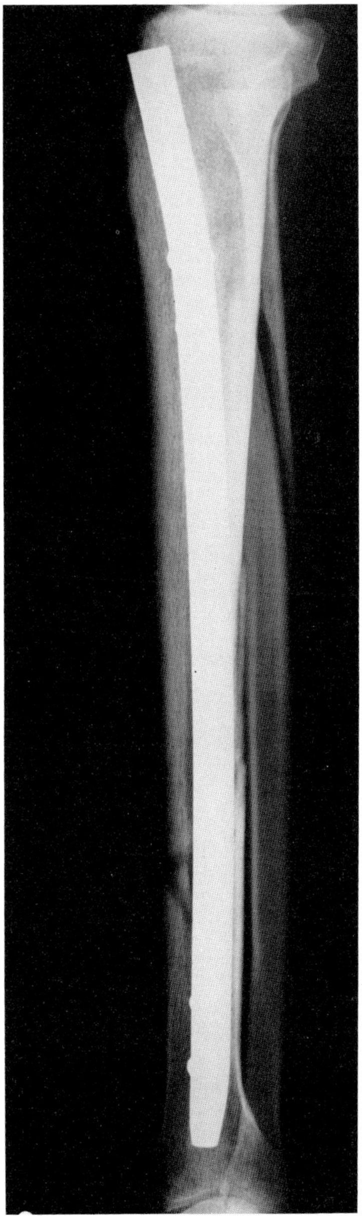

Figure 221

Figure 220 The same tibial fracture after completed nailing with a standard interlocking nail, AP view, three months after full weight-bearing, showing nearly complete bone healing.

Figure 221 The same case, lateral view.

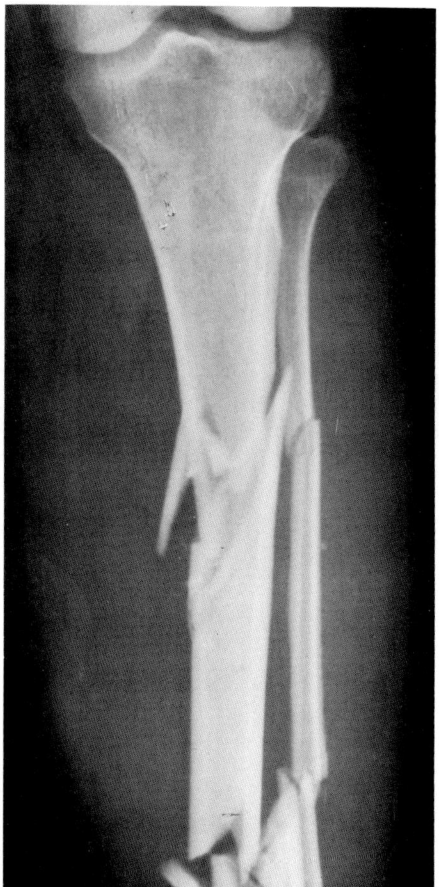

Figure 222

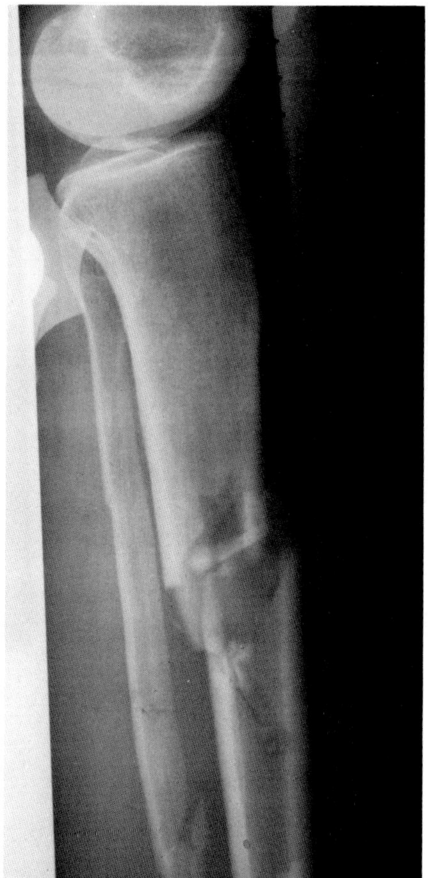

Figure 223

Figure 222 Fragmented tibial and fibular fractures in skeletal traction, AP view.

Figure 223 The same fragmented fractures, lateral view. Roentgenogram taken in traction with the superimposed x-ray scale used to determine the correct nail dimensions.

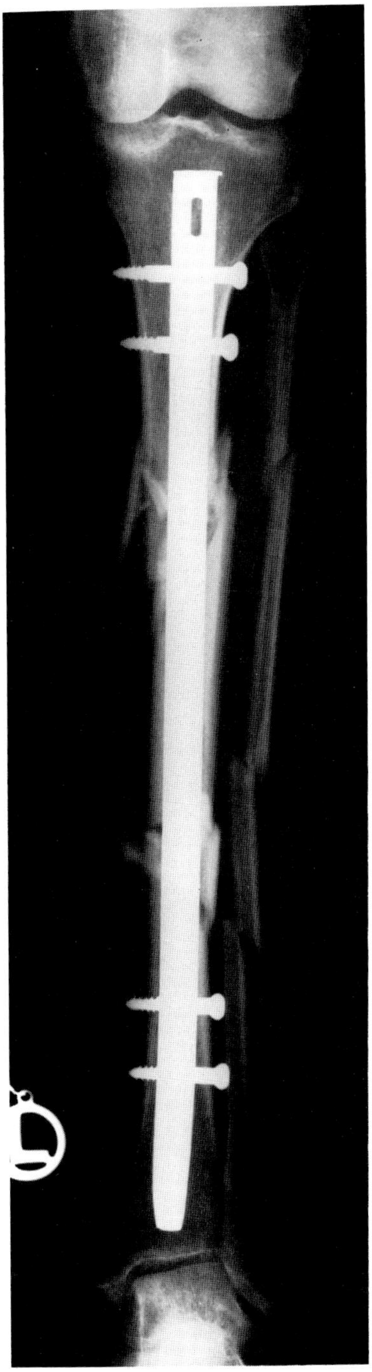

Figure 224

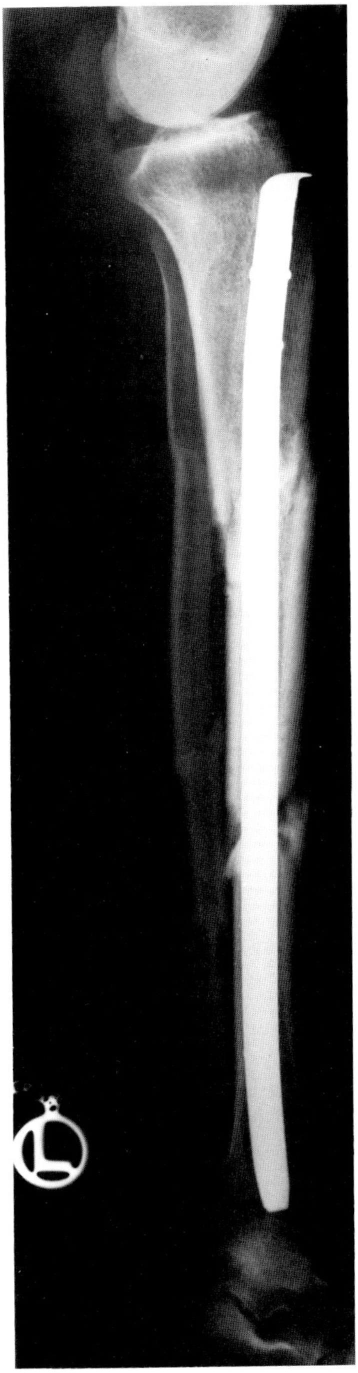

Figure 225

Figure 224 Fragmented tibial and fibular fractures, AP view. Completed nailing with custom-made interlocking nail.

Figure 225 The same fragmented fractures after interlocking nailing, lateral view.

Compression Nailing

Kaessmann compression nailing is a combination of intramedullary nailing and compression osteosynthesis. A special nail supplied with a mandrel is held by a transverse screw and maintains the axial compression, generated by the Kaessmann compression device.

Indications

Transverse fractures and short oblique fractures with satisfactory cortical support, localized in the wide areas of the medullary canal, where reaming cannot provide a locking of the nail with the cortex both proximally and distally of the fracture site, are candidates for compression nailing. Regular Küntscher nailing is the preferred method of osteosynthesis in all cases in which sufficient cortical support can be provided on both sides of the fracture after reaming. Comminuted fractures and long oblique fractures cannot be satisfactorily stabilized by compression nailing.

Instruments

The standard Küntscher instrument set for the corresponding bone is used in conjunction with the appropriate Kaessmann compression nail. Straight Kaessmann nails are used for the femur; bent ones are used for the humerus and tibia. These nails are available in varying lengths and diameters. A compression nail is comprised of a nail, a mandrel with a plate, a transverse screw, and a locking collar with a set screw. Additionally, several instruments are necessary; a Kaessmann compression device, a hexagonal screwdriver, a nail set with a conical end for the tibia and humerus compression nail, a nail set without a conical end for femur compression nail, a triangular awl (4.5-mm diameter for tibia and femur and 3.5-mm diameter for humerus compression nailing) with a handgrip, and a pin cutter to cut the mandrel.

Positioning and Reduction

The patient is in the same position on the fracture table as that described for the corresponding regular Küntscher nailing, and the fracture is also reduced in the same way.

Image Intensification

Preoperative roentgenograms and image intensification are identical to that which was described in the chapter of the corresponding Küntscher nailing.

Operative Technique

The type of skin incision, the opening of the medullary canal, and the insertion of a guide pin into the distal fragment are identical to the procedure described in the chapter on Küntscher nailing. If the medullary canal's narrowest point is not 0.5 mm larger than the chosen compression nail, the medullary canal must be reamed in the typical manner. The ball-point guide pin is then exchanged for a mandrel.In tibial fractures, the mandrel is inserted with a pin handgrip to about 1 cm above the talotibial joint. The length of the compression nail can be determined by superimposing the nail on the tibia when fluoroscoping. Home the selected nail under image intensification with the driver. If the nail length is correctly chosen, the mandrel with its plate will protrude approximately 5 cm from the nail tip.The mandrel's plate must be guided into the dorsally oriented slot of the advancing nail. The mandrel within the nail is thereby secured against rotation. The lip of the nail should rest firmly on the bone. Under fluoroscopy, a skin incision is made over the slotted hold in the mandrel. The canal for the fixating screw is prepared with the triangular awl. The length of the screw is determined with a depth gauge. The correct screw is then inserted through the proximal cortex, the hole in the mandrel, and then the distal cortex. A locking collar is inserted over the mandrel and rests on the nail's proximal end. The Kaessmann compression device is guided over the mandrel until contacting the locking collar. Firmly tighten the compression device by its locking screw to the mandrel. Increase the compression until the desired compression is indicated on the scale. The set screw of the locking collar is then tightened to maintain the desired compression on the fracture. Now loosen the locking screw of the compression device and remove the device from the mandrel. The mandrel is then cut just proximal to the locking collar.

When using the compression nail in the femur, the mandrel's transverse screw should not be more distal than the proximal end of the condyles. The length of the straight femoral compression nail is determined in the same fashion as that of the tibial compression nail. The transverse screw is inserted after making a lateral stab incision in the same manner as described for the compression nailing of the tibia. Further operative technique is identical to that of the tibia compression nailing; however, the shape of the locking collar is designed slightly differently. Humerus nailing uses the bent tibial nail. The operative technique is the same.

The longitudinal pressure to be applied is 60 kg for the humerus nailing, 80 to 90 kg for the tibia nailing, and 90 kg for the femoral nailing.

Common Mistakes

If the nail is rotated while driving, the mandrel's plate cannot enter the nail slot correctly. The nail thereby pushes the mandrel with it as it is being driven.

If the hole in the mandrel's plate is not exactly laterally oriented, the insertion of the transverse screw is very difficult.

If the locking disc is not firmly attached to the mandrel by its set screw, the compression immediately vanishes with the removal of the compression device.

Aftercare

The patient is able to exercise his injured extremity immediately after the operation. The timing of physiotherapy and weight-bearing depends on the condition of the soft tissue and the progress of the bone healing.

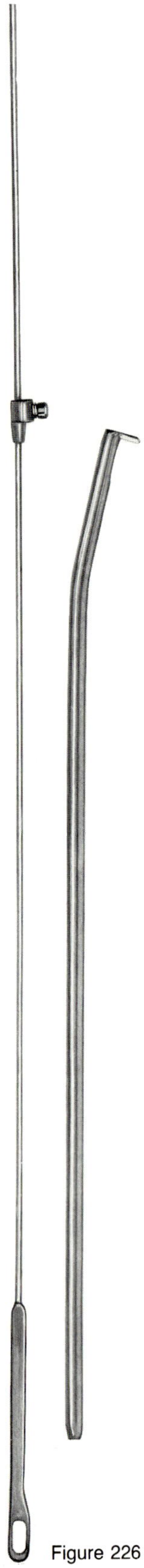

Figure 226

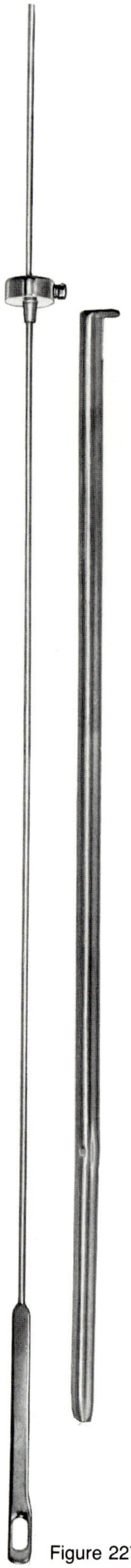

Figure 227

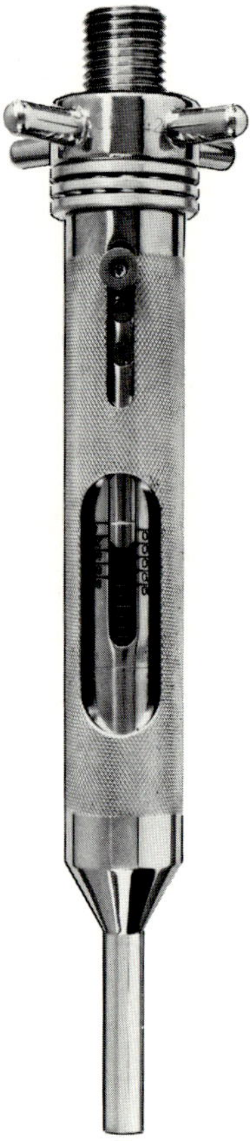

Figure 228 Compression apparatus for Kaessmann compression nailing.

Figure 226 Kaessmann tibial compression nail with mandrel.

Figure 227 Kaessmann femoral compression nail with mandrel.

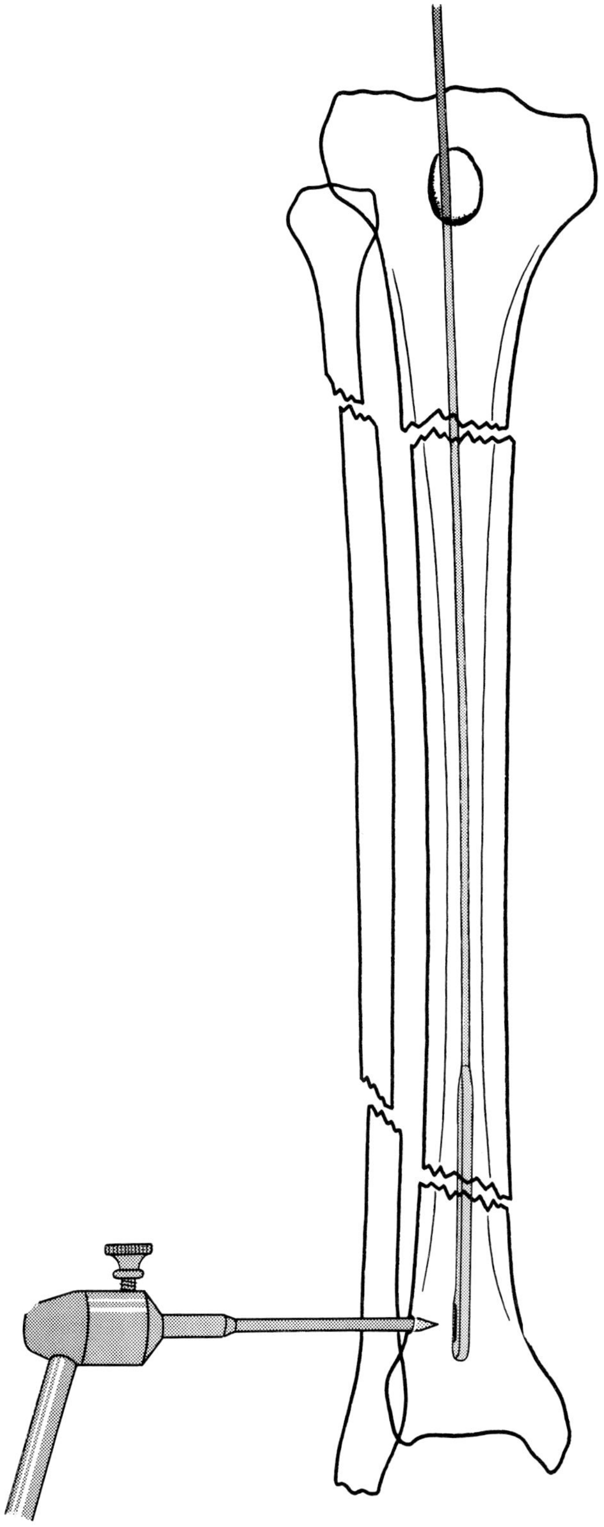

Figure 229 Fragmented tibial and fibular fractures with a mandrel positioned in the tibial medullary canal for Kaessmann compression nailing. Preparing the hole for the transverse screw.

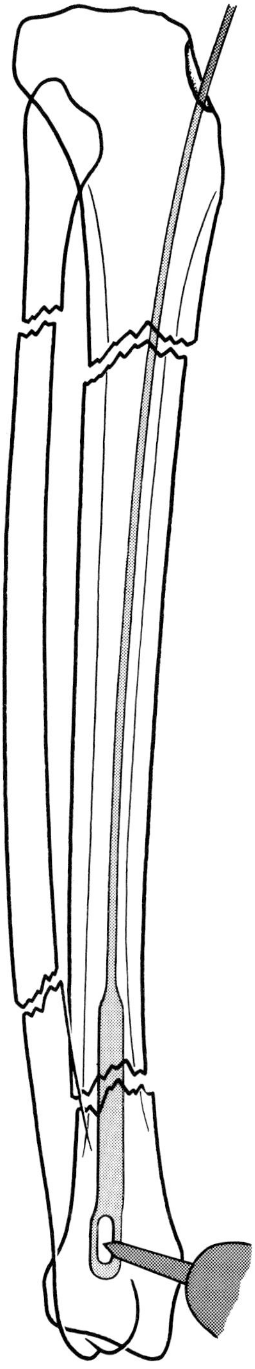

Figure 230 The same case, lateral view.

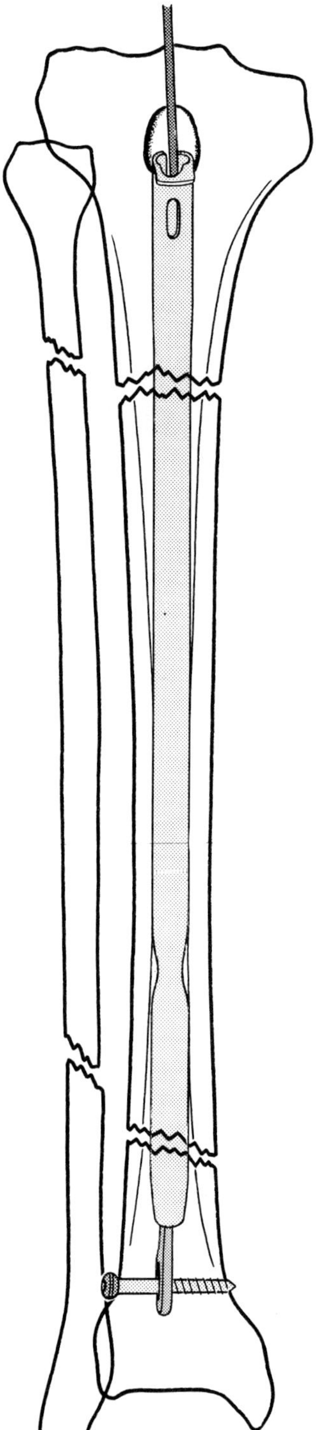

Figure 231 Fragmented fractures of the tibia and fibula, completed Kaessmann compression nailing. The transverse screw through the opening of the plate without any compression.

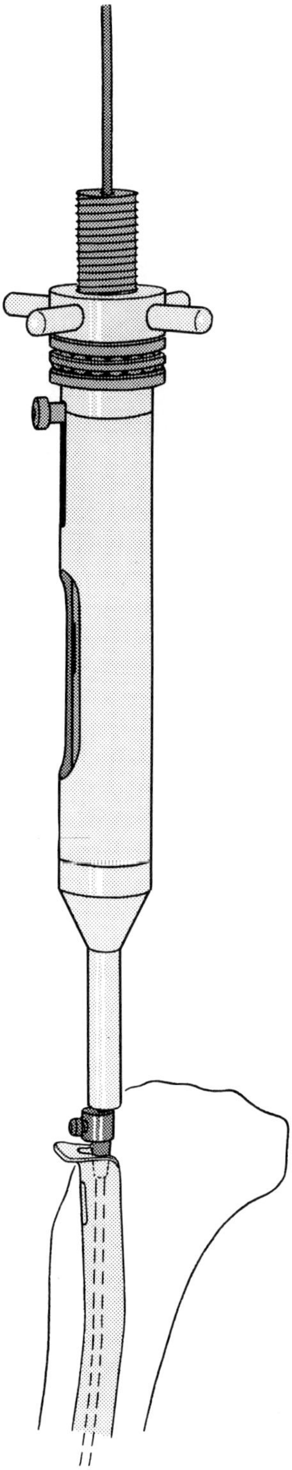

Figure 232 The Kaessmann compression apparatus supplying the compression.

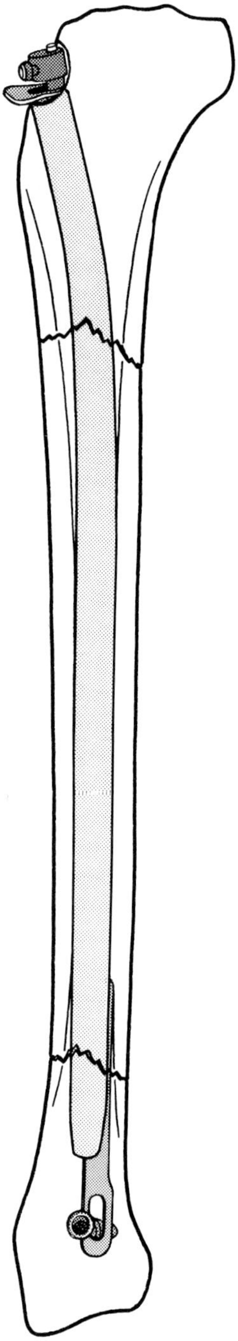

Figure 233 Completed Kaessmann compression nailing of the fragmented tibial fracture.

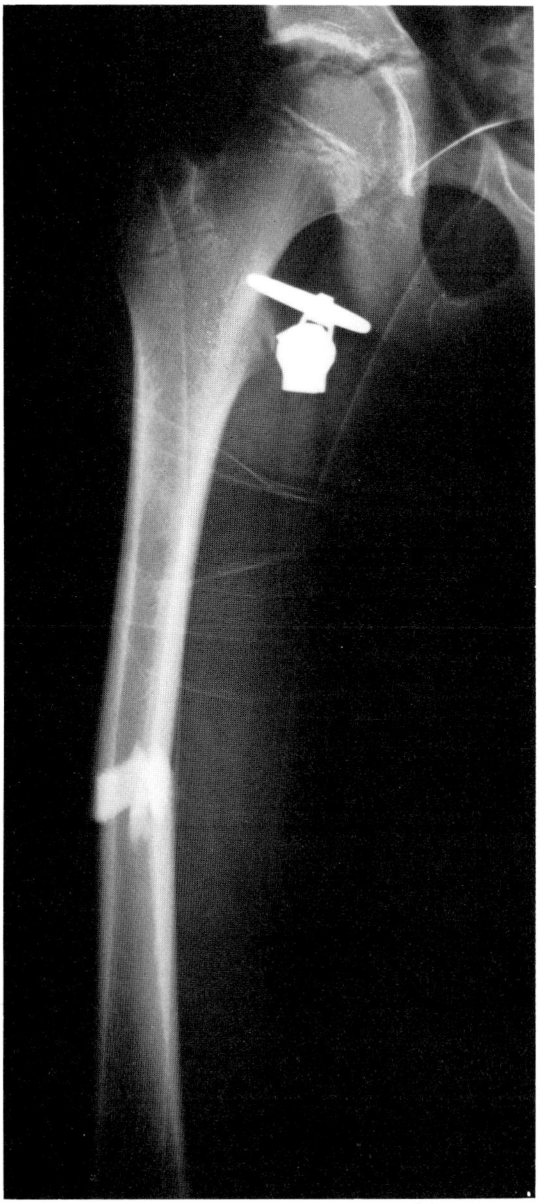

Figure 234 Fresh femoral fracture in a 13-year-old male, AP view.

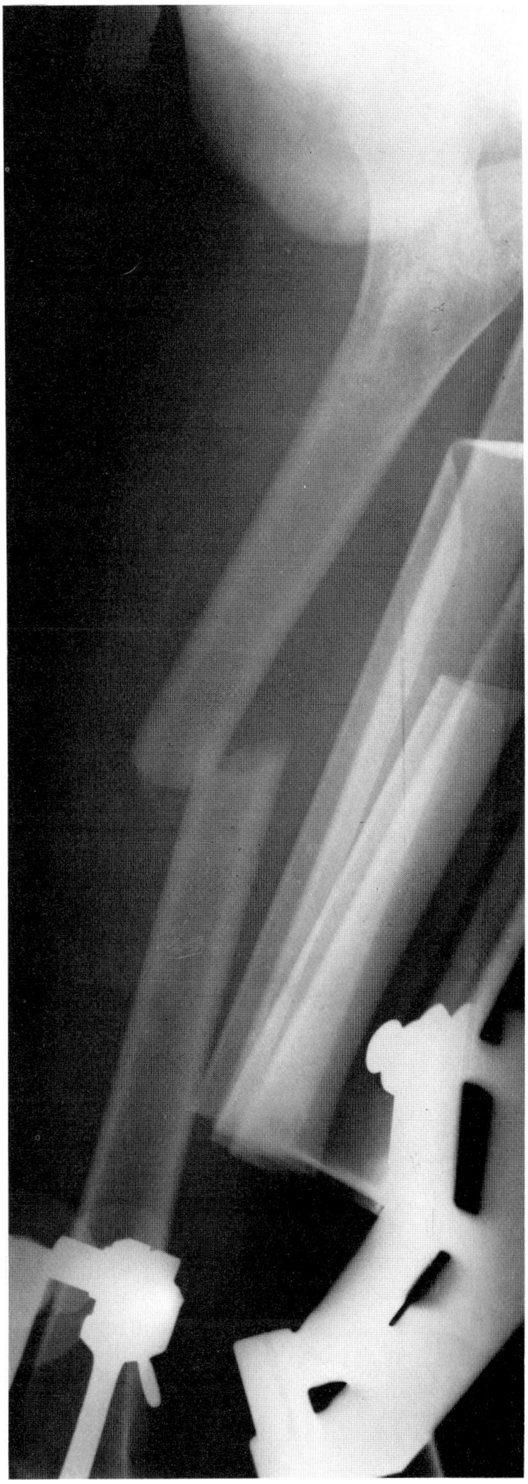

Figure 235 The same fresh fracture in supracondylar skeletal traction, positioned on a splint, lateral view.

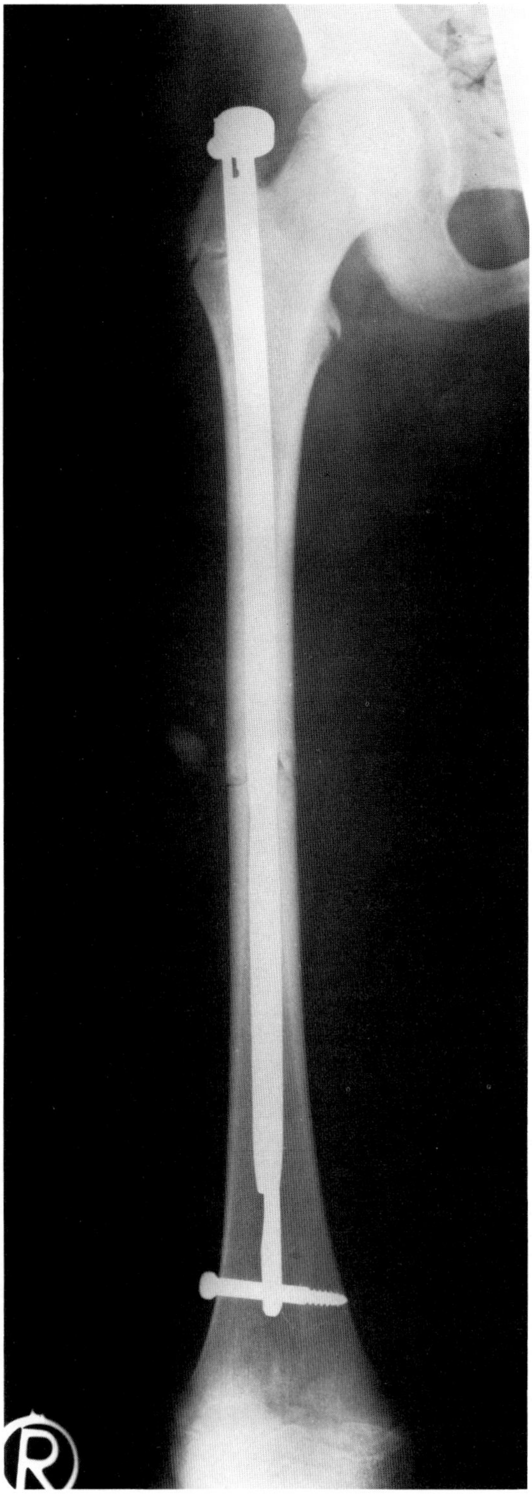

Figure 236 The same fracture after compression nailing, without prior reaming, AP view.

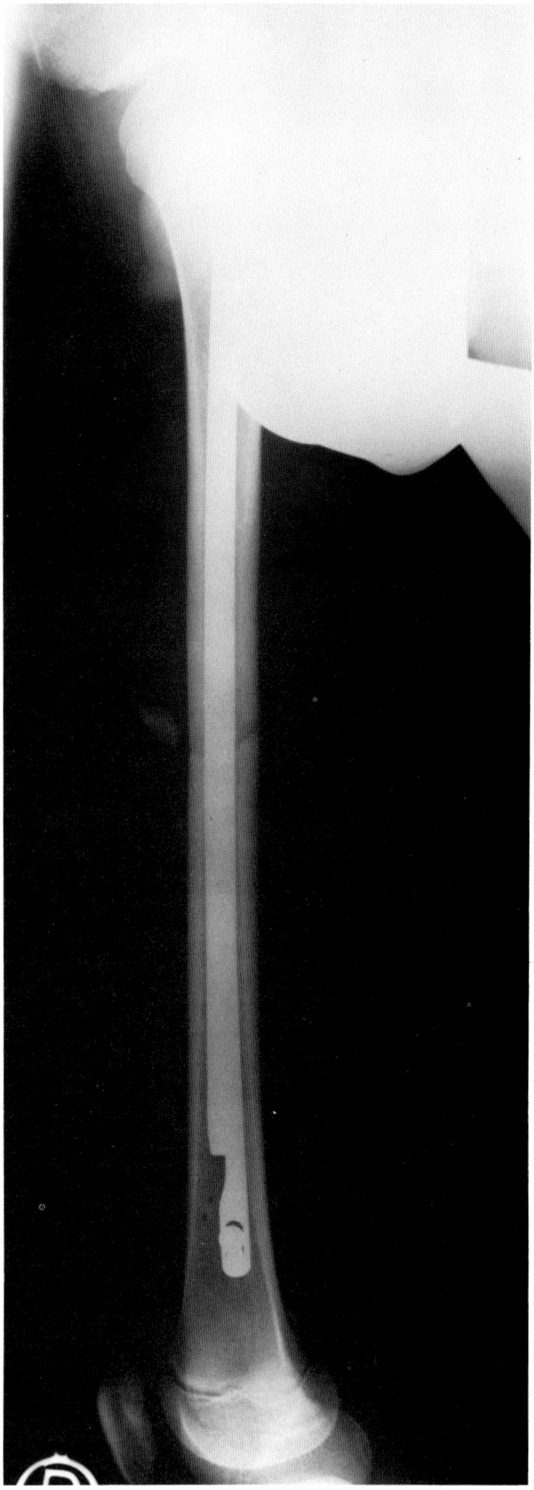

Figure 237 The same fracture after compression nailing, lateral view.

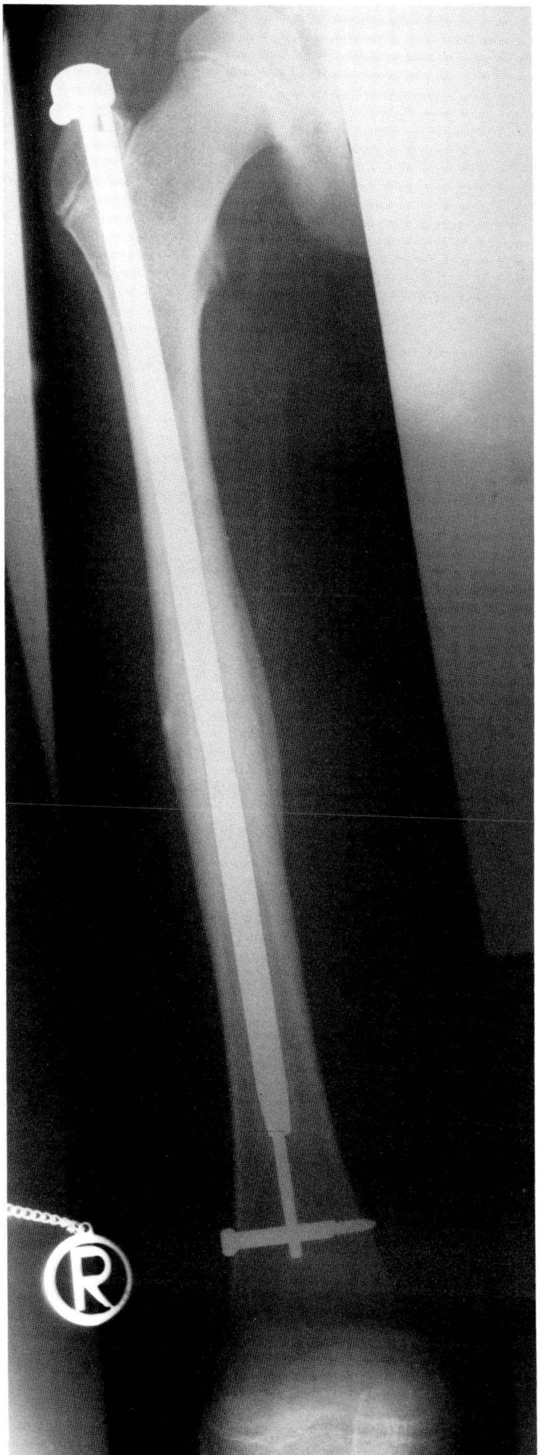

Figure 238 The same fracture six months later, fracture firmly healed, AP view.

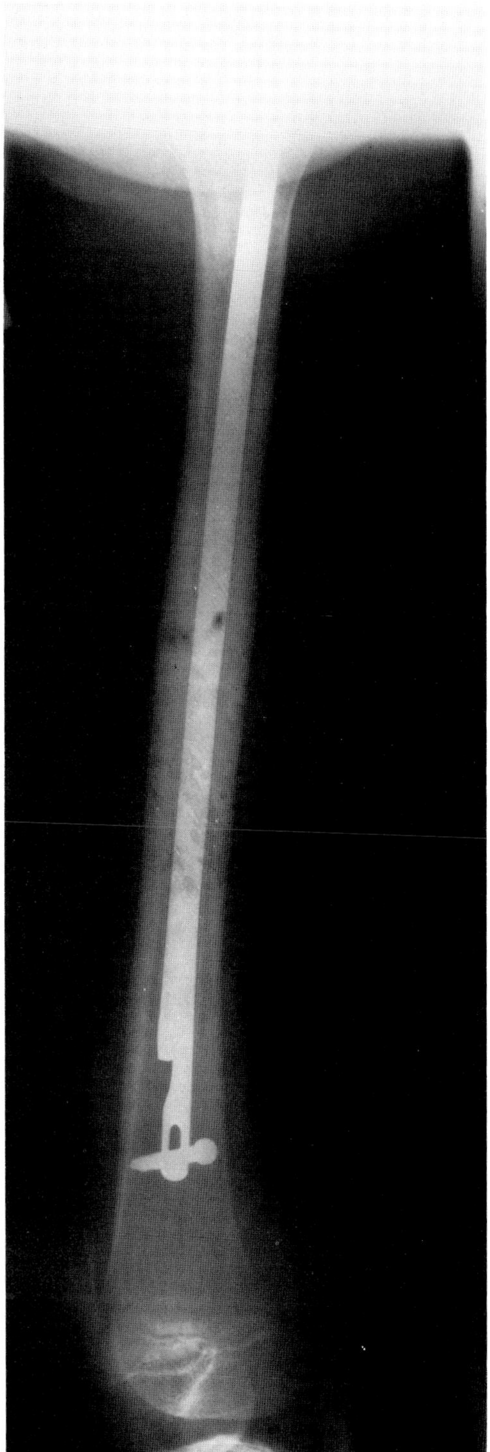

Figure 239 The same case in lateral view.

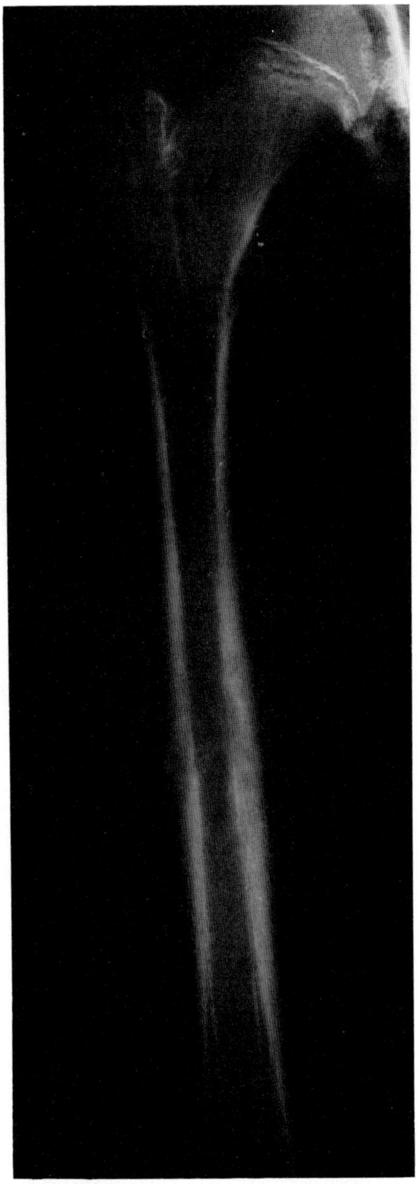

Figure 240

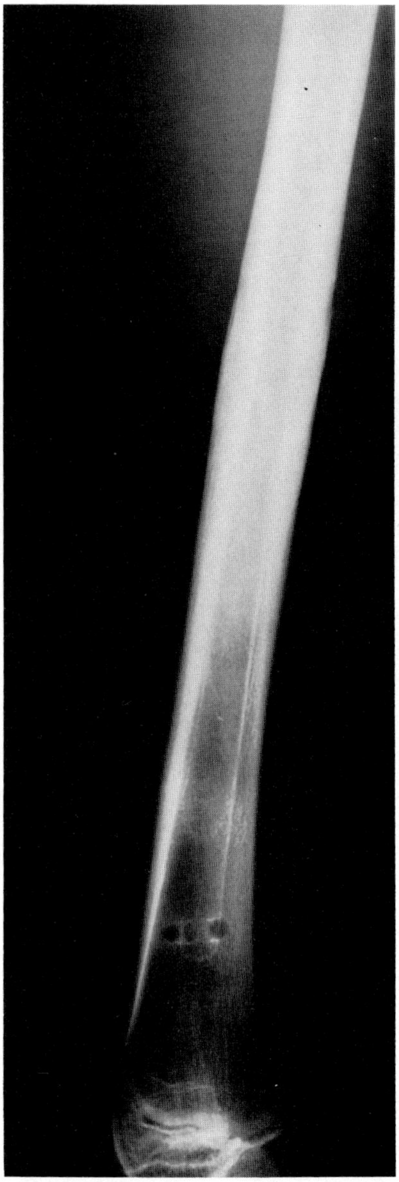

Figure 241

Figure 240 The same fracture, firmly healed, after nail removal 6½ months after the accident.

Figure 241 The same case, lateral view.

Closed Intramedullary Nailing of Pseudarthrosis

Intramedullary nailing of pseudarthrosis in long bones should always be closed, whenever possible. The intramedullary nailing must be locked in both fragments in the same fashion as in the nailing of fresh fractures. The indications for the nailing of pseudarthrosis are widened because of the changes of the bone. The medullary canal is narrowed or even completely closed by the transformations of endosteal callus into bone. For this reason, the locking of the intramedullary nail is often possible even in areas that otherwise would have too wide a medullary canal.

Rigid Pseudarthrosis

Each pseudarthrosis has a capsule of tough connective tissue, which varies in thickness and rigidity. Rigid pseudarthrosis by definition is a false joint with minimal motion. Slight malalignment of the fragments can easily be corrected on the fracture table despite the rigid capsule of connective tissue. The disruption of the pseudarthrosis capsule can be obtained with a distractor, rendering the fracture amenable for reduction. The distraction must be done slowly in small increments (see p. 11), because the vascular circulation and nerve function may be otherwise compromised. The distraction and the correction of a pseudarthrosis may take eight to ten days. Afterward the intramedullary nailing is always done with the distractor in place.

Instruments

The standard Küntscher nail set is used as described for the intramedullary nailing of the corresponding bone. In addition, pseudarthrosis-chisels are used in varying lengths and diameters.

Image Intensification

Preoperative roentgenograms of the entire bone and the adjacent joints are taken at a 1-m distance in two planes. The image intensifier is positioned as described in the chapter concerning the nailing of the corresponding bone. Postoperative roentgenograms of the entire bone are necessary in two planes.

Pseudarthrosis of the Femur

With sufficient narrowing of the medullary canal, pseudarthroses of the femur can be nailed between the subtrochanteric and the supracondylar locations. If the pseudarthrosis of the femur is reducible, the pseudarthrosis is nailed and reduced on a fracture table in the same manner as fresh fractures.

Once the medullary canal is opened, a drill point guide pin is used to penetrate into the distal fragment under image intensification. The bony covers are penetrated by the guide pin, occasionally necessitating hammer taps on the guide pin handgrip. If the pseudarthrosis cover is very hard and the medullary canal is closed for a relatively long distance, use a pseudarthrosis-chisel. Forceful hammer taps may be needed for the chisel to perforate the cover. The chisel must be intermittently withdrawn or rotated in order to avoid the trapping of the chisel's tip in the eburnated bone. The chisel is exchanged for a ball-point guide pin, once the chisel has perforated both covers and has entered the distal medullary canal. Thoroughly ream the medullary canal. The nailing is then performed in the usual fashion.

If the distractor was used for an irreducible pseudarthrosis of the femur, the patient should be positioned in the distractor on the fracture table. The distractor is removed only when the ball-point guide pin is positioned in the distal fragment. Hereafter, the operative technique is identical with that described above.

Pseudarthrosis of the Lower Leg: Pseudarthrosis of the Tibia

The indications for the nailing of the pseudarthrosis of the lower leg are dependent on the width of the tibial medullary canal. If the tibial medullary canal was narrowed at a considerable distance proximally or distally from the fracture, the indication for the typical Küntscher nailing can be widened (p. 23). A concurrent pseudarthrosis of the fibula, excluding that of the lateral malleolus, remains untouched during the operation.

The patient is positioned on the fracture table as described for the nailing of the fresh fractures of the tibia. Rigid but reducible pseudarthroses are reduced on the fracture table. If an intact fibula hinders the reduction, percutaneous osteotomy of the fibula should be performed. If the percutaneous procedure is not possible, as for instance in very distal pseudarthroses, an oblique osteotomy of the fibula must be done. In case a rigid pseudarthrosis of the lower leg is irreducible, the distractor must be used. In irreducible pseudarthrosis of the tibia with the fibula intact, osteotomy of the fibula is necessary before the distractor is applied.

The tibial medullary canal is opened in the usual way with an awl. A drill point guide pin is advanced into the distal medullary canal. The perforation of both pseudarthrosis covers is facilitated by hammer taps on the guide pin handgrip. If the pseudarthrosis covers are very hard and the medullary canal is closed for a relatively long distance, use a pseudarthrosis-chisel until its tip penetrates the distal medullary canal. Sometimes forceful hammer taps are necessary for the chisel to penetrate the covers. The chisel must be intermittently withdrawn or rotated in order to avoid trapping of the chisel in the eburnated bone. The chisel is exchanged for a ball-point guide pin after the chisel penetrates the distal medullary canal. The operative technique from here on is the same as that for fresh tibial fractures (p. 23). The reaming of pseudarthrosis is often much more laborious than that of fresh fractures. The reamer must be withdrawn and the reamer heads cleaned of bone debris more often. If the reduction of the pseudarthrosis of the lower leg necessitates the use of the distractor, the lower leg is positioned on the fracture table in the distractor. The distractor is removed only after the ball-point guide pin is placed into the distal medullary canal of the tibia. The operative technique from here on is identical with that of the reducible rigid pseudarthrosis.

Pseudarthrosis of the Humerus

The indications for the nailing of pseudarthrosis of the humerus are identical with those for the nailing of fresh fractures (p. 33). Rigid pseudarthroses of the humerus are rare. Rigid irreducible pseudarthroses of the humerus are extremely rare. The use of a distractor on the humerus is seldom necessary. The position and reduction are identical to those for fresh fractures (p. 33).

The medullary canal is opened either proximally or distally, depending on the location of the pseudarthrosis. A drill point guide pin is used to penetrate both pseudarthrosis covers until it is advanced into the farthest medullary canal. A pseudarthrosis-chisel is rarely used for the humerus. The drill point guide pin is exchanged for a ball-point guide pin. On those rare occasions when the distractor has to be used, the distractor is removed only after the ball-point guide pin has been advanced into both medullary canals. Hereafter, the operative technique is identical to that described for fresh fractures (pp. 33 and 34).

Pseudarthrosis of the Forearm

The indications for the nailing of pseudarthrosis of the forearm are identical to those for fresh fractures (pp. 47 through 49)

Pseudarthrosis of the Radius

Positioning and reduction usually necessitate the use of a distractor as described on page 47.

A small, sharp guide pin penetrates the pseudarthrosis covers after the medullary canal is opened in the conventional fashion. This sharp guide pin may be bent at its tip. If the pseudarthrosis cover cannot be perforated by this sharp guide pin, a Kirschner wire, attached to a power drill, can be used instead. The Kirschner wire or the sharp guide pin is exchanged for a small ball-point guide pin. If the distractor was used for the reduction, it should be removed only after the ball-point guide pin was advanced into both medullary canals.

The reaming and nailing is identical with that for fresh fractures. The reaming is especially laborious because of the extremely hardened bone and must be done very slowly and cautiously because the reamer head can break off easily. Pseudarthroses of the radius are preferably fixated with V-nails.

Pseudarthrosis of the Ulna

Pseudarthroses of the ulna are handled in exactly the same manner as fresh fractures (p. 47). The covers of the ulna are perforated in the same fashion as in radial pseudarthrosis. If the medullary canal is narrow, use a V-nail. A cloverleaf nail is used in a wider medullary canal.

Pseudarthrosis of the Radius and Ulna

Pseudarthroses of the forearm, which are maligned, must nearly always be reduced in a distractor. The distal skeletal wire must perforate both the radius and the ulna (Fig. 97). The positioning and the operative technique used are identical to that described for the isolated radius and ulna pseudarthroses. The distractor is removed only after the small ball-point guide pin is positioned in both medullary canals in each fracture.

Pseudarthrosis of the Clavicle

The pseudarthrosis of the clavicle is nailed like a fresh fracture (p. 86). The soft-tissue capsule of the pseudarthrosis is incised longitudinally to the clavicle and folded away from the clavicle with a periosteal elevator. The soft-tissue capsule is left intact. Use a small drill bit mounted on a handchuck to initially locate the medullary canal. The reaming of the pseudarthrosis is done cautiously so that the medullary canal is not missed or perforated. Incrementing the sizes of the twist drill diameters proves to be an effective method of reaming.

Flexible Pseudarthrosis

Flexible pseudarthrosis is characterized by extreme mobility of the fragments within the connective tissue capsule. For this reason, the pseudarthrosis is nearly always easily reduced, and seldom warrants the use of a distractor. The indication for the intramedullary nailing of a flexible pseudarthrosis is met if the satisfactory locking of the nail is possible in both fragments.

Positioning and reduction are accomplished as discussed in the description of the Küntscher intramedullary nailing of the corresponding bone.

Roentgenograms and image intensification are necessary, as described for the intramedullary nailing of fresh fractures of the corresponding bone.

The operative technique is also identical to that of a fresh fracture. The use of a pseudarthrosis-chisel is unnecessary, because the covers of the pseudarthrosis are usually soft. Traction should be reduced when inserting the nail into the distal fragment in order to compress the fragments longitudinally. Early weight-bearing in flexible pseudarthroses of the lower extremities is especially important.

If the prerequisites for the use of a regular intramedullary nail are not satisfied by the shape of the medullary canal, the pseudarthrosis can often be stabilized by other nails (interlocking nails, compression nails, conical nails) or by other systems of osteosynthesis.

Defect Pseudarthrosis

The defect in this type of pseudarthrosis must be filled as nearly completely as possible with autogenous cancellous bone. The autogenous cancellous bone should be brought into the defect through the medullary canal, if possible. Pseudarthroses in which the defect did not lead to a shortening of the extremity are nailed like fresh fractures when the medullary canal of both fractures provides sufficient locking of the intramedullary nail. If less than 2 cm of shortening occurred in a pseudarthrosis of the lower extremity, the fragments are nailed after longitudinal compression and the shortening is accepted. Even larger shortenings are accepted for the humerus. If the defect in the lower extremity is larger than 2 cm, an interlocking nail is used to avoid shortening. The defect is filled with autogenous cancellous bone.

Position, reduction, roentgenograms, and image intensification are all performed as for fresh fractures. The nailing is also indentical to the technique described in the chapters on intramedullary nailing of freshly fractured bones. The cancellous bone is placed into the defect through the reamed medullary canal by intramedullary gripping pliers under fluoroscopy. The cancellous bone may also be placed into the defect through an additional incision, made over the defect after the capsule is split longitudinally. Resecting the pseudarthrosis is superfluous.

Pseudarthrosis After Intramedullary Nailing

If a fresh fracture is nailed with an intramedullary nail too small in diameter, which is insufficiently locked in both fragments, the fracture site is not mechanically stabilized. Fracture healing does not ensue and a pseudarthrosis develops with the inserted intramedullary nail. These pseudarthroses are easily treated: The small intramedullary nail is removed, the medullary canal is reamed open as wide as possible, and an appropriately larger nail is inserted.

If the nail exchange is not done in this type of pseudarthrosis, the small nail will break. The nail exchange in this circumstance then becomes more difficult.

Pseudarthroses After Compression Plating and Screw Fixation

If a pseudarthrosis forms after compression plating or a screw fixation of a fracture, the implants must be removed. They should be removed through a stab incision whenever possible in order to avoid exposing the pseudarthrosis. A decision as to which of the several different nails to use (Küntscher nail, interlocking nail, Y-nail, or others) can be made only after the removal of these implants.

Positioning, reduction, x-ray examination, image intensification, and operative technique are all identical to those described for the fresh fractures of the corresponding bone. Because the cortex is often transformed into cancellous bone under the compression plate, reaming and nailing must be done carefully; otherwise, the bone can easily split.

Because avirulent infections in the individual screw canals are not always clinically recognizable, specimens for culture and sensitivity testing should be taken from the implants and bone debris. The pseudarthrosis should be weight-bearing shortly after the nailing.

Because of the difficulty in judging the stage of bone healing, premature removal of the implants in compression plating and screw fixation is possible, often causing a pseudarthrosis. These pseudarthroses are nailed by the technique just described

Infected Pseudarthroses

Even infected pseudarthroses can be nailed under certain circumstances: the infection must be avirulent (a nearly normal sedimentation rate, normal values of electrophoresis, and a normal white blood count). Sinus formation is no contraindication to nailing. One must remove the sequestra before the nailing if they sustain sinus formation. The culture and sensitivity results must also be known before nailing. An acute stage of the infection, if present, must be converted into an avirulent stage with appropriate measures before nailing. Bone healing is severely retarded in an infected pseudarthrosis. Therefore, absolute immobilization of the fragments must be secured for a considerable length of time. The bone should be reamed to the largest diameter possible, even in infected pseudarthrosis. A nail with an appropriately large diameter should be used. The nail must interlock in a large area of both fragments. If a defect pseudarthrosis is infected, the defect is meticulously debrided and filled with autogenous cancellous bone, as described on page 127. The skin incision for the nail entry point in an infected pseudarthrosis is left open and a drain is inserted.

If the avirulent infection becomes acute after the nailing, the appropriate antibiotics (according to results of the culture and sensitivity tests) are administered intravenously. Suction drainage through the intramedullary nail is also advised.

If the nail becomes loose during the lengthy healing period in an infected pseudarthrosis, the nail must be exchanged for one with a larger diameter in order to restore absolute mechanical stability in the fracture area. The healing of the infection and the closure of the sinuses usually take place only after the complete bone healing of the pseudarthrosis and after the final removal of the intramedullary nail. The operative technique for the nailing of the infected pseudarthrosis is the same as that of fresh fractures of the corresponding bone.

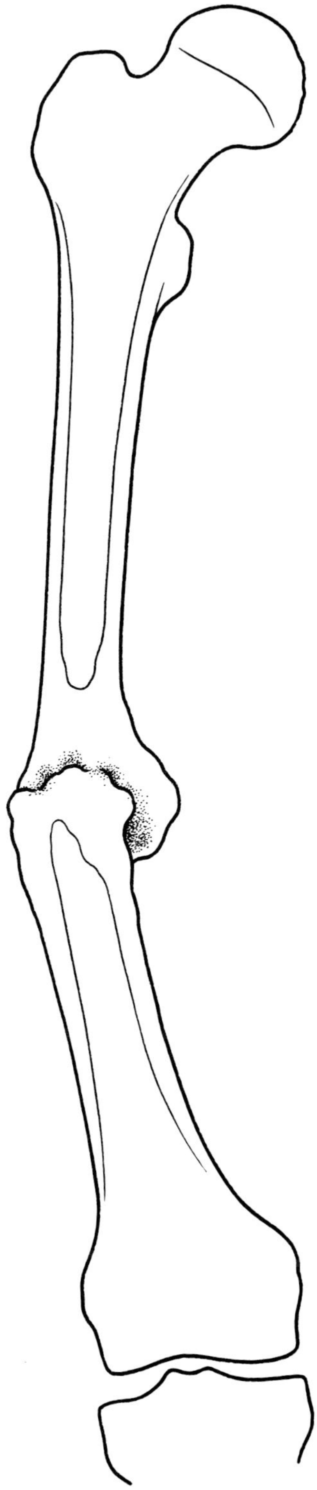

Figure 242 Femoral pseudarthrosis with deformity. Bony sealing of the medullary canals of both fragments.

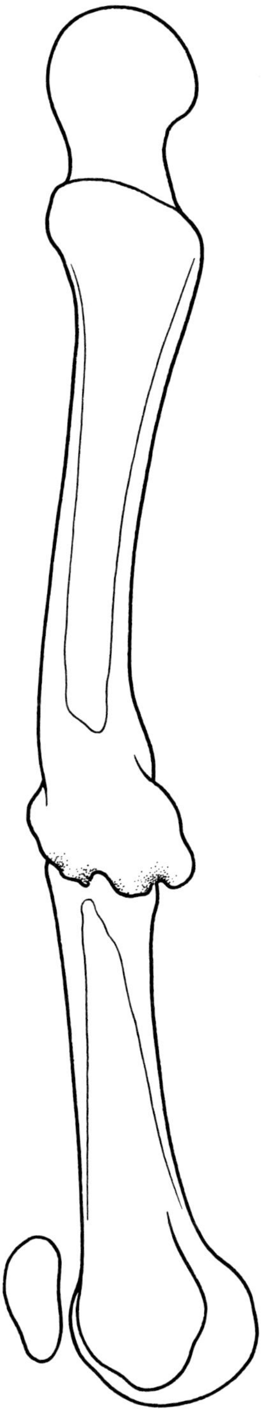

Figure 243 Femoral pseudarthrosis, lateral view.

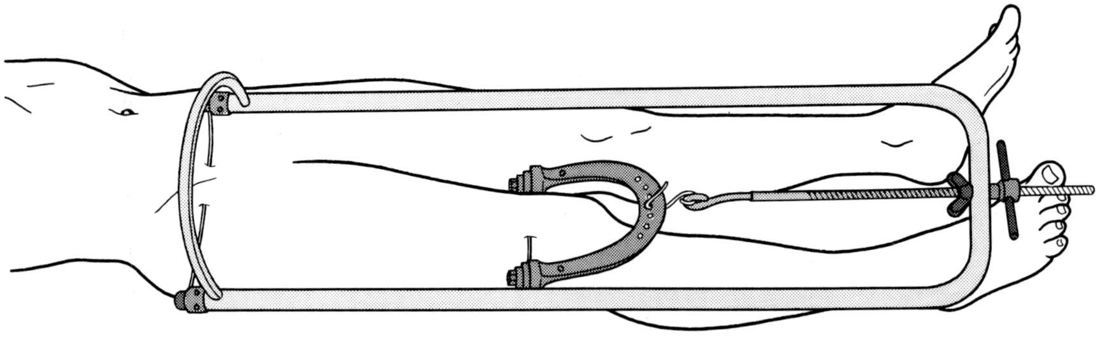

Figure 244 Distractor for the femur. Proximal Kirschner wire through the iliac crest, with supracondylar distal Kirschner wire.

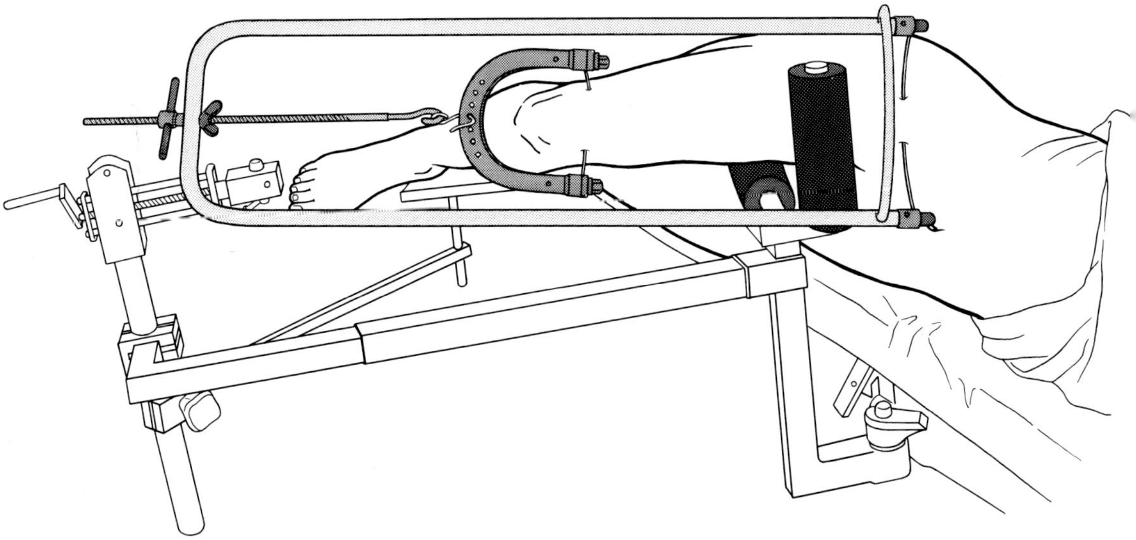

Figure 245 The correct position of the patient on the fracture table in a femoral distractor, lateral position.

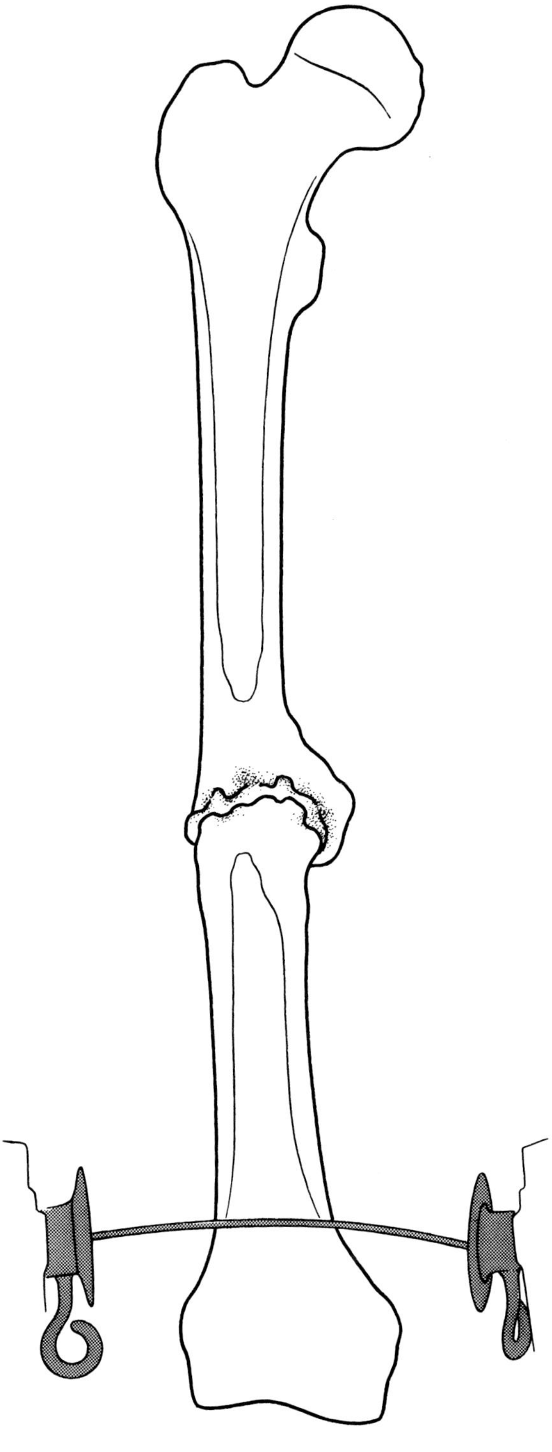

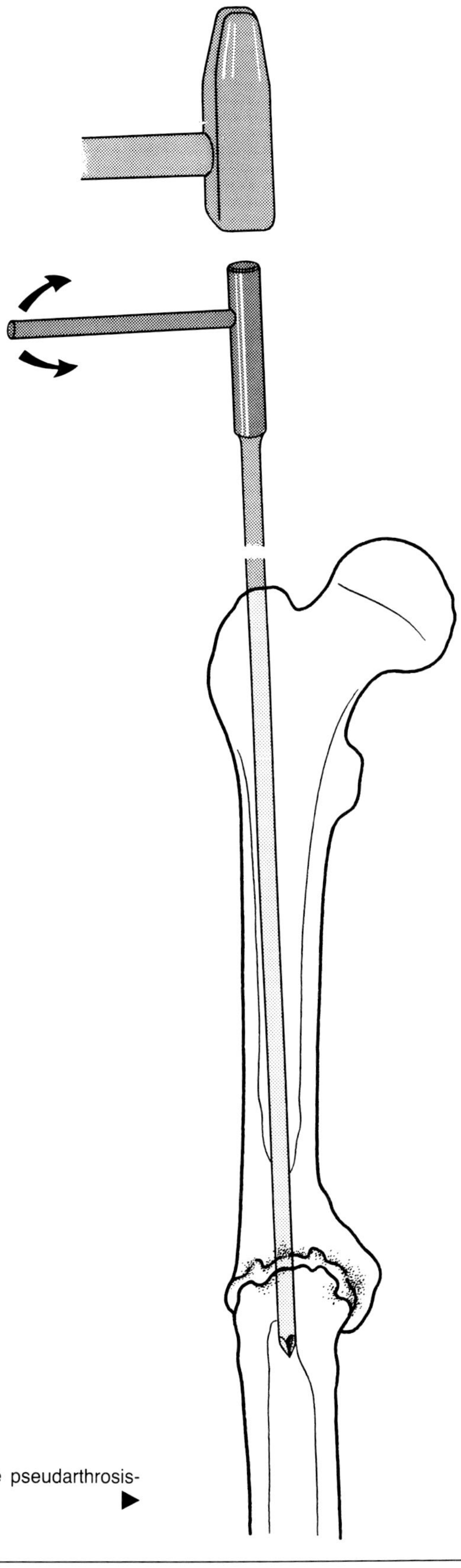

Figure 246 Reduction of the femoral pseudarthrosis in the distractor.

Figure 247 The pseudarthrosis cover is perforated by the pseudarthrosis-chisel to open the medullary canal. ▶

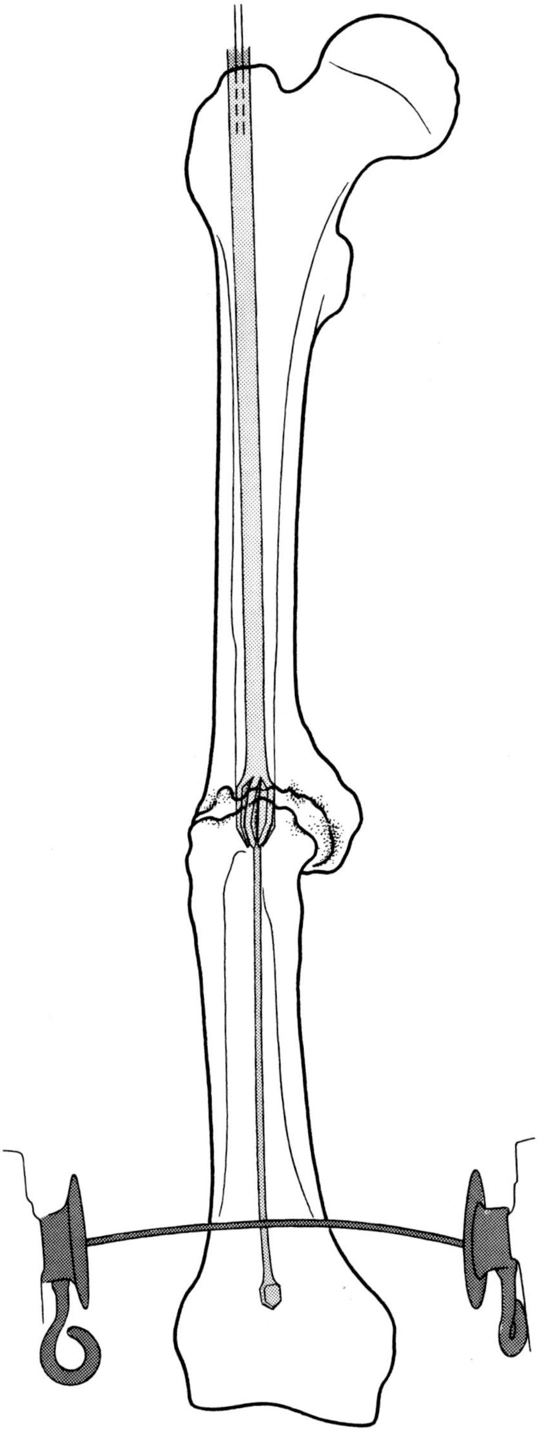

Figure 248 After the insertion of a drillpoint guide pin, the pseudarthrosis cover is perforated, and the medullary canal of both fragments is reamed. The supracondylar skeletal traction is still in place.

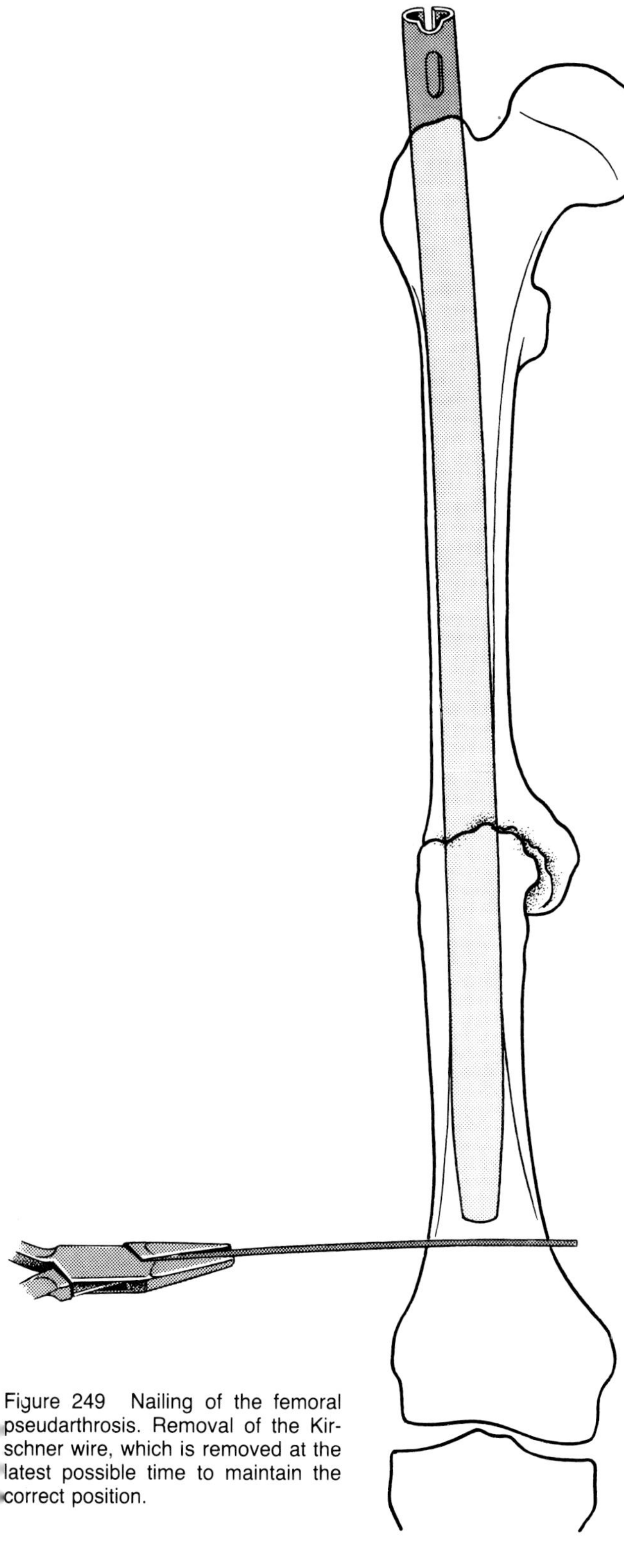

Figure 249 Nailing of the femoral pseudarthrosis. Removal of the Kirschner wire, which is removed at the latest possible time to maintain the correct position.

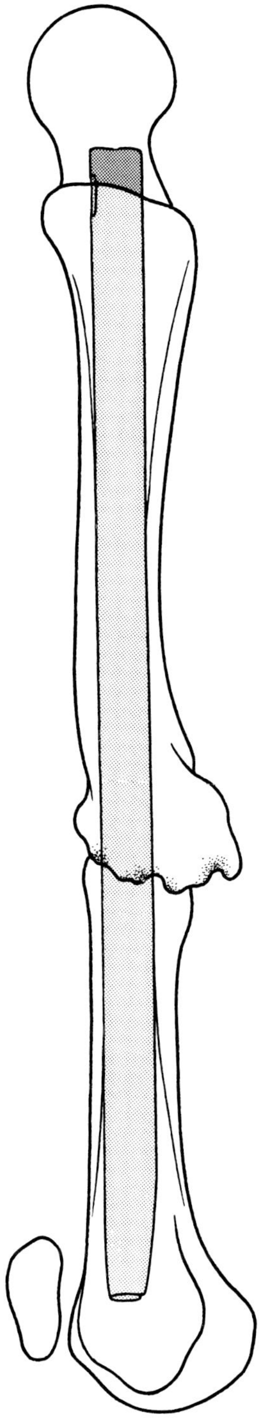

Figure 250 Completed nailing of femoral pseudarthrosis, lateral view.

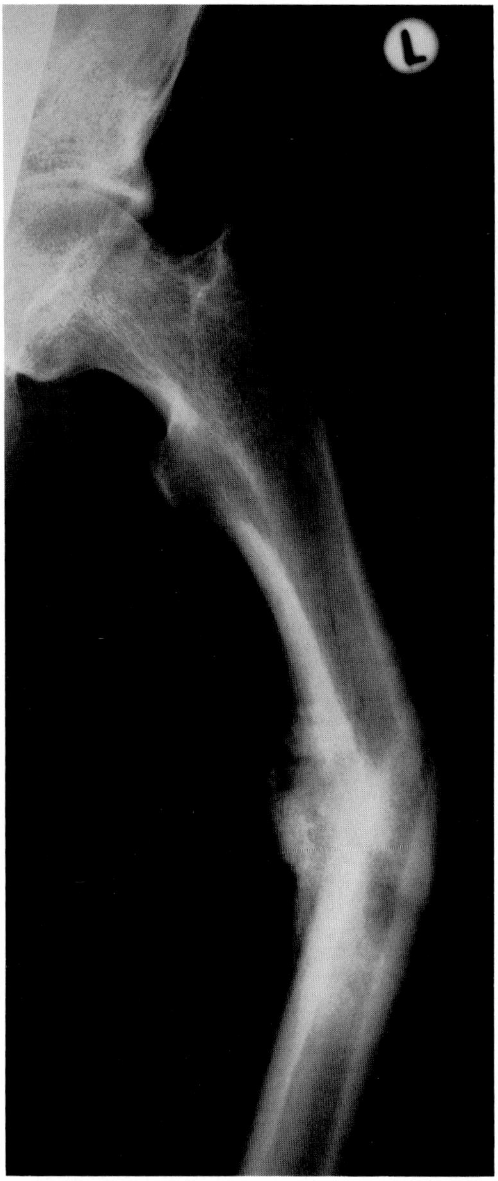

Figure 251

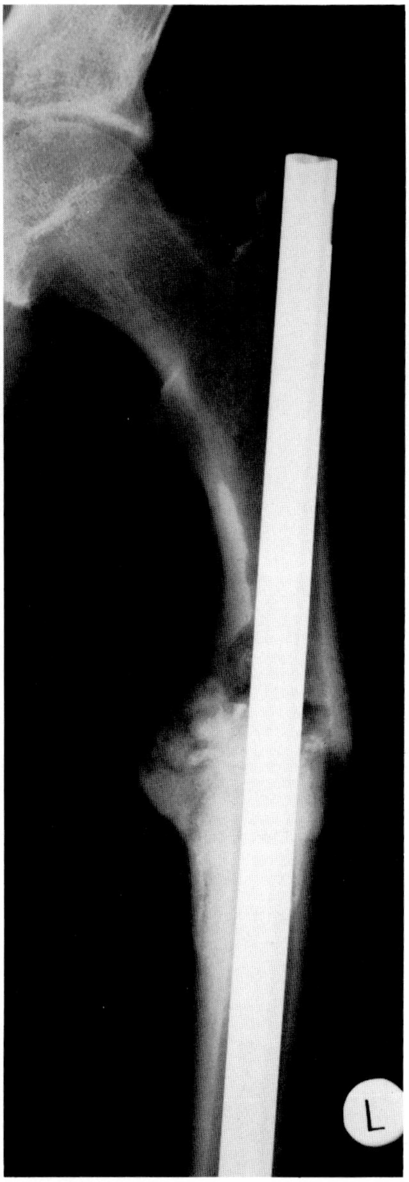

Figure 252

Figure 251 Femoral pseudarthrosis with severe angulation, AP view.

Figure 252 The same pseudarthrosis after correction of the deformity and nailing, AP view.

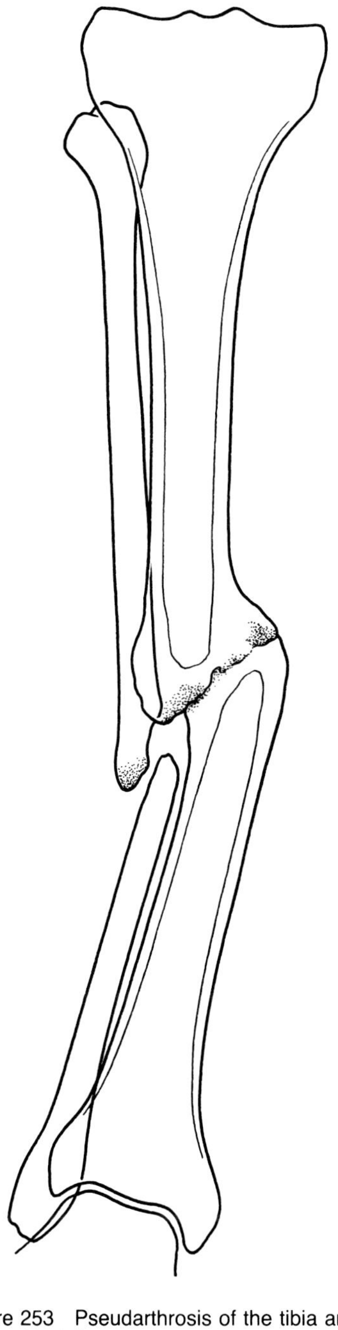

Figure 253 Pseudarthrosis of the tibia and fibula with deformity and bony sealing of the medullary canals of the tibia.

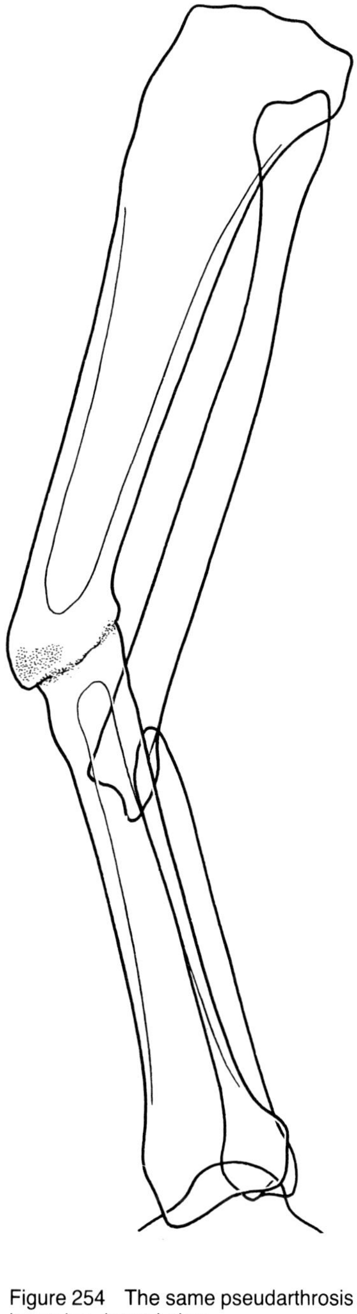

Figure 254 The same pseudarthrosis of the lower leg, lateral view.

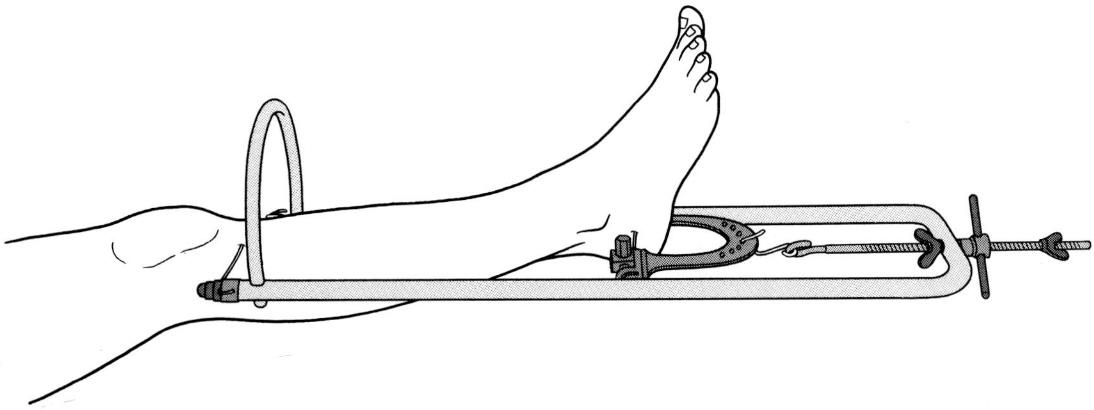

Figure 255 Distractor for the lower leg. Proximal Kirschner wire through the tibial tubercle, distal wire through the os calcis.

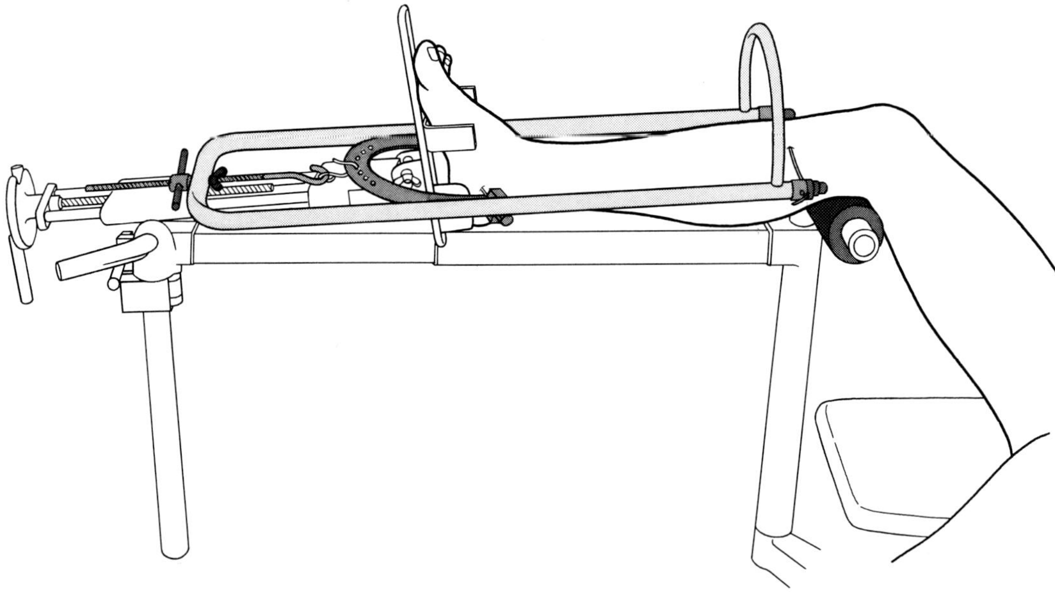

Figure 256 The correct position of the patient on the fracture table in a lower leg distractor.

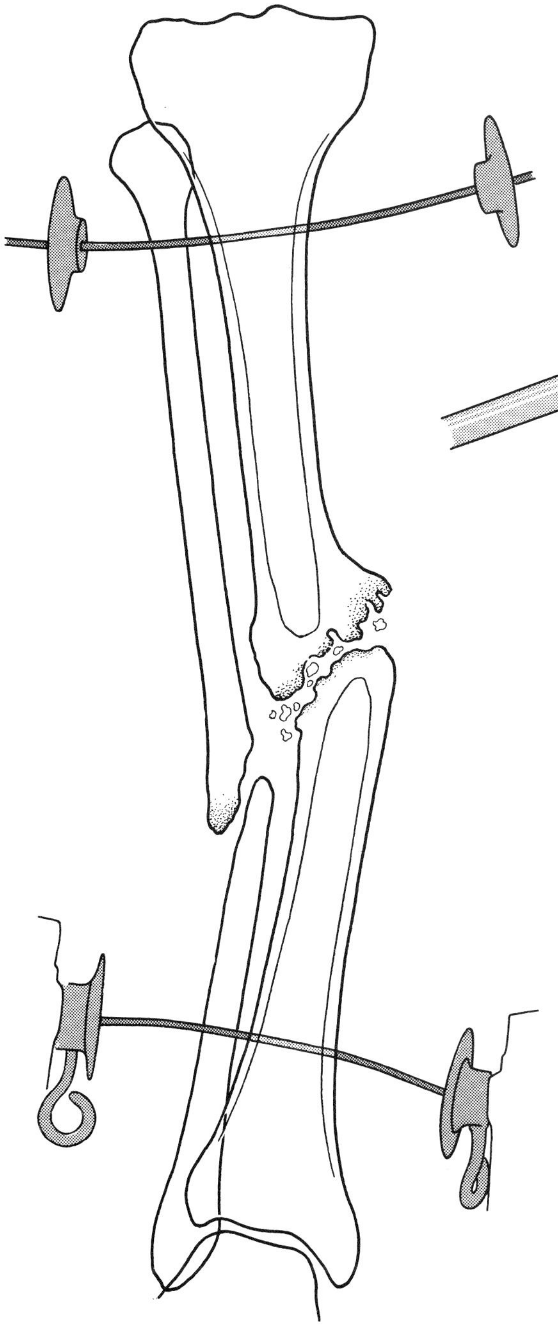

Figure 257 Separation of the pseudarthrosis by the distractor. Distal Kirschner wire through the distal tibia.

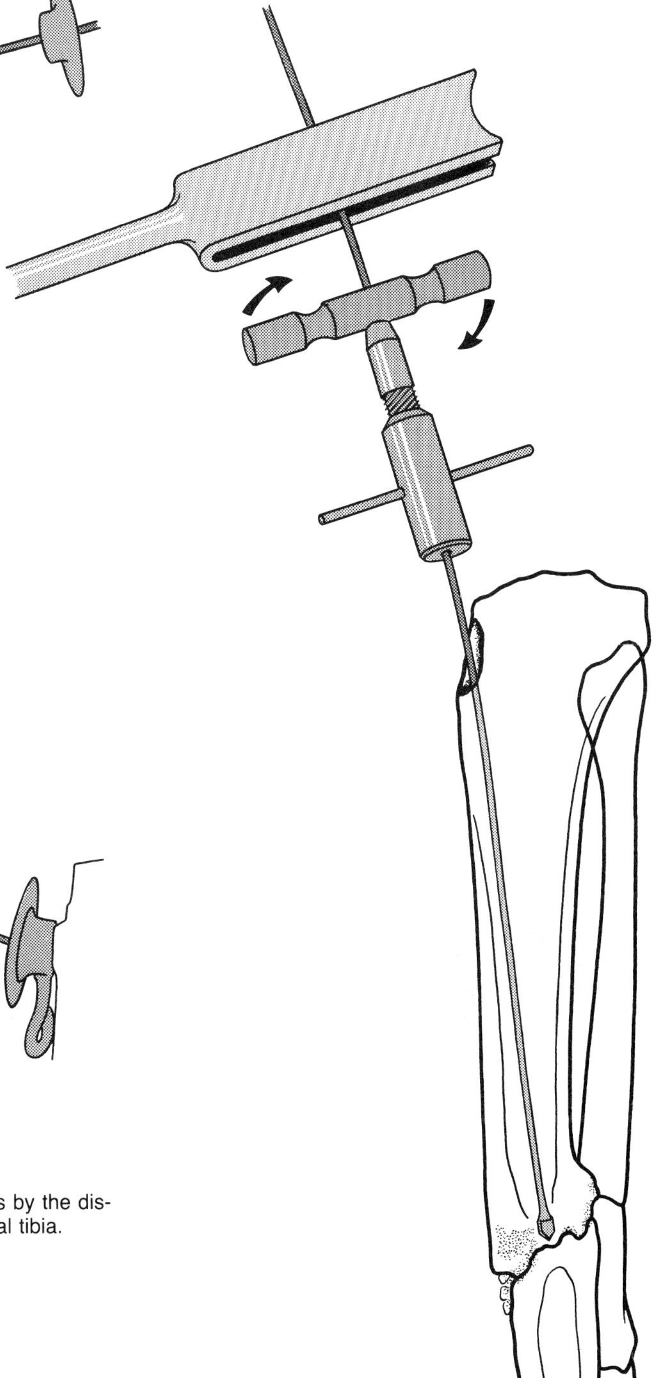

Figure 258 Perforation of the pseudarthrosis cover by a drill point guide pin after the correction of the deformity.

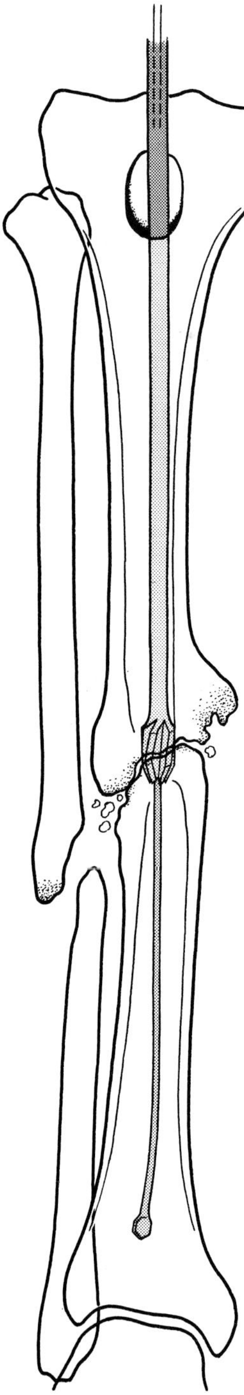

Figure 259 Reaming of the medullary canal of the tibia over the guide pin.

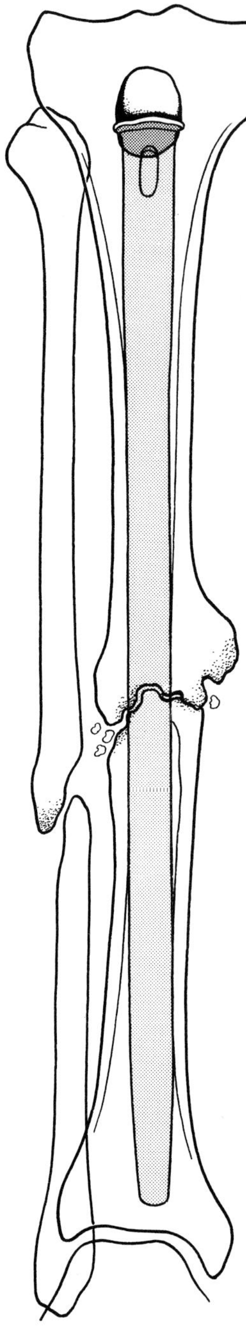

Figure 260 Completed nailing of the tibial pseudarthrosis, AP view.

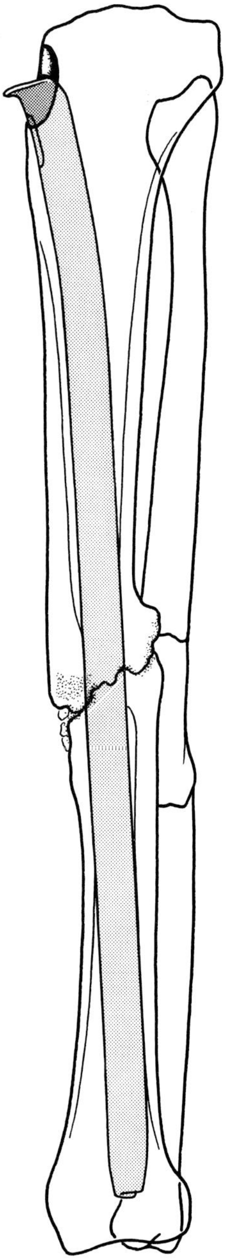

Figure 261 Completed nailing of the tibial pseudarthrosis, lateral view.

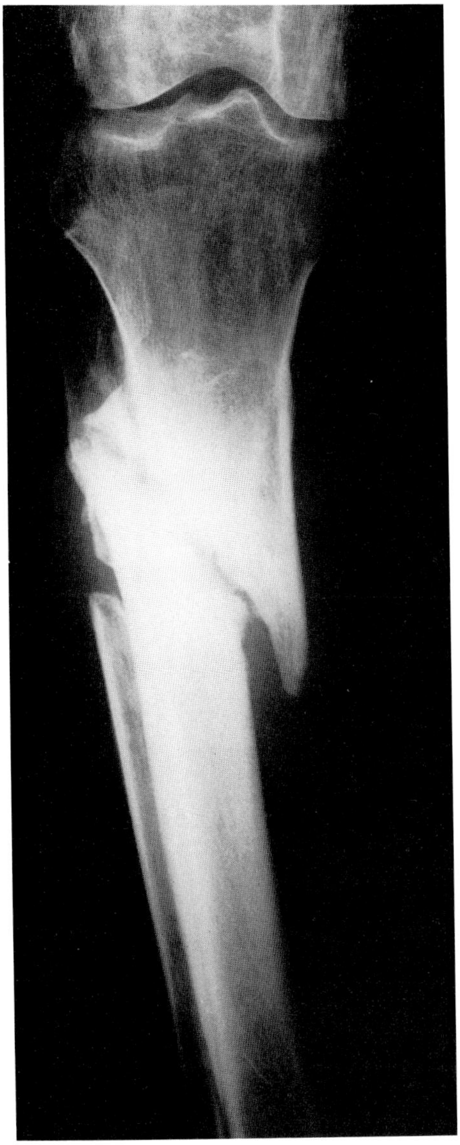

Figure 262

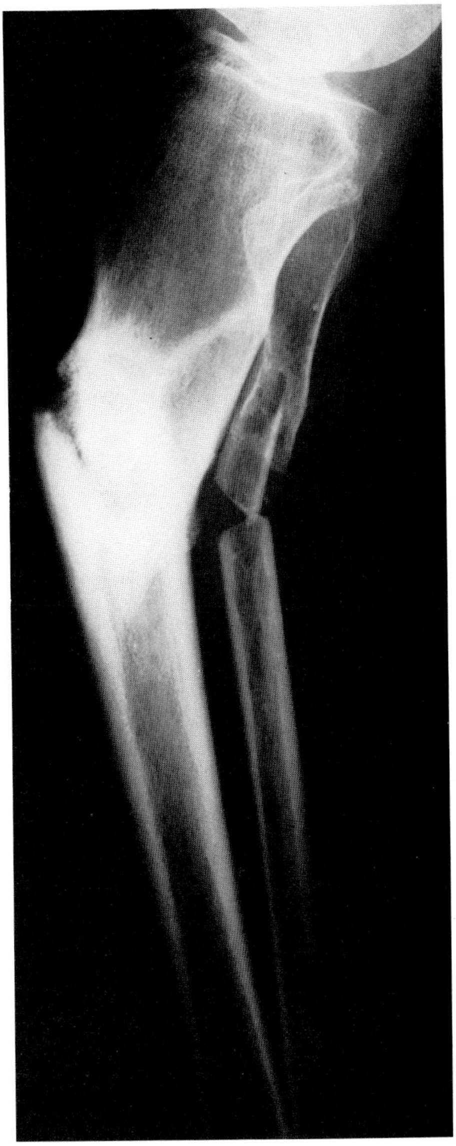

Figure 263

Figure 262 Rigid pseudarthrosis of the tibia with antecurvature deformity. Condition after unsuccessful resection of the fibula, AP view.

Figure 263 Same pseudarthrosis, lateral view.

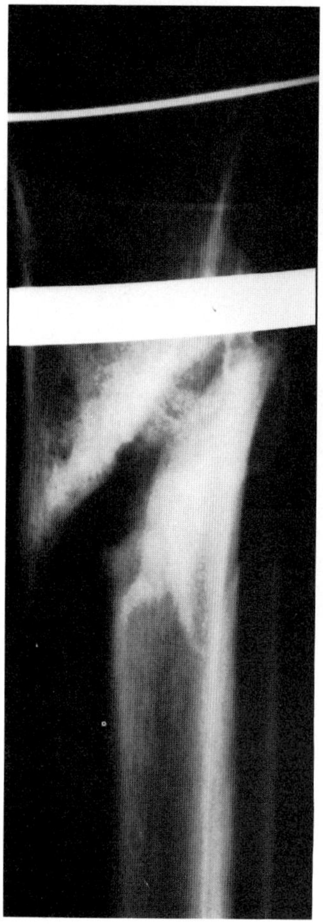

Figure 264

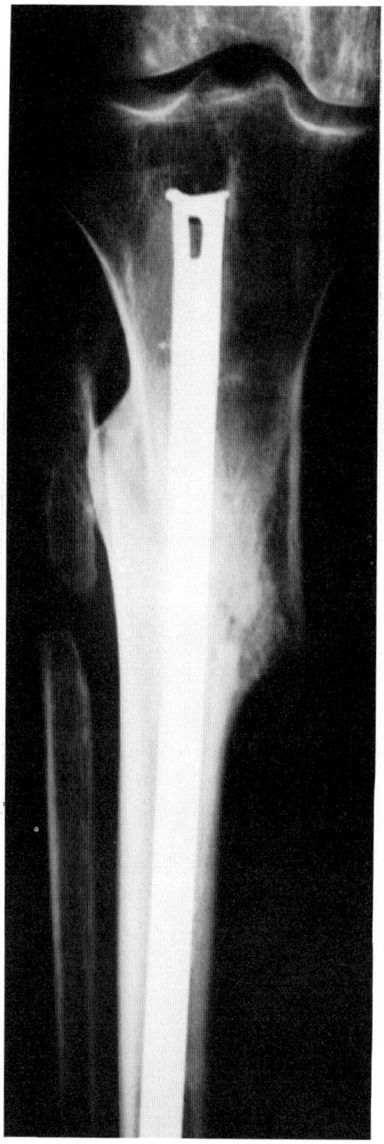

Figure 265

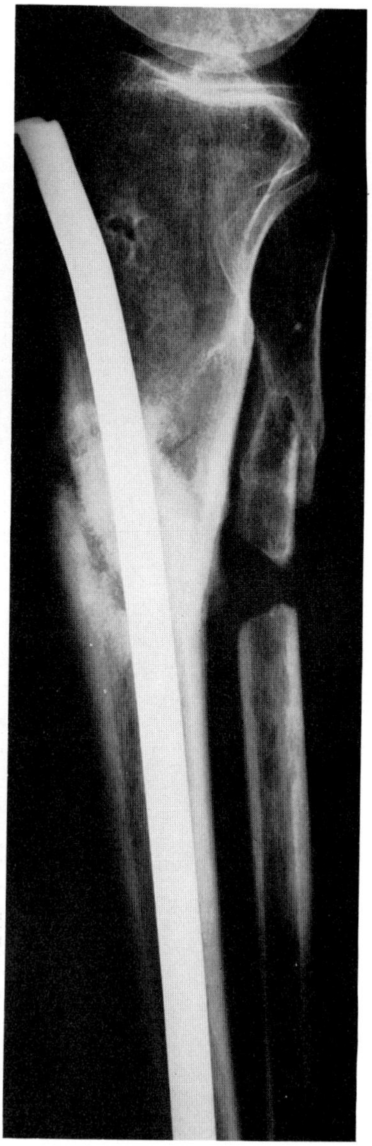

Figure 266

Figure 264 Magnified view of the pseudarthrosis gap after separation by distractor.

Figure 265 The same pseudarthrosis after nailing and complete bone healing, one year later, AP view.

Figure 266 The same case, lateral view.

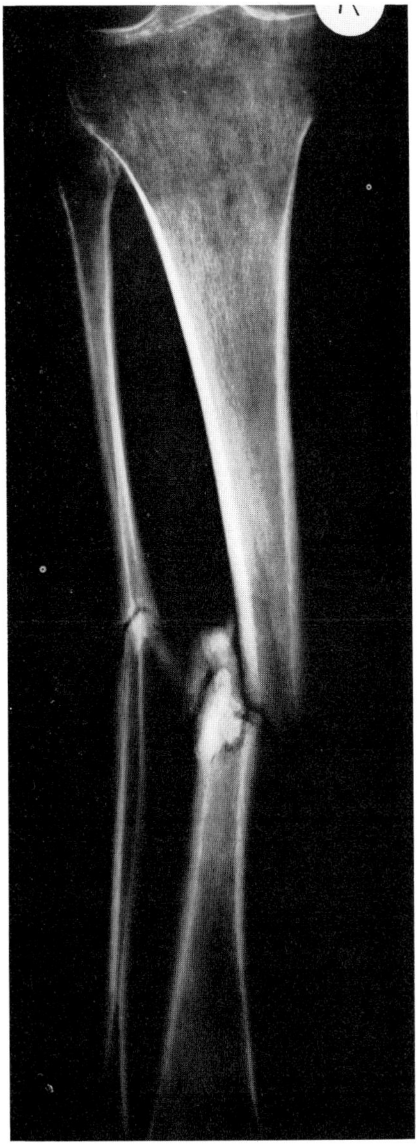

Figure 267

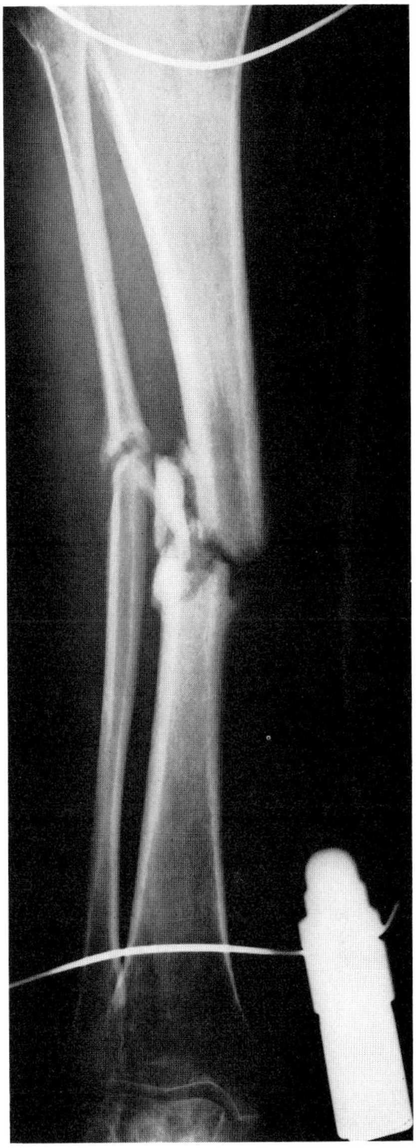

Figure 268

Figure 267 Flexible pseudarthrosis of the lower leg. Multiple fragments at the fracture site make this pseudarthrosis difficult to reduce, AP view.

Figure 268 The same pseudarthrosis positioned in a distractor for reduction, AP view. Distal Kirschner wire through the tibia.

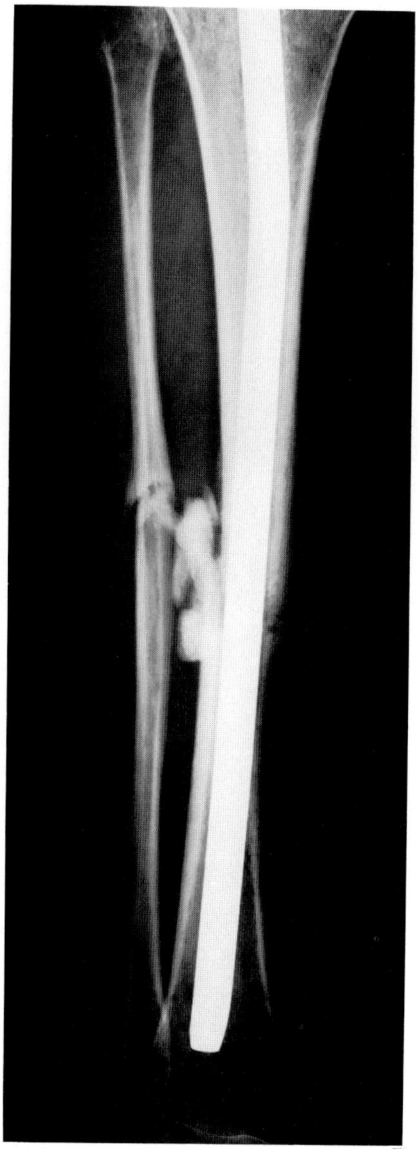

Figure 269

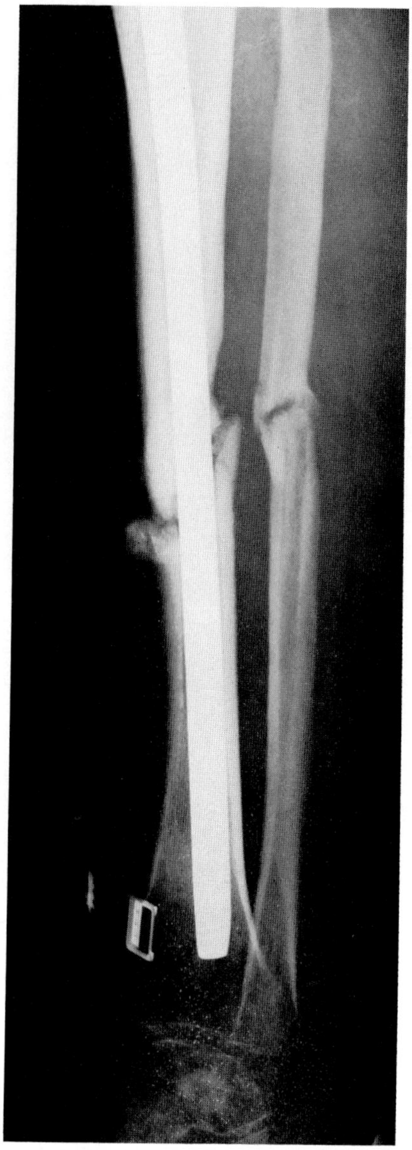

Figure 270

Figure 269 Pseudarthrosis after the reduction and nailing, 14 days postoperatively, AP view.

Figure 270 The same case, lateral view.

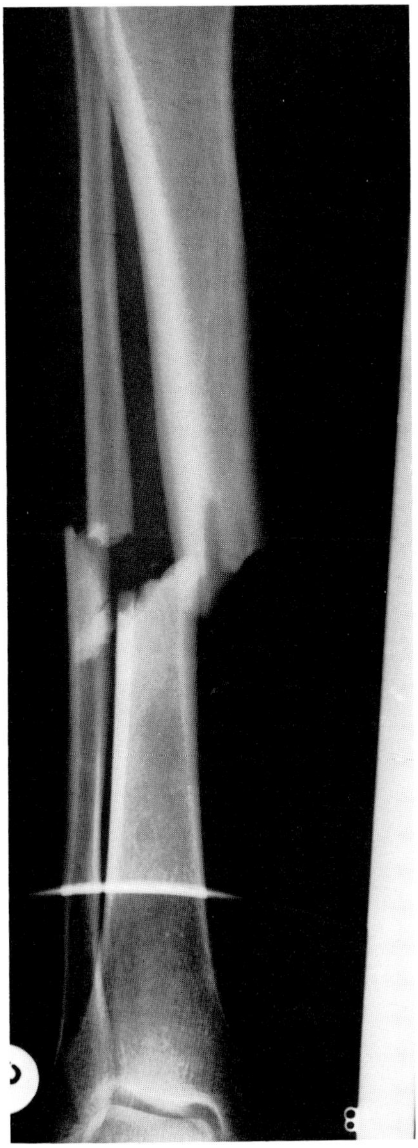

Figure 271

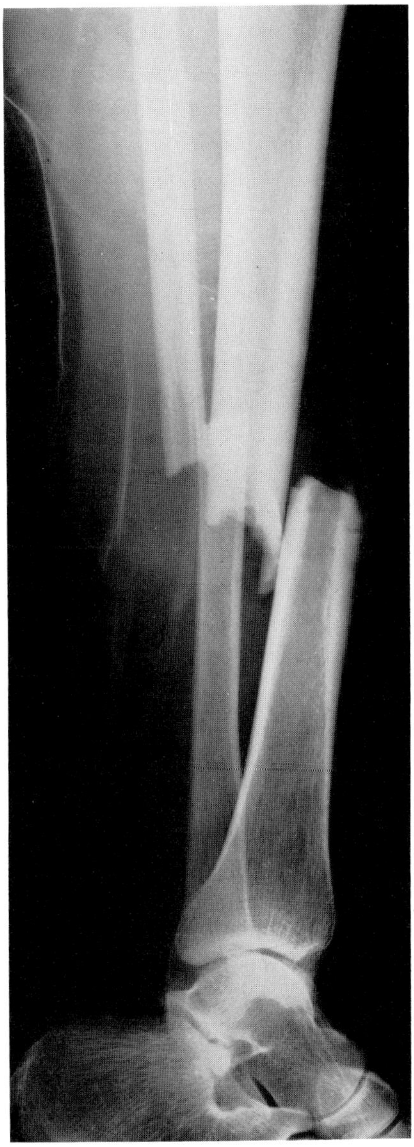

Figure 272

Figure 271 Fresh fracture of the lower leg, AP view.

Figure 272 The same fractures, lateral view.

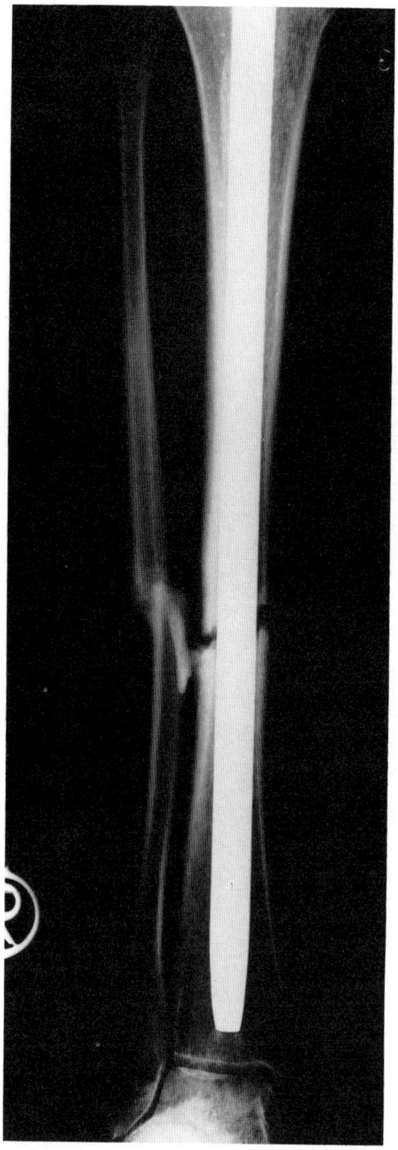

Figure 273

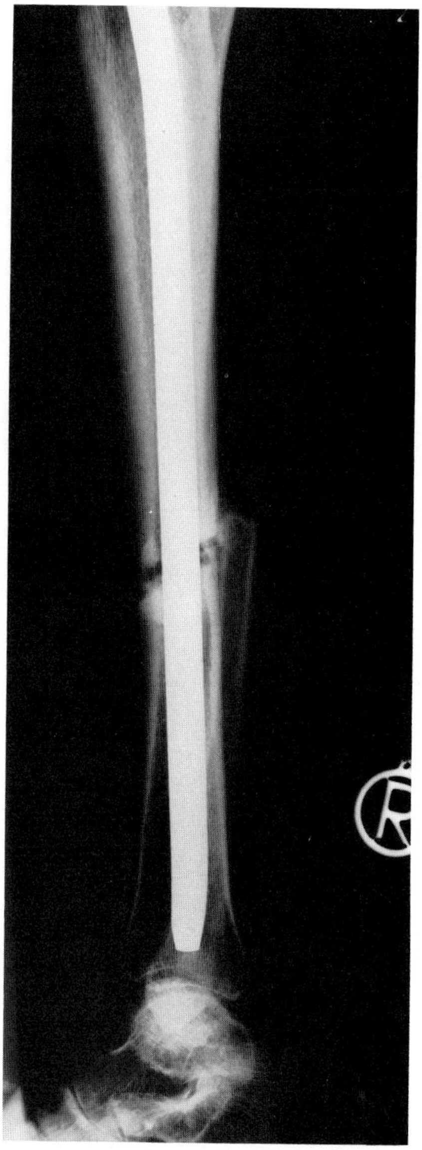

Figure 274

Figure 273 The same fractures, six months after the nailing. Formation of a tibial pseudarthrosis caused by using too small a nail. Bone healing of the fibula, AP view.

Figure 274 The same pseudarthrosis of the tibia, lateral view.

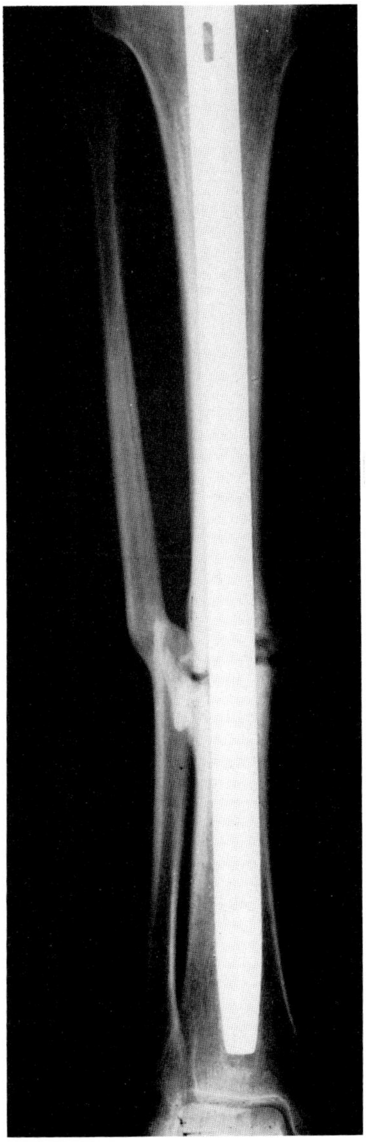

Figure 275

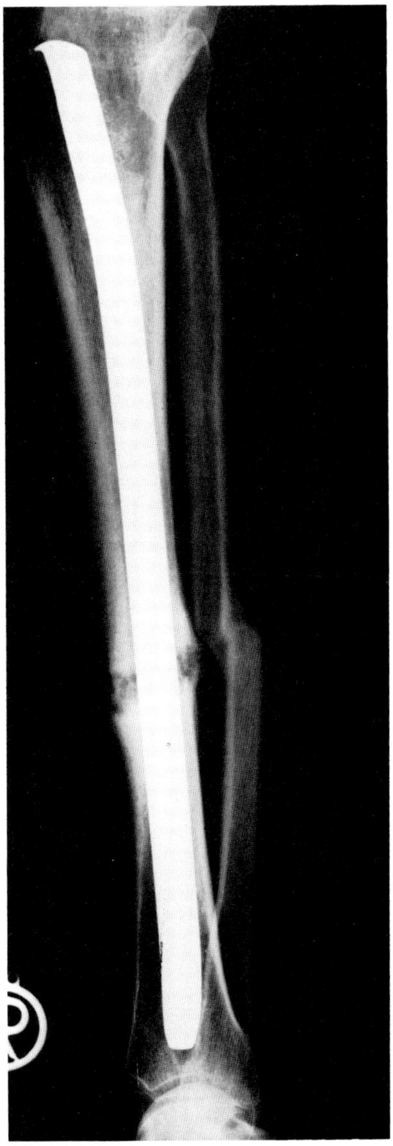

Figure 276

Figure 275 The same pseudarthrosis 12 months after the accident. Condition after the exchange of the tibial nail for one that is 2 mm larger in diameter.

Figure 276 The same condition, lateral view.

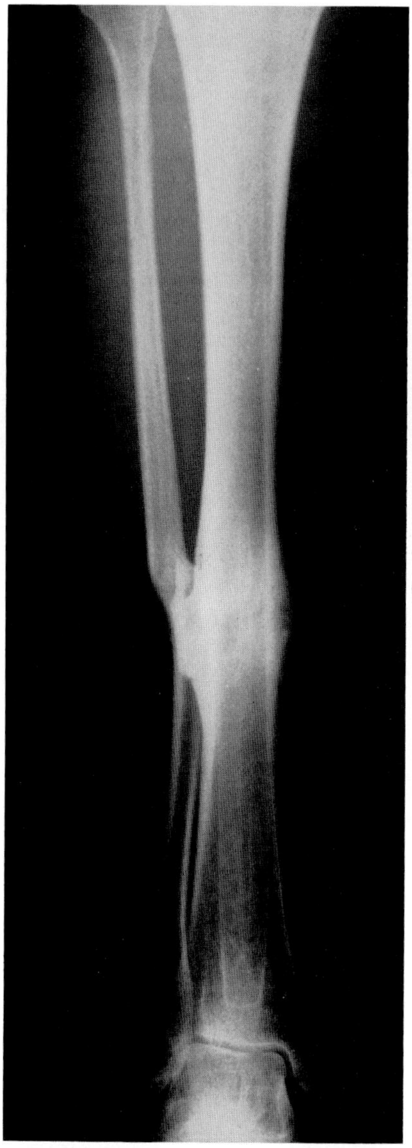

Figure 277

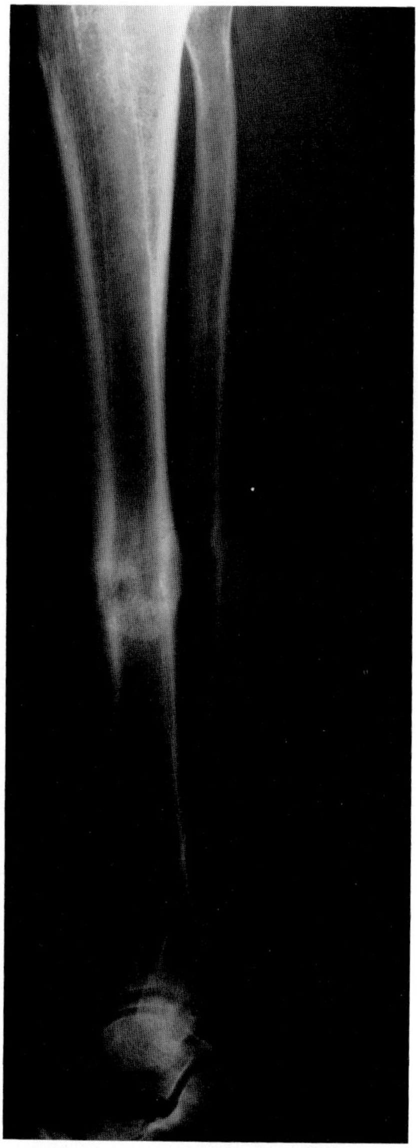

Figure 278

Figure 277 Twenty-four months after the accident and 12 months after the nail exchange. The healing of the fracture is complete. Condition after nail removal, AP view.

Figure 278 The same case, lateral view.

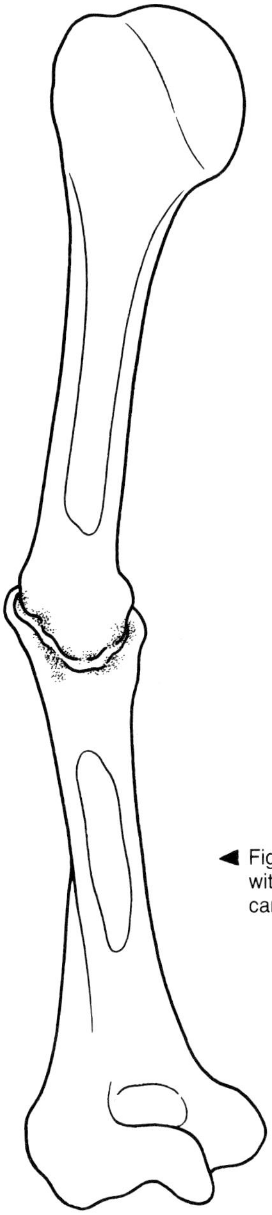

◀ Figure 279 Pseudarthrosis of the humerus with deformity and sealing of the medullary canals of both fragments.

Figure 280 Pseudarthrosis of the humerus with sealing of the medullary canals, lateral view. ▶

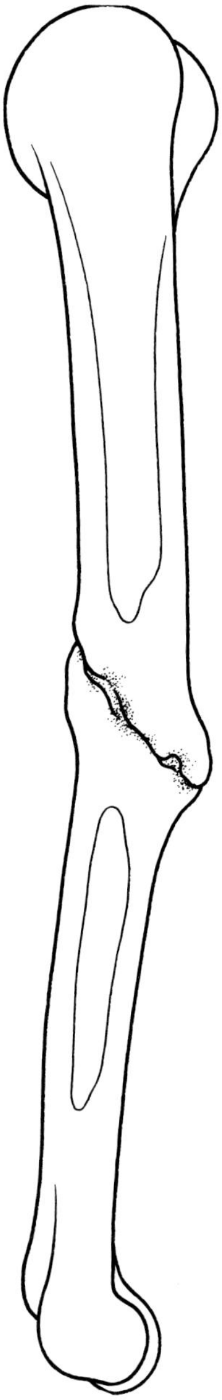

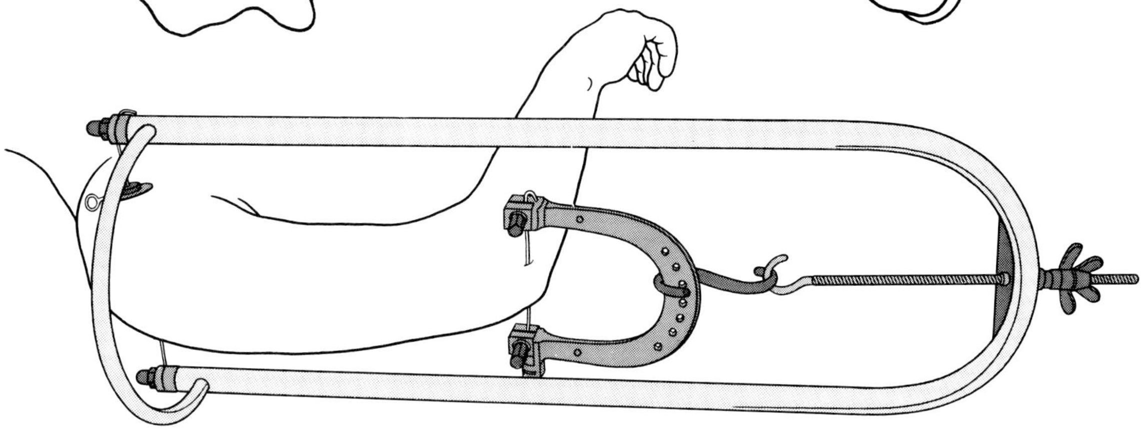

Figure 281 Distractor for the humerus. Proximal Kirschner wire through the head of the humerus, distal Kirschner wire through the olecranon.

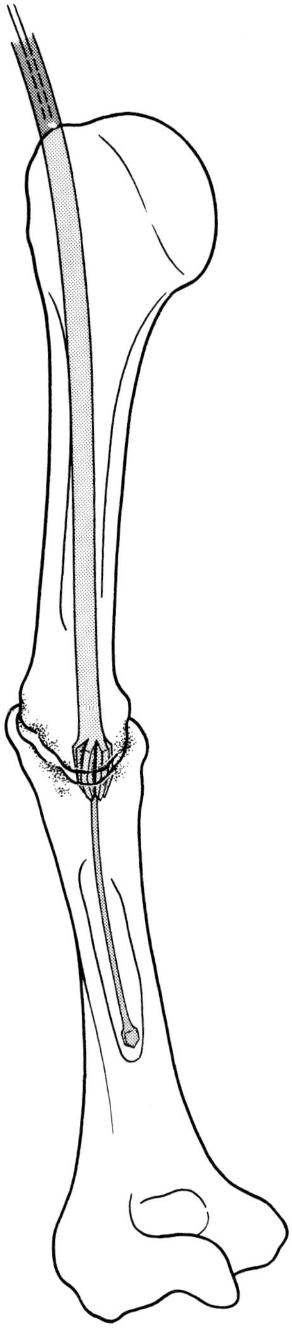

Figure 282 Reaming of the medullary canal after perforation of the pseudarthrosis cover by a drill point guide pin.

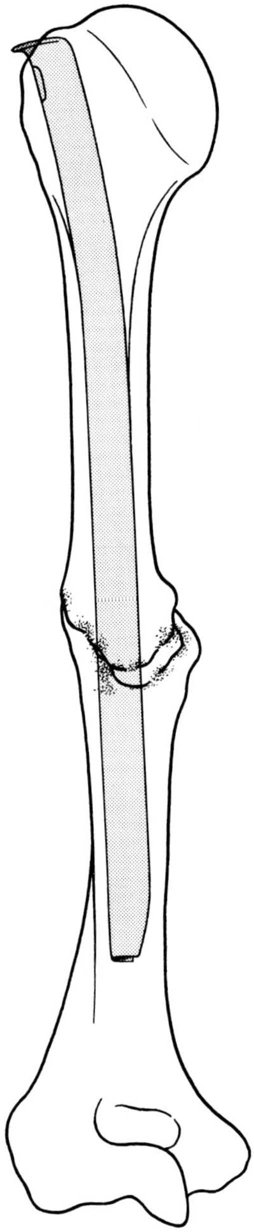

Figure 283 Completed nailing of the pseudarthrosis of the humerus.

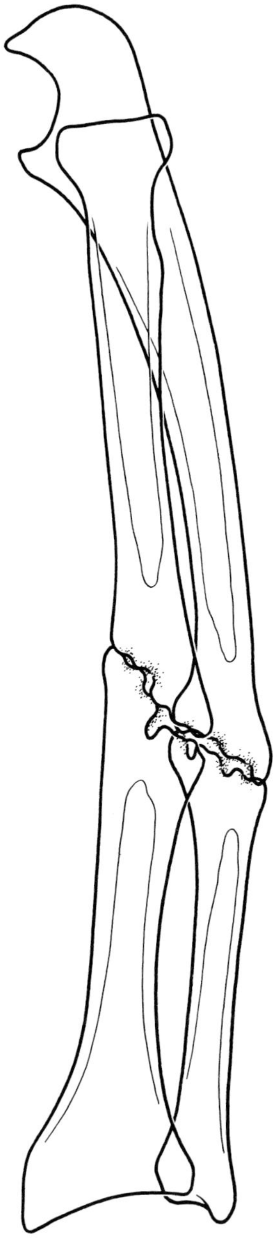

Figure 284 Pseudarthrosis of the forearm with deformity and sealed medullary canals.

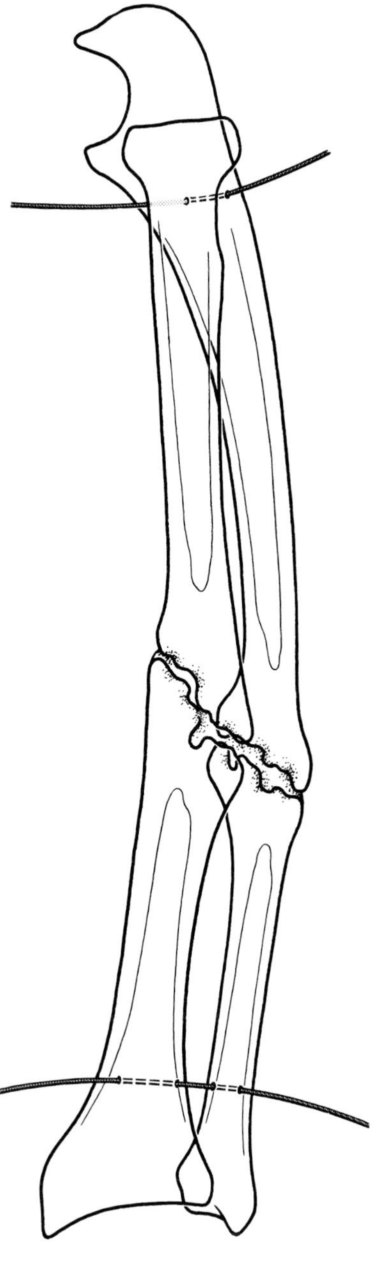

Figure 285 Pseudarthrosis of the forearm in the distractor. Distal Kirschner wire through the radius and ulna.

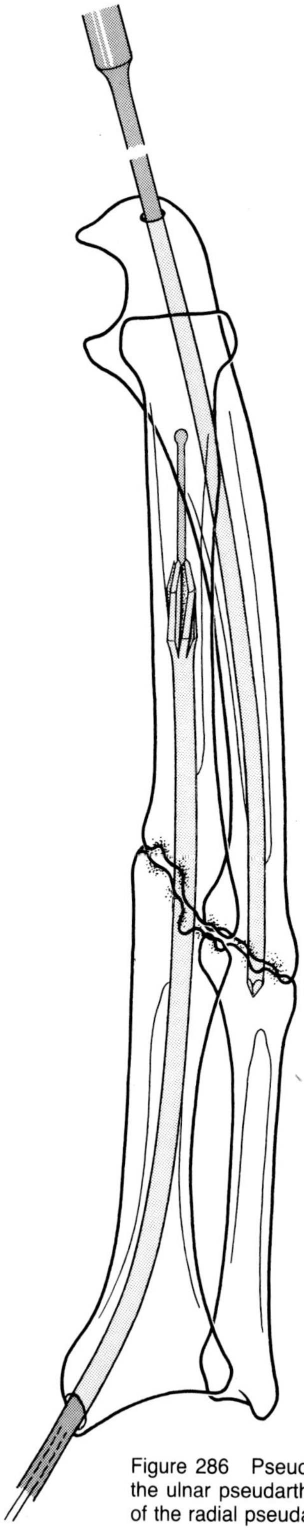

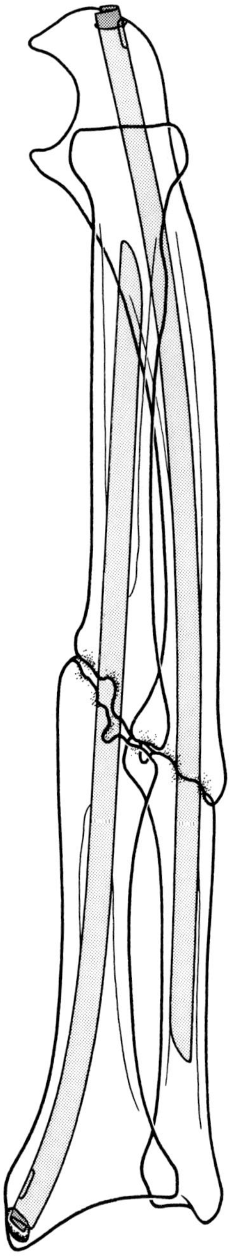

Figure 287 Completed nailing of a pseudarthrosis of the forearm.

Figure 286 Pseudarthrosis of the forearm. Perforation of the pseudarthrosis cover of the ulnar pseudarthrosis with a pseudarthrosis-chisel. Reaming of the medullary canal of the radial pseudarthrosis over a guide pin.

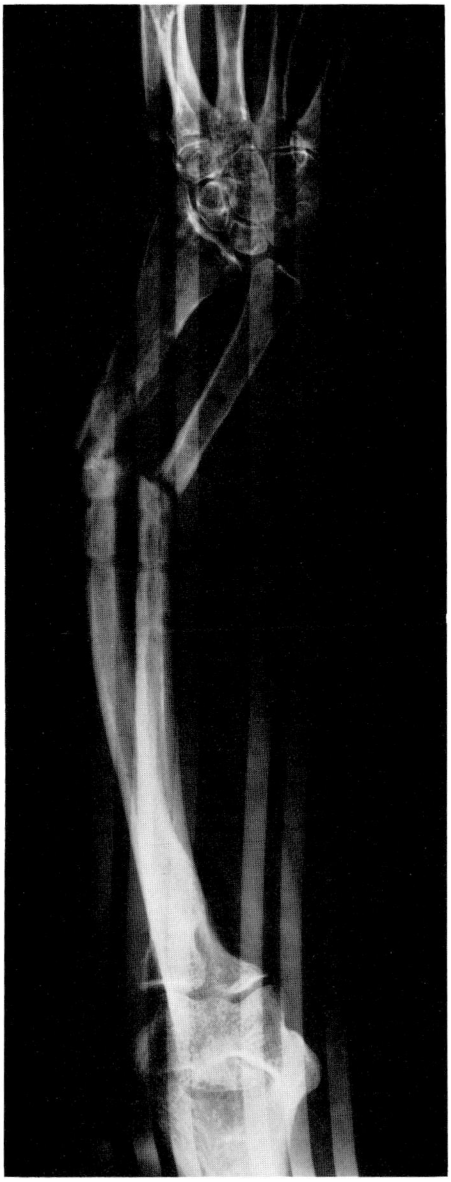

Figure 288

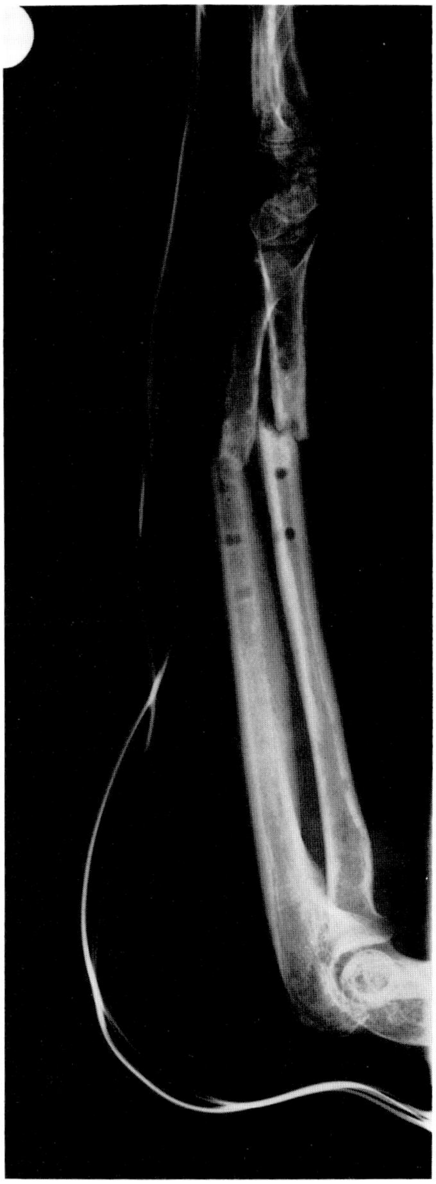

Figure 289

Figure 288 Pseudarthrosis of the forearm, condition after compression plating and removal of the implants, AP view.

Figure 289 The same case, lateral view.

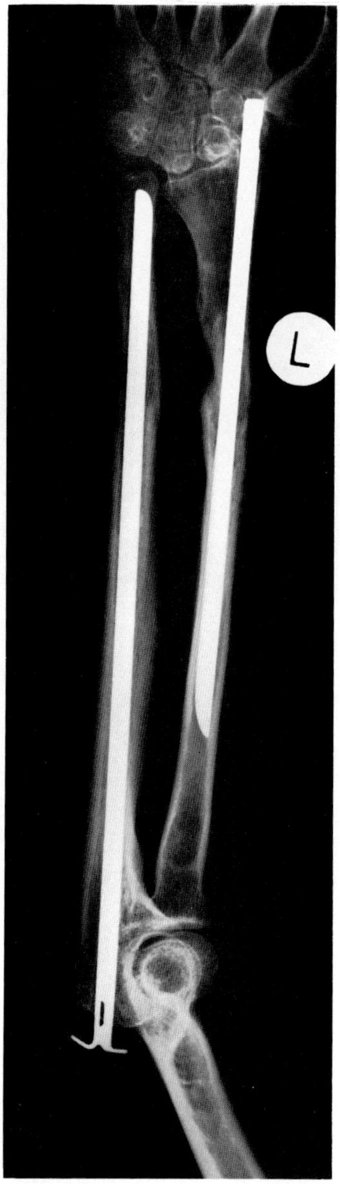

Figure 290 Completed nailing and the bone healing of the same pseudarthrosis. The ulnar nail protrudes out from the olecranon.

Closed Intramedullary Nailing of Infected Fractures

Bone infection can be caused by soft tissue damage in compound or closed fractures. More often, the infection occurs after surgical treatment of the fractures. The callus formation is retarded considerably in infected fractures, and the danger of forming a pseudarthrosis is increased. Any movement in the fracture area will maintain the infection and tends to form a pseudarthrosis. Therefore, the stability of the osteosynthesis must be maintained for a long period of time. This can best be done with a rigid intramedullary nailing. If the type and localization of the fracture lend themselves to intramedullary nailing, an infection is no contraindication for the nailing procedure. The infection, however, must not be in an acute stage; the patient cannot have septic temperatures, no abscess may be present in the extremity, the white blood count must not be significantly increased, the sedimentation should be close to normal, and the sequestra should not be visible on the preoperative roentgenograms. An acute bone infection with clinical symptoms must be converted into an avirulent stage by the appropriate measures, as determined by results of culture and sensitivity tests. The presence of a sinus is no contraindication to the nailing of an avirulent bone infection. Specimens for culture and sensitivity tests should be taken from the bone dust during the operation. If the avirulent infection becomes acute postoperatively, the results of the culture and sensitivity tests are helpful in combatting the postoperative flare-up of the infection. However, the nailing of an infected fracture usually passes without remarkable temperature elevations. The nailing of the fracture is performed as described for fresh fractures. The medullary canal is, of course, reamed open to as large a diameter as possible.

The skin incision at the nail's entry portal should not be closed. If the nail becomes loose

should not be closed. If the nail becomes loose as a result of the infection before any solid healing of the bone occurs, the nail must be exchanged for one with a larger diameter in order to secure complete mechanical stability at the fracture site. The medullary canal is re-reamed during the nail exchange.

Suction drainage can be inserted into the medullary canal to combat the infection further. A string of gentamycinpalacos beads may be inserted into intramedullary nails with large diameters in order to enhance the fight against the infection. Abscesses, if they arise, are incised.

If a bone infection arises after the nailing of a fresh, noninfected fracture, the nail is left untouched as long as it is firmly lodged in the medullary canal. The incision should be reopened in all infected cases. The nail inherently drains the medullary canal very effectively. The further treatment of the infection and of the fracture is as previously described.

If an infection arises after compression plating and screw fixation of a fracture that lends itself to intramedullary nailing, the implants are not removed if the osteosynthesis is stabilized. The incision is completely opened. If the implants become loose, they are to be removed. If the bone infection is avirulent, intramedullary nailing should be done in the same session (of course, after reaming the medullary canal). The treatment of the infection and of the fracture is as previously described.

An interlocking nail may prove to be effective when the fracture cannot be stabilized by an intramedullary nail because of the location of the fracture. The indications and the technique for the interlocking nail are discussed on pages 92 through 115. The incision is also left open after the insertion of the interlocking nail.

Open Intramedullary Nailing

Open intramedullary nailing, by definition, implies the visualization of the fracture site during the reduction and nailing procedures. The opening of the fracture site and the open reduction of the fracture are no longer necessary since the advent of image intensification. Only fractures of the clavicle are still reduced and nailed openly. The reduction and nailing of all compound fractures are also medically termed open procedures if done immediately after the trauma. However, it is not advisable to nail a compound fracture immediately. Instead, the laceration should be debrided, the fracture reduced, and the laceration closed, thus converting the compound fracture into a closed fracture. The fracture is immobilized, either by splint or by skeletal traction, until the laceration is healed. A closed intramedullary nailing then can be performed after uneventful wound healing.

Indications

Open intramedullary nailing of long bones should not be done routinely. It should be the exception rather than the rule. For example, either vascular or nerve damage close to a fracture site are candidates for open reduction and nailing. The same indications are valid for open intramedullary nailing as for closed intramedullary nailing of the corresponding bone.

Positioning and Reduction

Depending on the concomitant laceration, the patient is positioned either on a regular operating table (vascular laceration) or a fracture table. The reduction is facilitated by the visualization of the fracture.

Image Intensification

Preoperative roentgenograms of the fractured bone comprising both adjacent joints must be taken at a 1-m distance in two planes. These films will act as gauges for the determination of the dimensions for the reamers and the nail. If an image intensifier is also used, it is positioned as described for the closed intramedullary nailing of the corresponding bone. Postoperative roentgenograms of the entire bone must be taken in two planes.

Operative Technique

The nail entry points for open nailing are the same as in closed intramedullary nailing. After the awl opens the medullary canal, a guide pin is inserted until it reaches the fracture site. The fracture is then visually reduced and the guide pin advanced into the distal fragment. However, fractures of the femur and ulna are handled differently. A sharp guide pin is inserted from the fracture into the proximal fragment until the nail's entry point is reached. In fractures of the femur, the trochanter tip is then perforated with the sharp guide pin. In fractures of the ulna, the sharp guide pin is used to pierce the olecranon. A skin incision is made over the protruding tip of the guide pin. In femoral fractures, the reamer awl is placed over the guide pin and enlarges the nail's entry portal. The sharp guide pin is then withdrawn. A ball-point guide pin is guided through the reamer awl into the proximal fragment and is advanced until it reaches the fracture. After the removal of the reamer awl, the fracture is visually reduced, and the ball-point guide pin is advanced into the distal fragment. The operative technique thereafter is identical with that for closed nailing of the femur.

A square head reamer is used in the open nailing of the ulna. It is advanced over the exposed tip of the guide pin in order to enlarge the nail's entry point. The sharp guide pin is exchanged for a ball-point guide pin, which is then advanced until it reaches the fracture site. After the fracture is visibly reduced, the ball-point guide pin is inserted into the distal fragment. The operative technique from this juncture is identical to that for closed ulnar nailing.

The medullary canal must always be reamed in open nailings. The soft tissue and the periosteum must be delicately handled when exposing the fracture. The fragments with sufficient soft tissue connection and vascularization are ignored during the reduction. The wounds are closed in the usual fashion.

Aftercare

The aftercare is identical to that in the closed nailing of the corresponding bone. In our opinion, prophylactic antibiotic treatment is unnecessary.

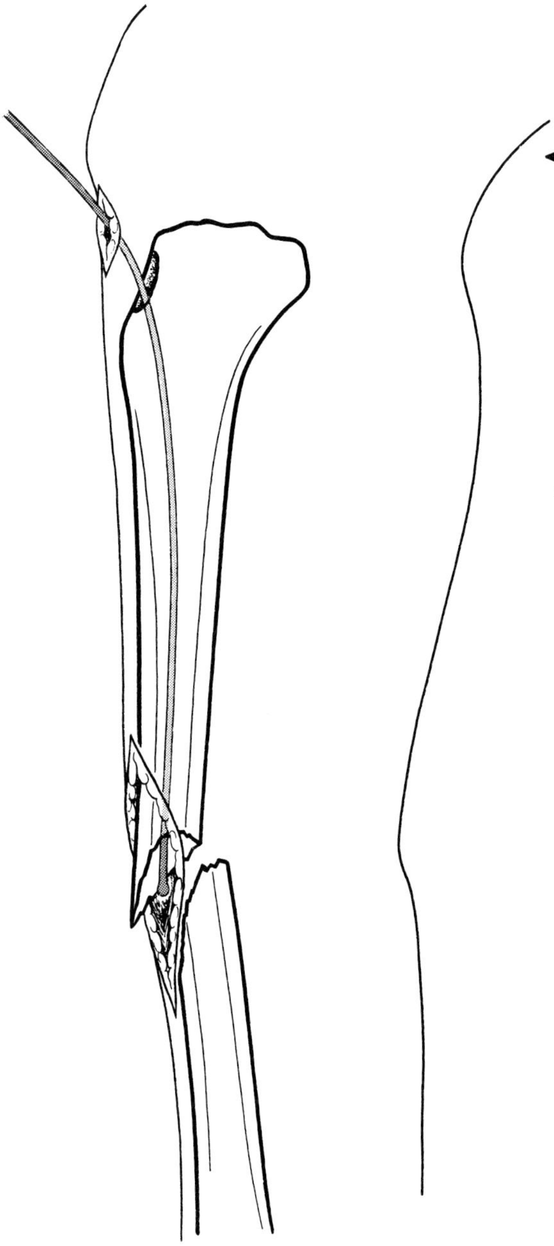

◀ Figure 291 Compound fracture of the tibia. Stab incision over the nail entry point. The guide pin is advanced to the fracture site.

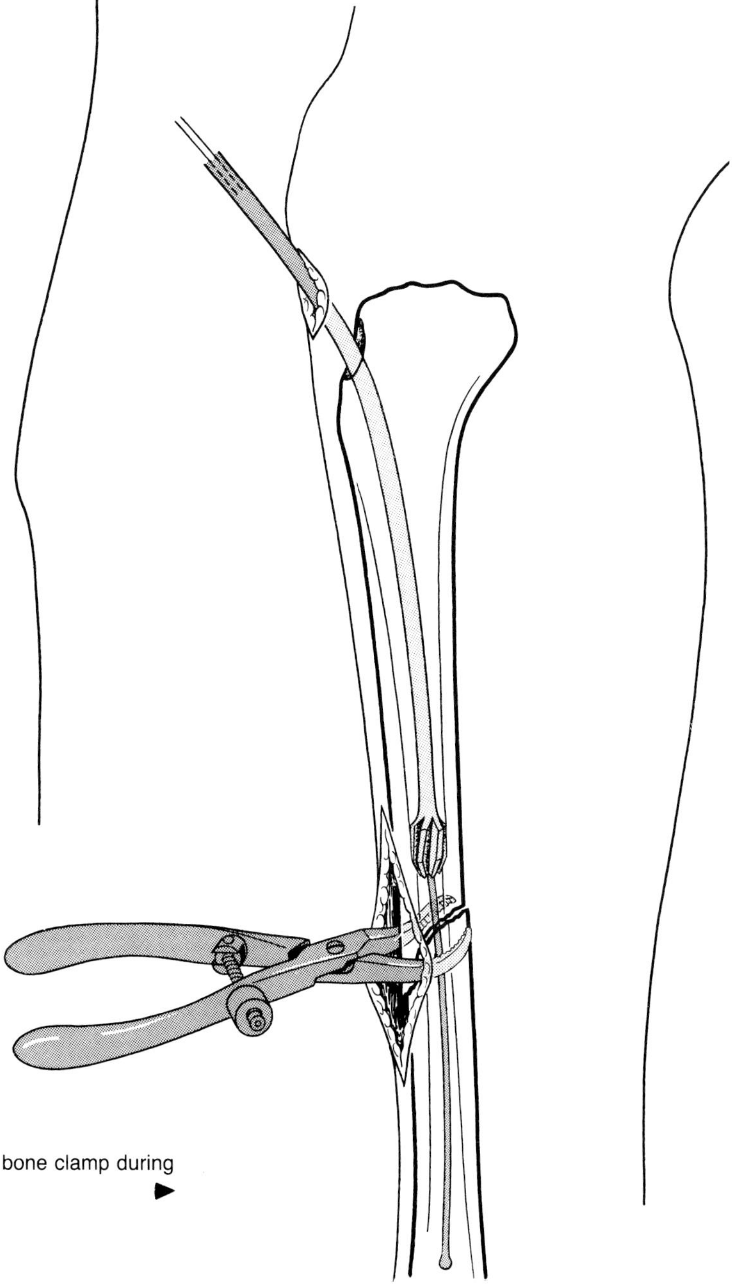

Figure 292 The fracture is held by a bone clamp during the reaming procedure. ▶

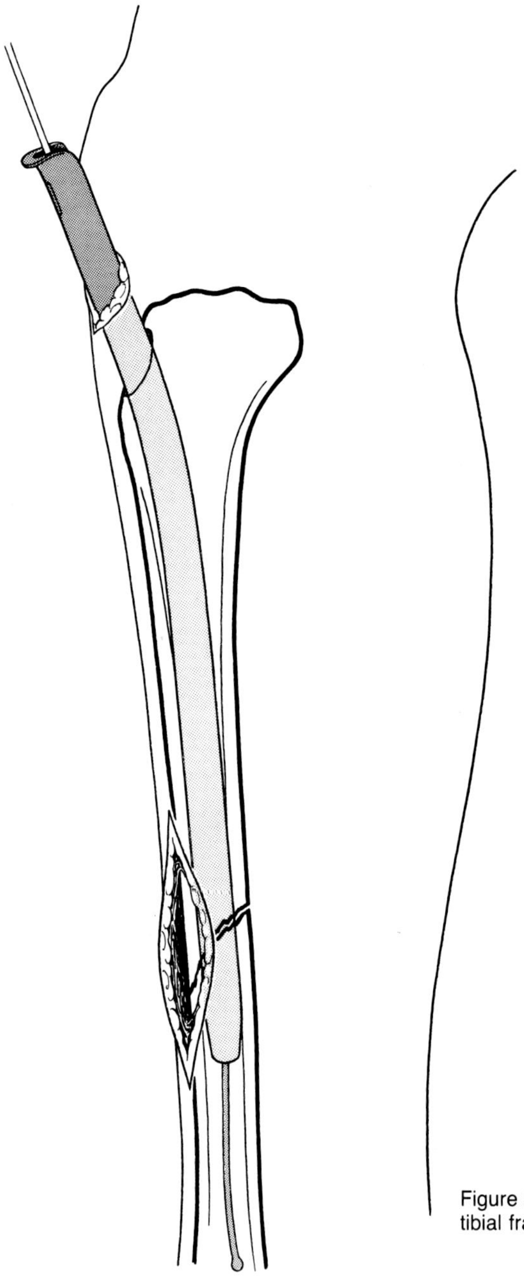

Figure 293 Nailing of the compound tibial fracture.

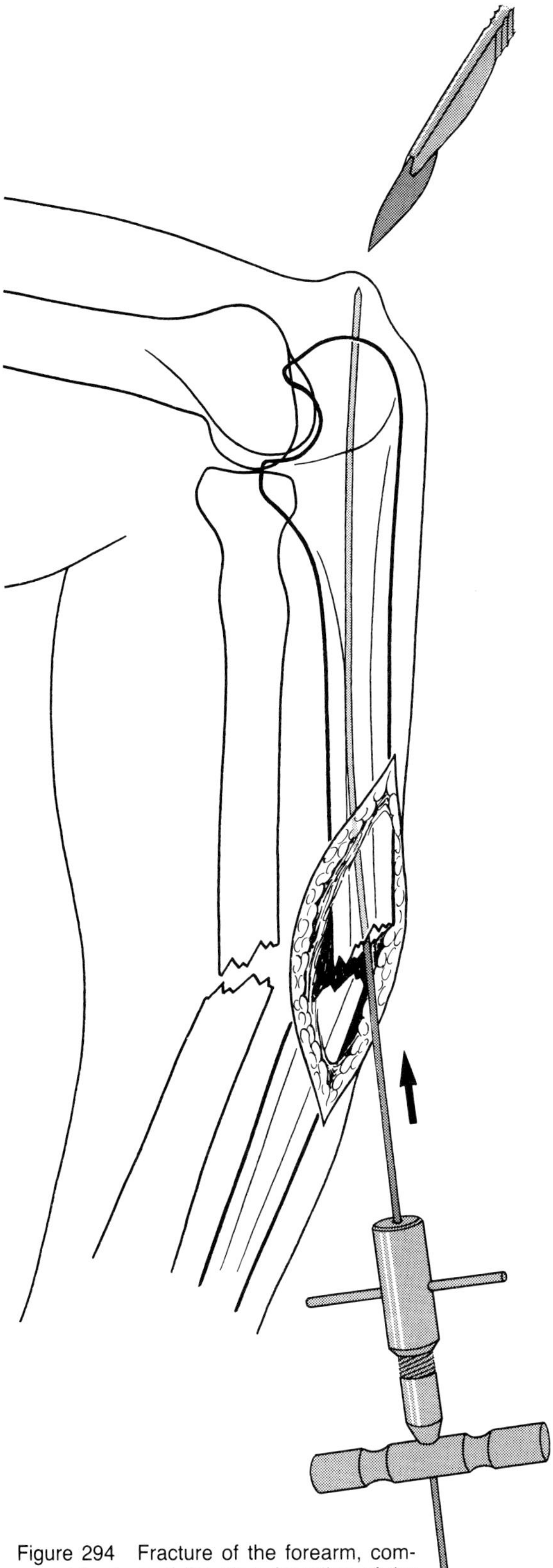

Figure 294 Fracture of the forearm, compound fracture of the ulna. Insertion of the guide pin through the fracture site into the proximal ulnar fragment to ascertain the proper nail entry point.

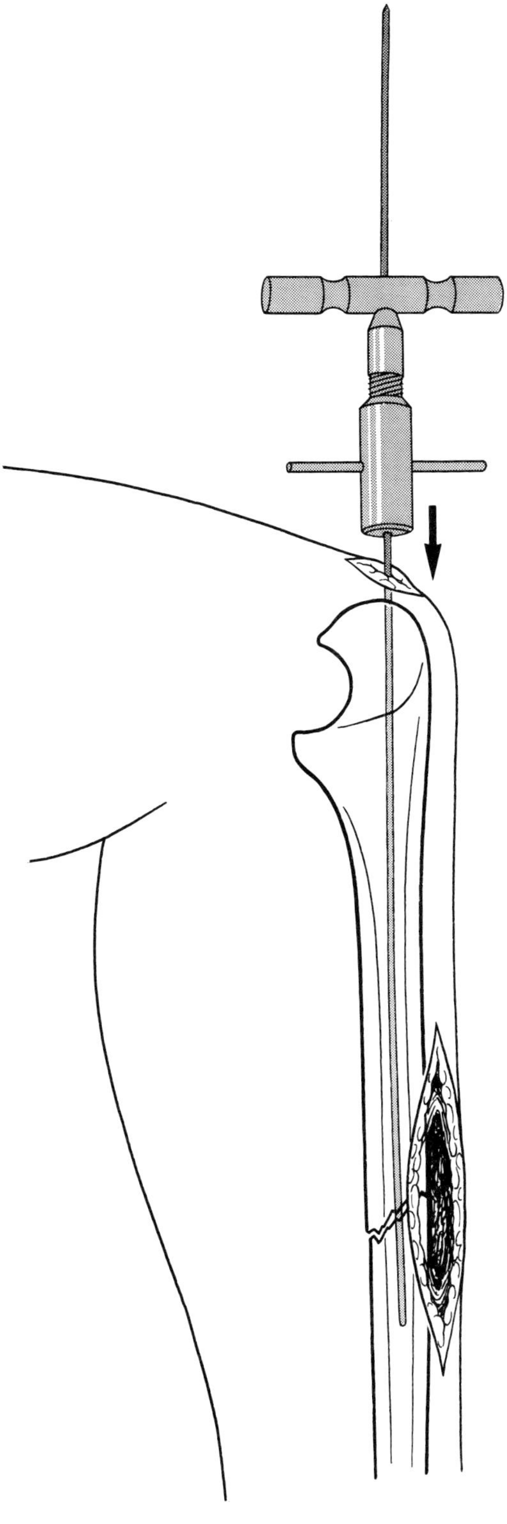

Figure 295 After the reduction of the ulnar fracture, the guide pin is advanced into the distal medullary canal from proximal entry, through the nail entry point.

Nail Removal

Timing of the Nail Removal

The nail can be removed from fractures, osteotomies, or pseudarthroses after bone healing. The stage of bone healing is determined radiographically. Because x-ray findings cannot supply definitive information about the stability of the callus, experience is necessary in judging the extent of the bone healing. The nail must never be removed from the long bones, like the femur, tibia, and humerus, until one year after the operation. Bone healing is considerably retarded in infected fractures and pseudarthroses. The nail should be left in situ for a long period of time, because the determination of the stage of bone healing is extremely difficult in these cases. These timing guidelines are not valid in growing bones. If, in an exceptional case, a nailing of a juvenile patient is performed, the nail must be removed immediately after bone healing. Otherwise, the bone will grow over the nail and the nail removal will be much more difficult. It is recommended that the nail be removed after bone healing in young patients; removal is unnecessary in the elderly. If the nail causes discomfort, however, it should be removed.

Operative Technique of Nail Removal

For this procedure, the patient is placed in the same position as for the original nailing. Preoperative roentgenograms of the nail's entry point are necessary in two planes. These indicate whether or not the nail is enclosed in bone, or whether or not the end of the nail is capped with bone. The end of the nail is usually palpable under the skin if the nail protrudes from the bone. The incision is made here. If this location is identical with the original incision, the scar is excised. If the nail is not palpable, its position is verified by fluoroscopy and the appropriate skin incision is made. If the nail has a bony cap, the awl is used to perforate the cap until the nail is felt. Parts of the bony cap must occasionally be excised. The awl can also destroy any ingrown bone tissue in order to free the slot of the nail. A sufficiently large extractor hook is maneuvered into the slot, under fluoroscopy if necessary. The nail is removed by blows to the extractor's handle with a slotted hammer (figs. 297 through 299).

If the ingrown bony tissue obstructs the slot, thereby making the insertion of a large extractor hook impossible, a smaller extractor hook should be used for the first few hammer taps. When the nail (and thereby its slot) is extracted several millimeters out of the bone, the small extractor hook should be exchanged for a larger one. Otherwise, the hook may break off from the small extractor. Removal of the bone tissue that has grown into the longitudinal nail slot is facilitated by a sharp guide pin. A nail that is firmly locked may be loosened by first minimally driving the nail further into the bone and then using the extractor hook.

If the nail is completely buried in the bone, one must free the end of the nail by using an awl or a chisel. In tibial nail removal, only the lip of the nail must be freed and the nail removal can be started by blows to a tamp positioned under this lip. A nail can thus be removed far enough so that the extractor hook can be inserted into the nail slot. Special extractor devices are necessary in the rare case in which the nail cannot be removed in the manner just described.

If the nail slot is destroyed, the nail can still be removed. The bone surrounding the nail end must be sufficiently removed to accommodate an extractor bush. An extractor bush is then attached to the nail, and the nail is removed by a conventional extractor.

Griessmann pliers also facilitate the removal of nails without slots.

An extraction device with self-cutting threads can also be attached to the end of the nail, which is then removed with the conventional extractor and slotted hammer.

A slotless nail may be driven retrograde with the aid of a nail catcher, until an extractor bush can be attached. The nail catcher is guided through the nail's canal under fluoroscopy, until it is seen to be under the tip of the nail. The nail catcher is then turned in such a way that the hook catches the nail tip. The distal part of a broken nail is removed in the same manner with the nail catcher.

As a last resort, a new slot can be drilled into the nail with a special drill bit.

If all the foregoing procedures are unsuccessful, the operation is aborted and the nail should be left in the bone; nail removal certainly should not cause a new fracture. If the nail is partly removed and deadlocks in such a way that it cannot be moved forward or backward, the protruding end must be sawed off. The remaining portion of the nail is left in the bone. Postoperative roentgenograms of the involved bone are necessary in two planes in all nail removal procedures.

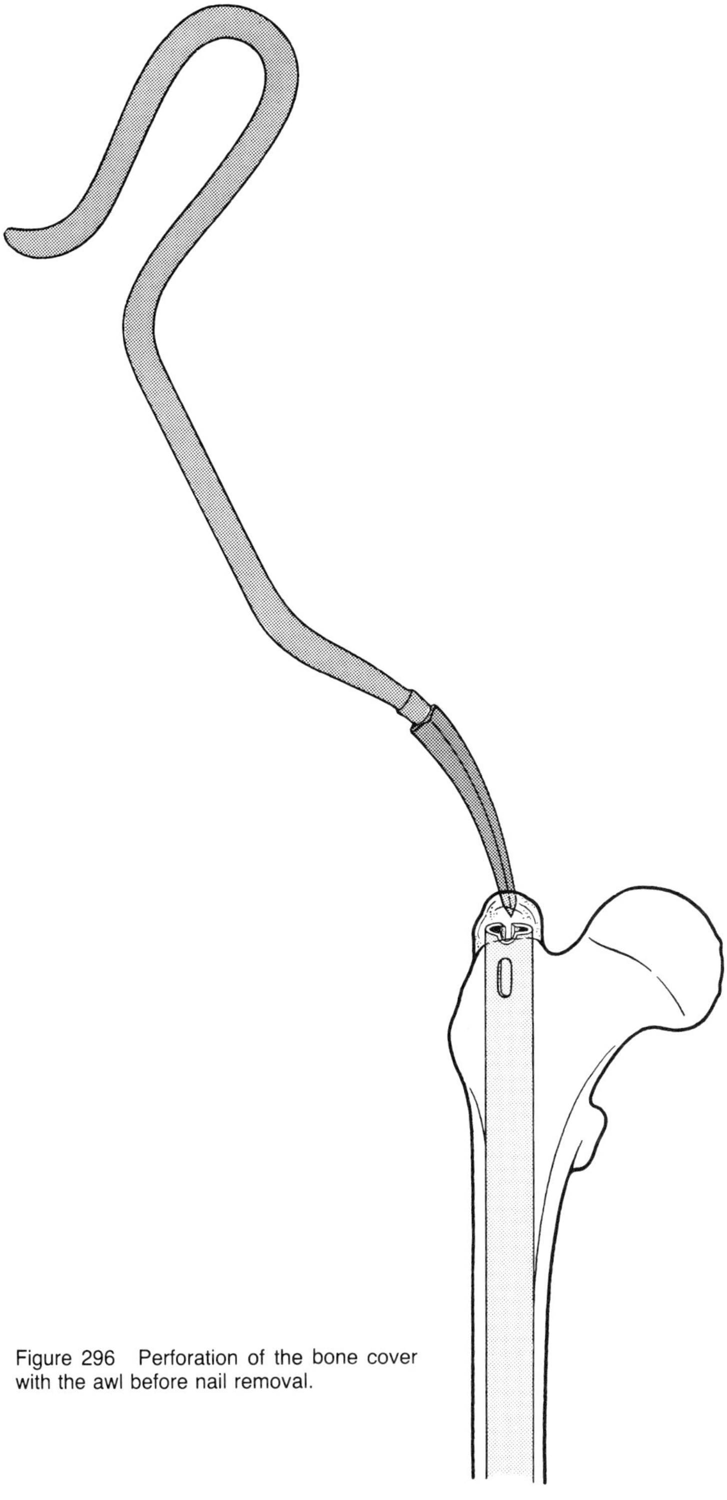

Figure 296 Perforation of the bone cover with the awl before nail removal.

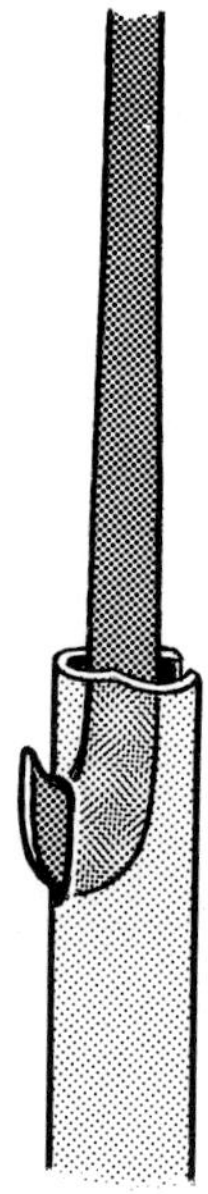

Figure 298 Nail extractor hook in the nail slot.

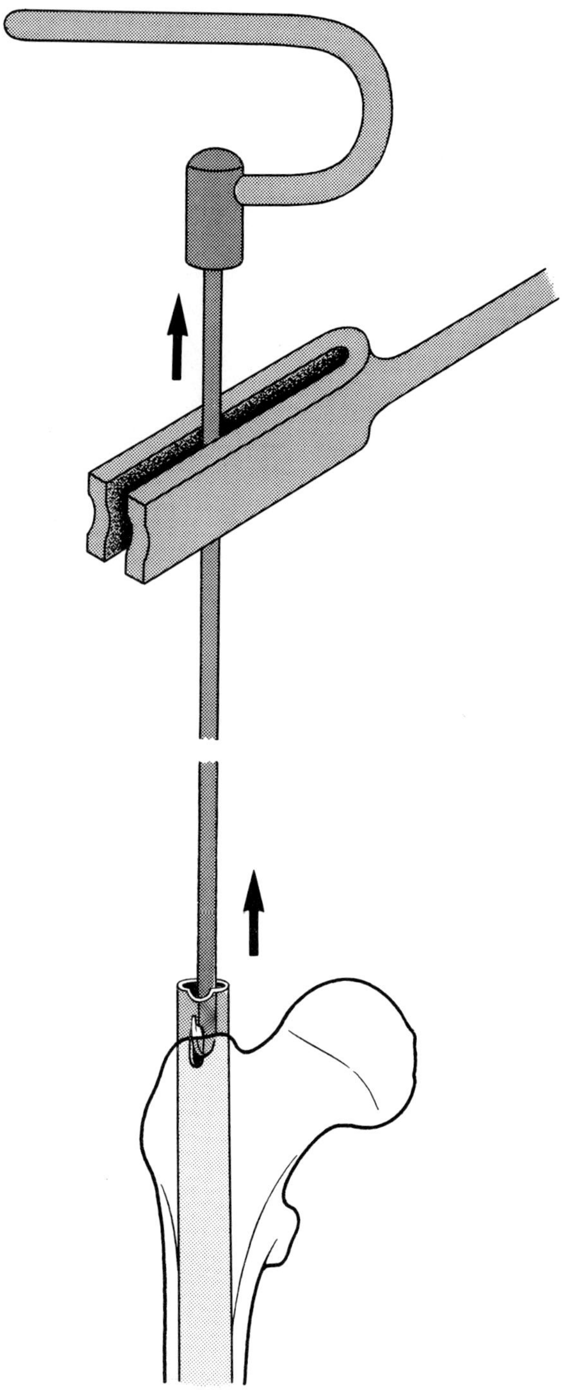

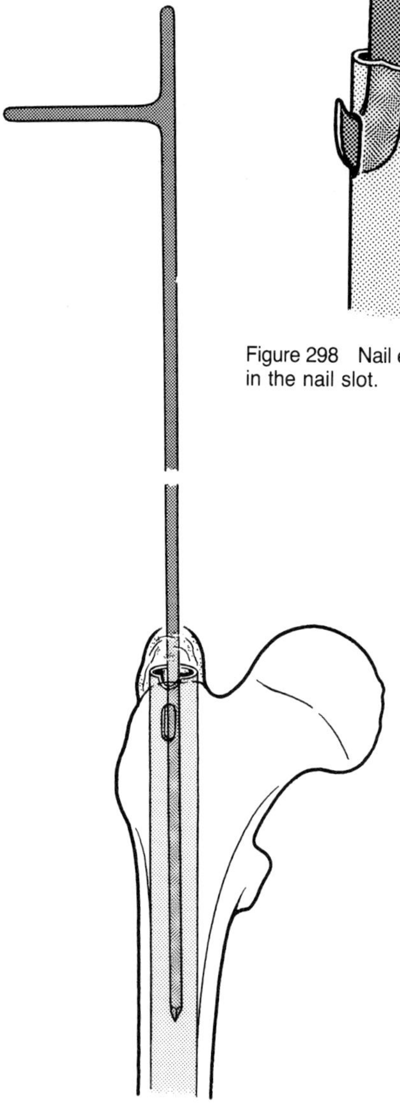

Figure 297 Loosening of the ingrown nail by perforating with a large sharp guide pin.

Figure 299 Nail removal with a nail extractor.

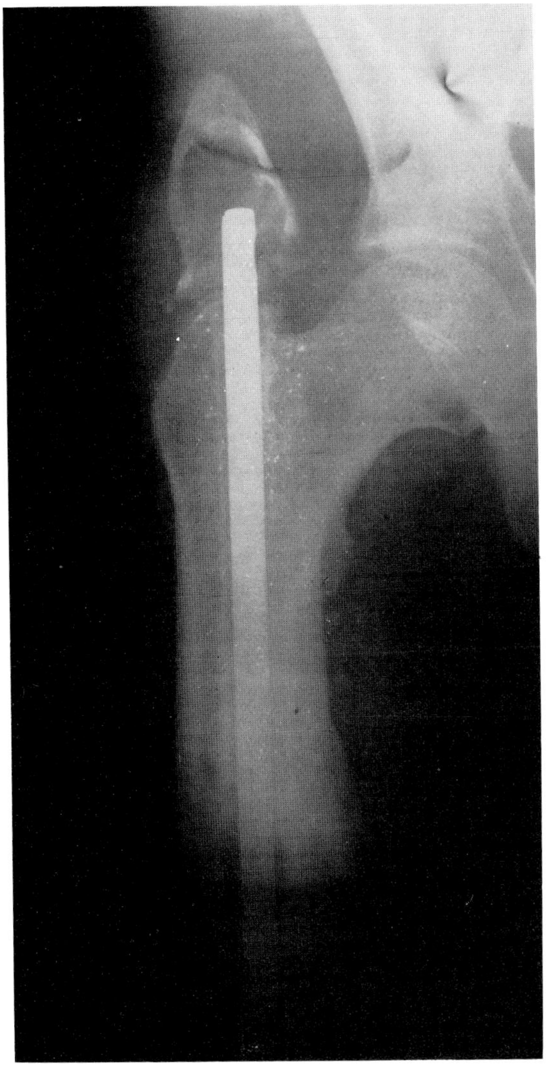

Figure 300 Large bony cap over the end of too small a femur nail. Fracture healed with massive callus formation, AP view.

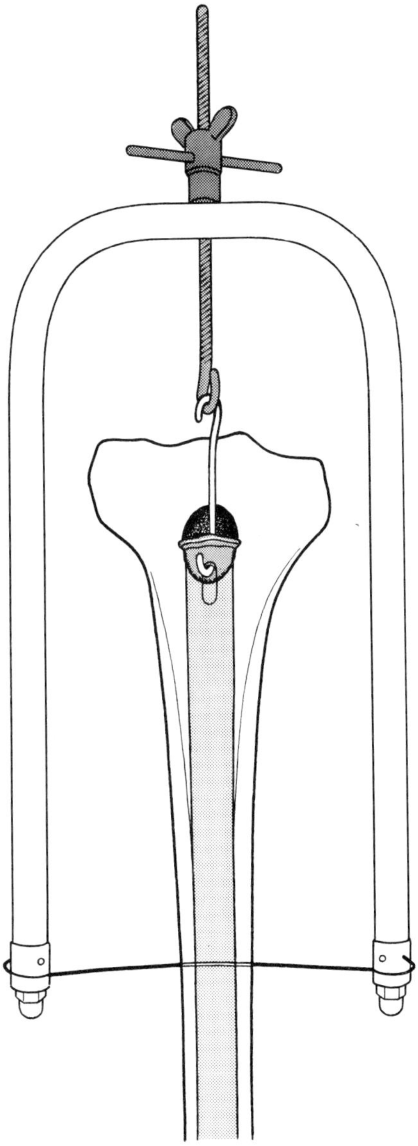

Figure 301 Use of a distractor for nail removal. The Kirschner wire is inserted through the bone as counterfixation.

Arthrodesis by Intramedullary Nailing

Closed intramedullary nailing can be advantageously used in arthrodesis of the knee and talo-tibial joints. If a knee arthrodesis is indicated, one should use an arthrodesis nail. The arthrodesis nail is an extra long curved nail. The nails are available in varying diameters. Preoperative roentgenograms of the femur and tibia in two planes are used to determine the correct dimensions of the nail.

The patient is positioned on the fracture table with the involved leg extended as described for the femoral intramedullary nailing (p. 13). The operative technique is initially identical to that described for femoral intramedullary nailing (p. 13). A long drill point guide pin is introduced into the femoral medullary canal until it reaches the condyles. Under fluoroscopy, the sharp guide pin then perforates the cortex of the intercondylar notch and is guided through the intercondylar eminence or, slightly anterior, into the tibial medullary canal. The guide pin should then be advanced into the middle of the tibia. Narrow tibial medullary canals must be reamed. The selected nail (its dimension determined by the preoperative roentgenograms taken at a 1-m distance) is then driven over the guide pin and through the knee joint into the tibial medullary canal. Small accessory incisions over both the medial and lateral interspaces of the knee joint are made through which a chisel can be used under fluoroscopy to destroy any remaining cartilage cover of the joint. Slightly curved arthrodesis nails are used to stiffen the knee joint in a slightly flexed angle. Once the leg is nailed, it can bear full weight. If the cartilage cover was not satisfactorily destroyed, bone fusion will not ensue, and one must expect a fracture of the nail.

Arthrodesis by intramedullary nailing of the knee joint is a relatively short procedure with little blood loss and stress for the patient. The method of arthrodesis by intramedullary nailing can also be used effectively for fracture treatment, especially for patients who cannot tolerate any other type of osteosynthesis (i.e., elderly patients in generally poor condition, and patients with a femoral supracondylar fracture or a proximal tibial fracture in a previously damaged leg). In the latter cases, of course, the cartilage cover of the knee joint is left intact. One should try to drive the guide pin and the nail ventral to the intercondylar eminence into the tibial medullary canal. The operative technique hereafter is identical to that already described. The arthrodesis nail is removed after the healing of the fracture. The knee joint mobility is satisfactorily restored after nail removal and appropriate physiotherapy.

Intramedullary nailing can also be used for the arthrodesis of the talo-tibial or the talocalcaneal joint if indicated. A long tibial intramedullary nail is used for this type of arthrodesis. The positioning and the operative technique are identical to those for closed tibial intramedullary nailings. In the arthrodesis of the talotibial joint, the guide pin is advanced into the talus. In the arthrodesis of both the talotibial and the talocalcaneal joints, the guide pin is advanced into the calcaneus. The selected nail (determined by the preoperative roentgenograms taken at a 1-m distance) is driven into the involved bones after satisfactory reaming of the medullary canals. Any existing cartilage cover of the talotibial joint is destroyed, under fluoroscopy, by a chisel introduced through a ventrolateral incision over the articular interspace. The nail is removed after the bony fusion of the arthrodesis.

The Kaessmann compression nail also can be used for the arthrodesis of the talotibial joint. The operative technique is identical to that described for the compression nailing of the tibia. In this case, however, the transverse screw through the mandrel is located in the talus. After the destruction of the cartilage cover, the fusion of the talotibial joint can be enhanced by the interposition and the apposition of an autogenous cancellous bone graft.

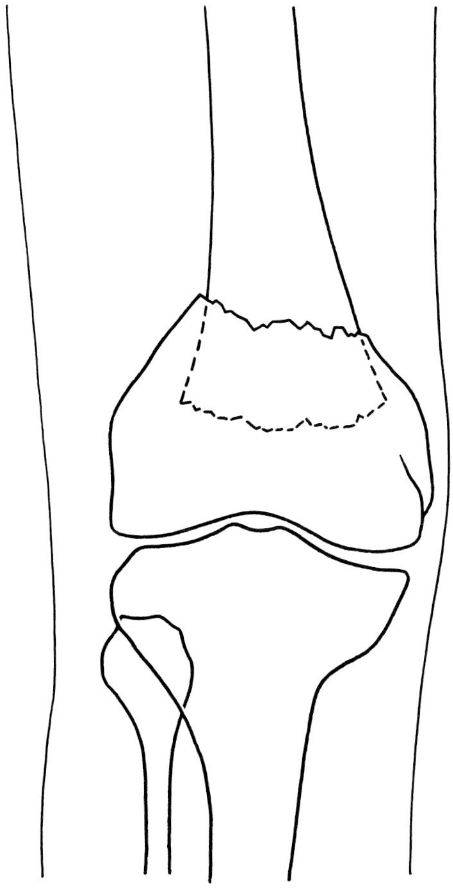

Figure 302 Supracondylar fracture of the femur in a paralyzed extremity.

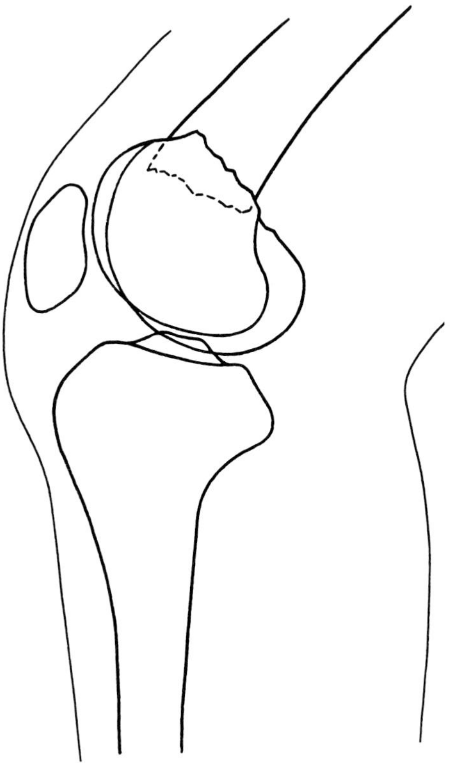

Figure 303 Same fracture, lateral view.

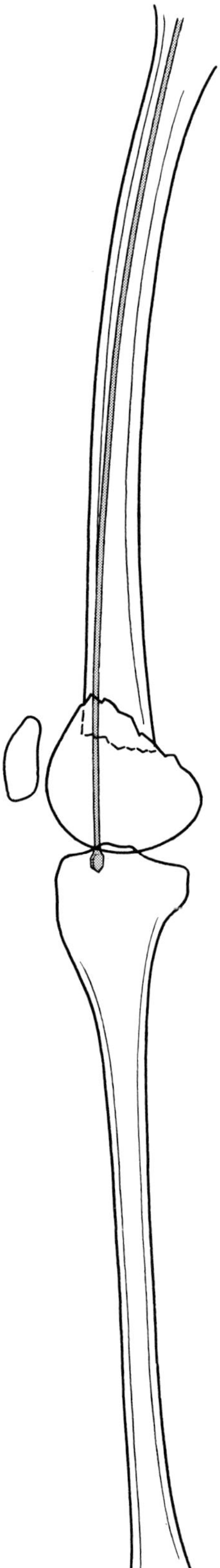

Figure 304

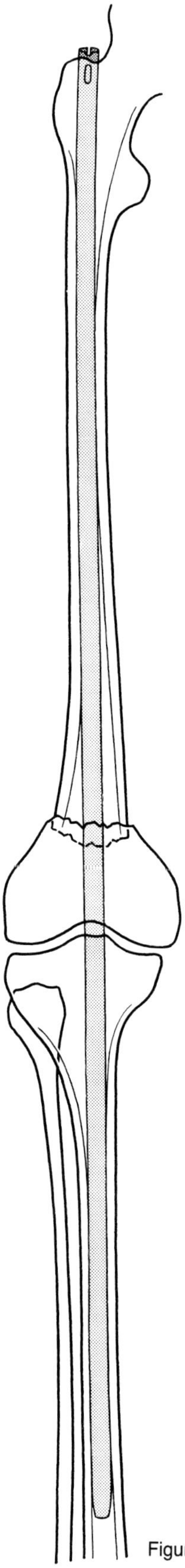

Figure 305

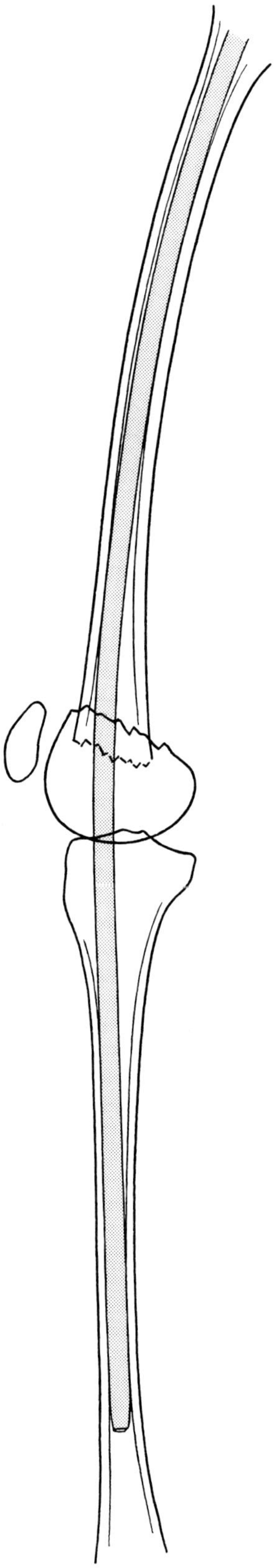

Figure 306

◀ Figure 304 Insertion of a drill point guide pin beyond the fracture site, through the knee joint into the medullary canal of the tibia. The guide pin passes in front of the intercondylar eminentia.

◀ Figure 305 AP view after completed nailing with a long arthrodesis nail.

◀ Figure 306 Lateral view.

Figure 307 Supracondylar femoral fracture, fixated with an arthrodesis nail, extremity damaged by poliomyelitis, AP view. ▶

Figure 308 The same fracture after arthrodesis nailing, lateral view. ▶

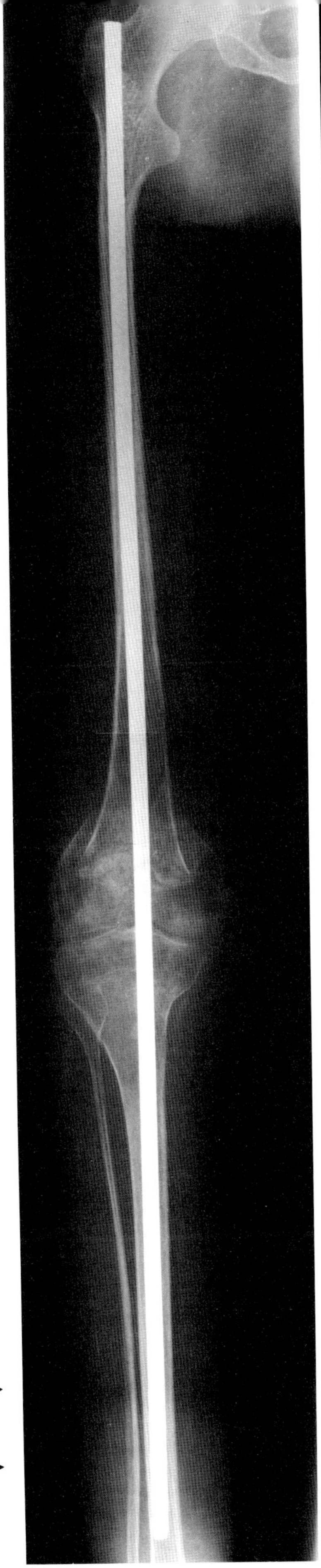

Figure 307

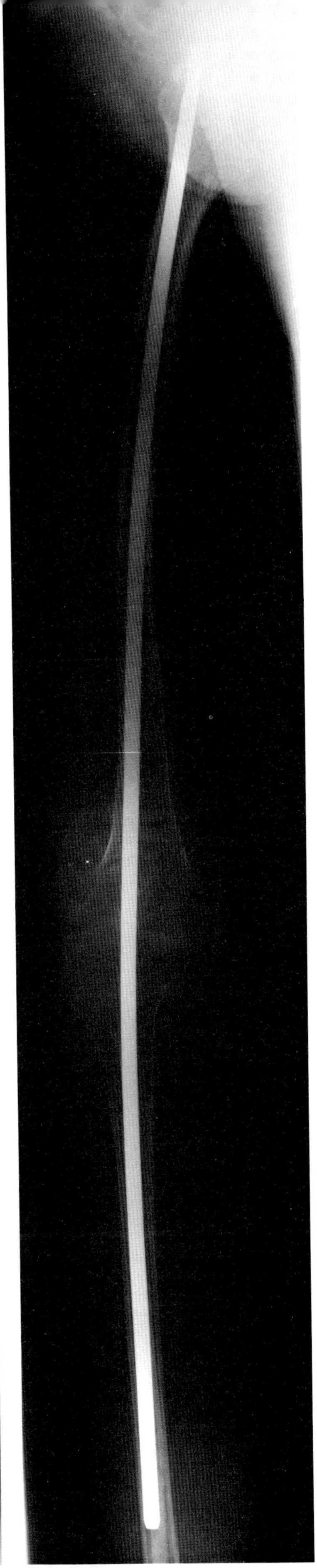

Figure 308

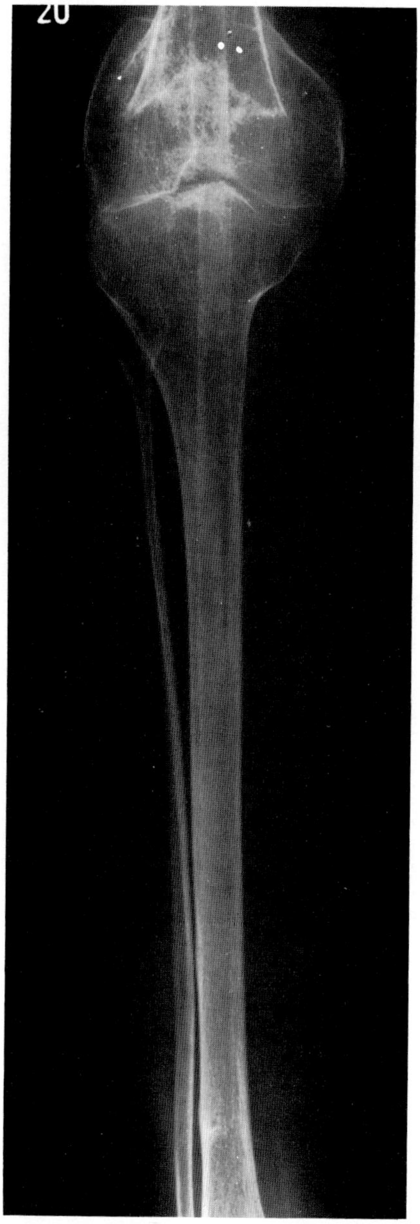

Figure 309

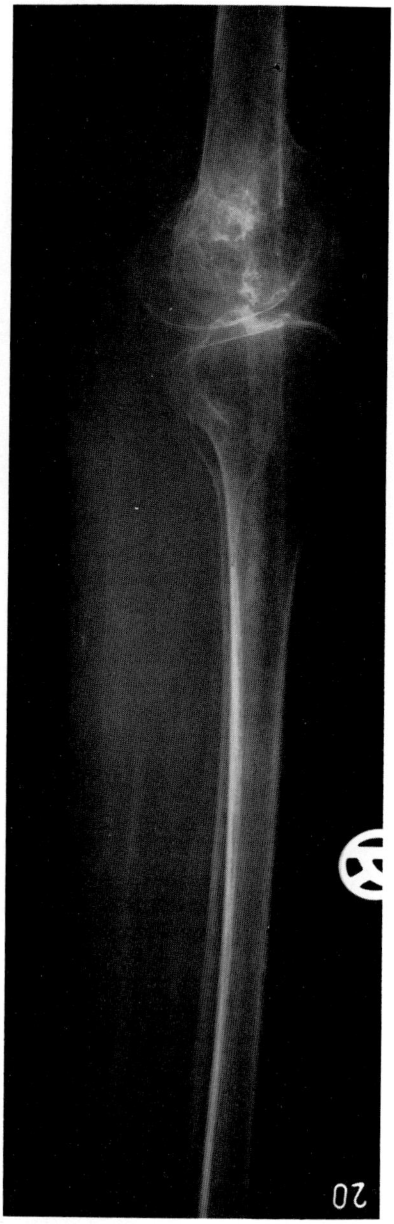

Figure 310

Figure 309 The same fracture after completed bone healing and nail removal, twelve months later, AP view.

Figure 310 Completed bone healing and nail removal, lateral view.

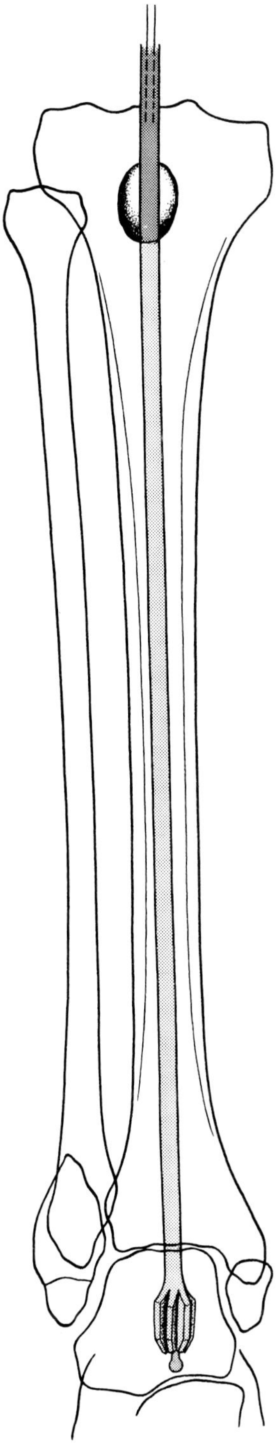

Figure 311 Painful arthrosis of the talo-tibial joint, after a healed bimalleolar fracture with deformity. Reaming until well into the talus for intramedullary arthrodesis.

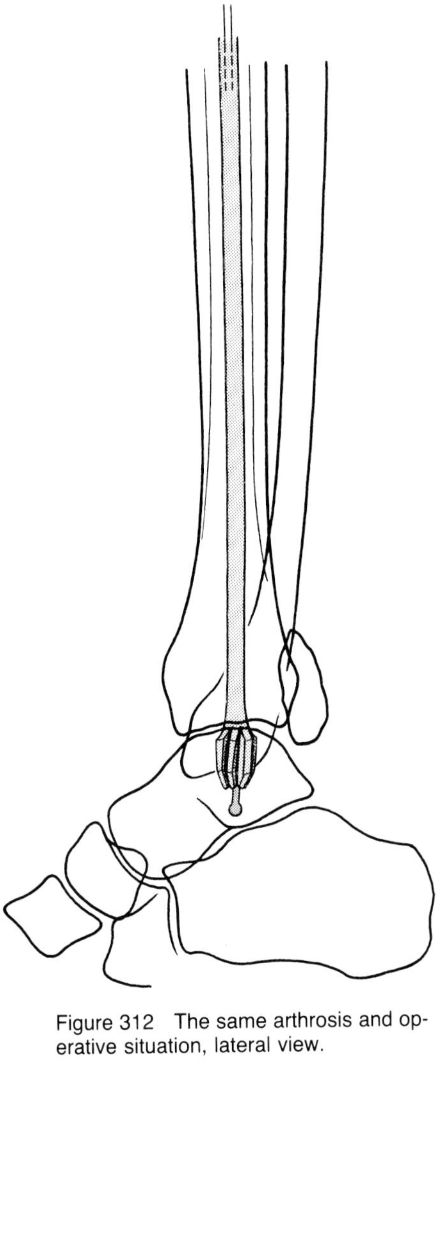

Figure 312 The same arthrosis and operative situation, lateral view.

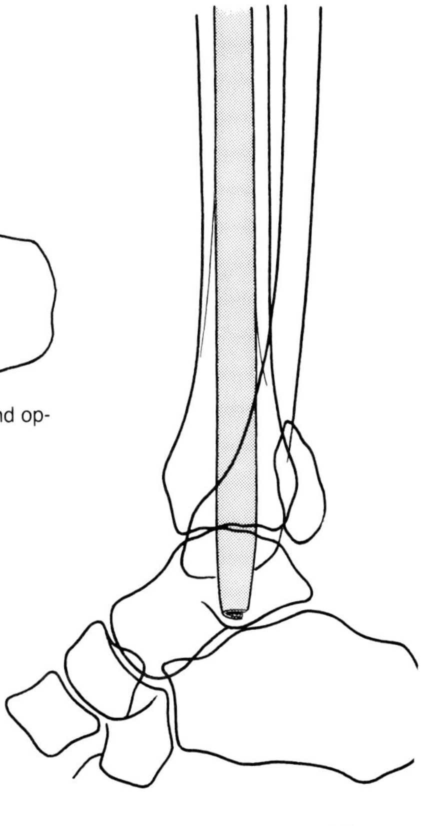

Figure 313 Completed intramedullary arthrodesis of the talo-tibial joint with a Küntscher nail.

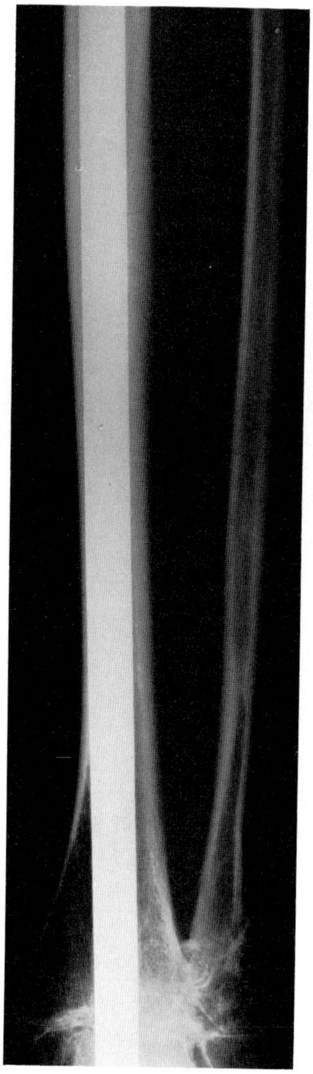

Figure 314

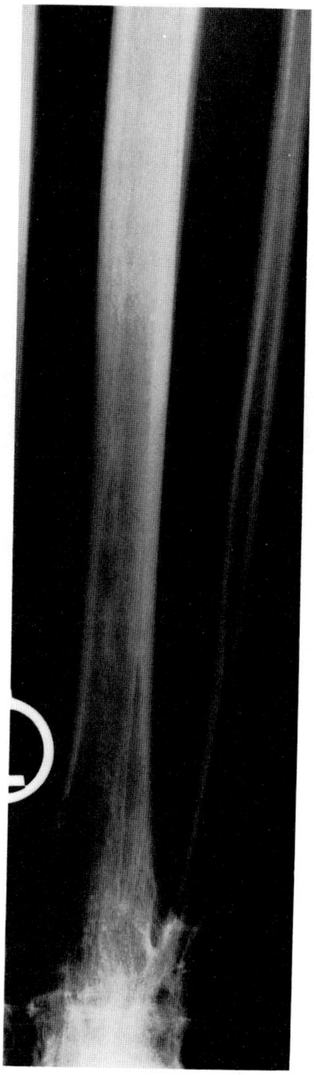

Figure 315

Figure 314 Completed intramedullary arthrodesis of the talo-tibial joint, AP view.

Figure 315 Condition after intramedullary arthrodesis of the talo-tibial joint. Bony bridging of the articular interspace. Nail removed.

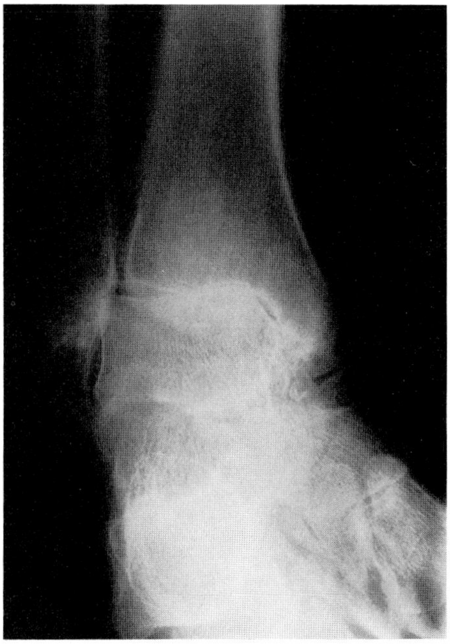

Figure 316

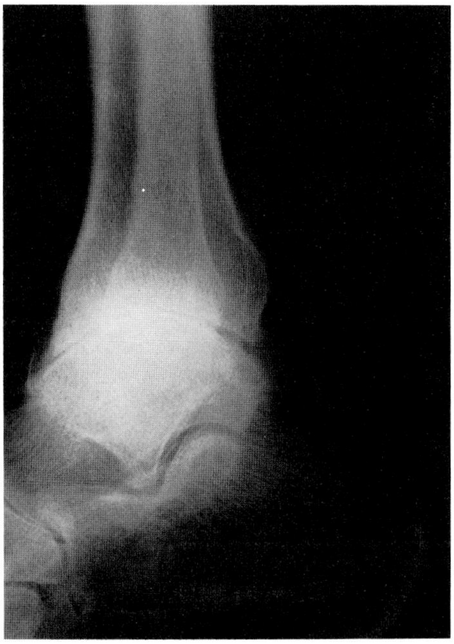

Figure 317

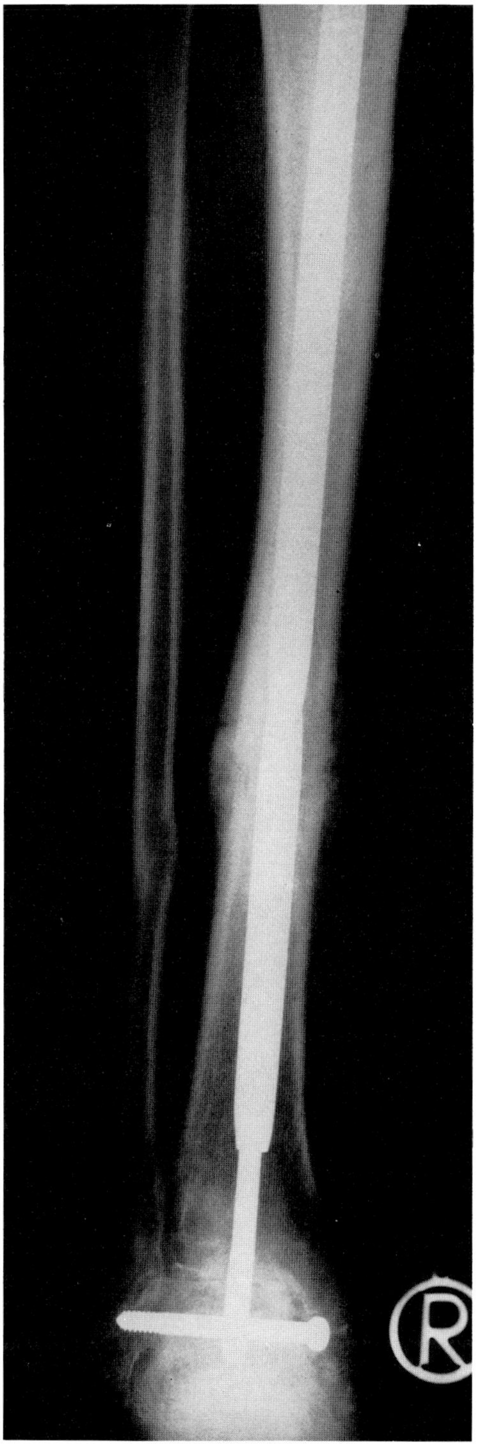

Figure 318

Figure 316 Arthrosis of the talo-tibial joint, AP view, after bimalleolar fracture of the ankle and an old fracture of the lower leg.

Figure 317 The same talo-tibial joint, lateral view.

Figure 318 The same talo-tibial joint after arthrodesis by Kaessmann nailing and spongiosa grafting. Articular interspace with bony bridging, AP view.

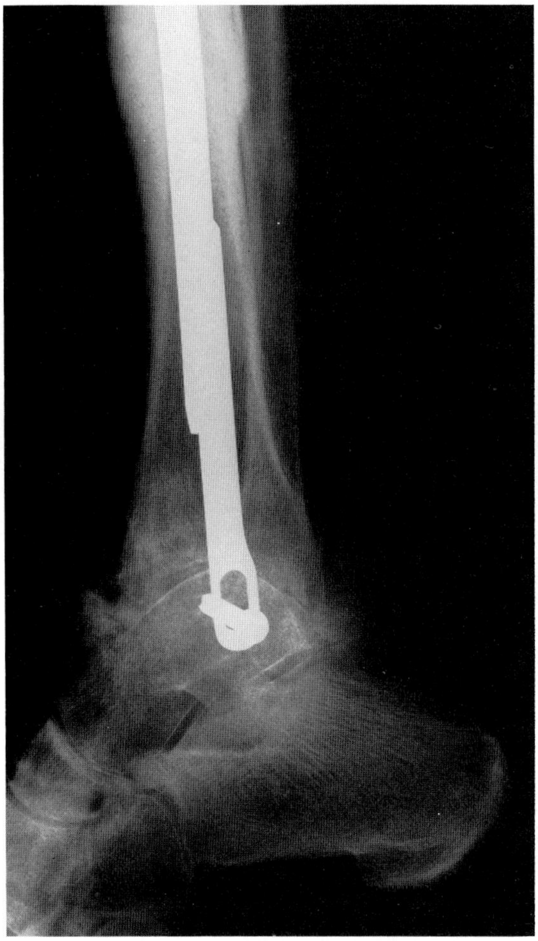

Figure 319 The same talo-tibial joint after bony bridging, lateral view.

Closed Osteotomy of Long Bones

Formerly, osteotomies required wide visualization of the involved bone. In 1962, however, Gerhard Küntscher designed the first internal bone saw, which made the closed osteotomy of long bones possible. Through this, the obvious advantages of closed intramedullary nailing could be applied to the osteotomy of long bones. The closed osteotomy is stabilized by a closed intramedullary nailing in the same session. The operation is done through the same stab incision through which the regular intramedullary nailing is done. Major involvement of the soft tissue is thereby avoided. The closed osteotomy was further simplified by refinements made in the instruments and techniques in the last few years.

Indications

A closed osteotomy can be performed in each long bone in which intramedullary nailing would be indicated if fractured. Closed osteotomy is designed to correct any angulation and rotational deformities. It is capable of correcting shortenings or lengthenings of different origins. Closed osteotomies are most often performed on the femur and tibia.

Obstacles to the reduction of fresh fractures and pseudarthroses, such as bony spikes at the fracture site, can be removed by the internal saw. The use of the internal saw is seldom indicated in the upper extremities and necessitates a special technique (to be discussed).

Instruments

The same instrument set is used as described for the closed intramedullary nailing of the corresponding bone. In addition, an internal saw with varying eccentric discs, a set of saw blades, an oscillating saw gear, and a rotating saw motor are necessary for the regular closed osteotomy. In osteotomies for shortenings, the internal saw is used in conjunction with a special measuring device, a set of saw blades, a set of internal ball reamers, a motor for the rotating saw, a gear for the oscillating saw, and various osteotemy hooks. The preoperative roentgenograms taken at a 1-m distance provide the correct nail dimensions for the following intramedullary nailing.

Positioning

For the closed osteotomy, the patient is positioned on the fracture table as described for the intramedullary nailing of the corresponding bone.

Image Intensification

Preoperative roentgenograms are taken, at a 1-m distance, of the involved bone and its adjacent joints in two planes, as is done for closed intramedullary nailing of fresh fractures. For the closed osteotomy, the image intensifier is positioned in the same way as for intramedullary nailing of the same bone. The head of the image intensifier must be easily maneuverable around the involved extremity. Postoperative roentgenograms of the entire bone are to be taken in two planes.

Operative Technique

Closed Osteotomy for the Correction of a Rotational Deformity

A Kirschner wire is inserted through the distal end of the bone before the osteotomy in order to later measure the angle of correction. A Kirschner wire tractor may be attached to the Kirschner wire and used for traction. The skin incision is made in the typical location described in the intramedullary nailing of the corresponding bone. The reaming is performed until the diameter indicated by the preoperative roentgenograms is reached. The medullary canal is reamed to the greatest extent possible to allow for the use of a saw blade with a large diameter. The osteotomy site is always at the narrowest section proximal or distal of the previous fracture site in order to avoid sawing through the thickened condensed cortex of the fracture. An appropriate disc with an eccentric hole is placed over the end of the internal saw's shaft. The largest possible saw blade is inserted into the medullary canal, followed by the saw's shaft with the disc. The saw is guided under fluoroscopy into the medullary canal with its shaft until the saw blade reaches the predetermined osteotomy site. The shaft with its eccentric disc is then withdrawn approximately 3 cm from the saw blade. The drive shaft for the rotating saw is then attached to the rotating gear driven by the motor. Under fluoroscopy, the bone is cut by slowly increasing the revolutions. The eccentric disc, attached to the shaft, must be slowly rotated in order for the saw to penetrate the varying thicknesses of the cortex. An additional measuring device attached to the saw's shaft and supported on the bone at the nail's entry portal can hinder the rotating saw blade from leaving the saw track. Any remaining cortical spikes can be removed by using the oscillating gear drive. Manual pressure can often break these spikes as well. The remaining bony bridge usually snaps off by itself owing to the weight of the extremity. The saw is withdrawn and a ball-point guide pin is placed into the distal fragment. The rotational deformity is corrected, as one visually notes the angular deviation of the long bone. A special protractor can be used to determine the change of rotation exactly to one-degree angle increments. The tip of the protractor is introduced through the nail's entry portal into the distal medullary canal, where it is anchored by opening a spreader. The sliding scale is attached to the trochanter and immobilized by its teeth. The rotation of the distal fragment is transmitted to the protractor, and the pointer indicates the corrected angle exactly. After the rotational deformity is corrected, the extremity is stabilized in the corrected position by the fracture table. From here on, the operative technique is identical to that for the intramedullary nailing.

Correction of an Angulation Deformity

Initially, the operative technique is identical to that described for the intramedullary nailing of the corresponding bone. The ball-point guide pin is inserted until it reaches the angulation. The medullary canal is reamed up to the angulation in the usual manner. The internal saw is then introduced in the manner previously described. The saw track should be made close to the vertex of the angulation. The osteotomy is performed as previously described. The saw is then withdrawn, and the angulation deformity is corrected by adequate traction. The ball-point guide pin is then inserted into the distal fragment under flurosсopy. If a Kirschner wire was previously inserted into the distal portion of the bone, it must be removed. The distal portion of the medullary canal is reamed open to the same diameter as in the proximal portion.The selected intramedullary nail is then inserted in the typical manner.

Correction of a Shortened Deformity by a Lengthening Osteotomy

Lengthening procedures are limited to 2.5 cm in one session because of the danger of vascular and neurologic damage. Lengthenings of greater magnitude must be done in several operative sessions. The operative technique is identical to that for osteotomy for rotational correction up to and including the point at which the ball-point guide pin is inserted after the separation of the bony portions. The desired lengthening is obtained by strong traction applied to the distal portion of the bone. The length is maintained by an interlocking nail or by a spacer-nail. The operative technique of interlocking osteosynthesis is described on pages 92 through 105.

The use of a spacer-nail for the lengthening procedure involves the insertion of a regular Küntscher nail and a special metal strip with a spacer. The spacer-nail is especially manufactured for each case. The ball-point guide pin is exchanged for a special thin guide pin. The spacer-nail is guided by the special thin guide pin through its eye. Under fluoroscopy, the spacer of the spacer-nail is maneuvered into the gap between the distracted portions of the bone. The special thin guide pin is then exchanged for a regular nail driving guide. The selected regular Küntscher nail is then driven in next to the spacer-nail. One should monitor to check whether the spacer's position changes when driving the regular Küntscher nail. The guide is then withdrawn and the incision is closed.

The bony bridging of the gap can be accelerated by filling the gap with autogenous cancellous bone inserted through the medullary canal.

Correction of a Length Deformity by a Shortening Osteotomy

A cylindric piece of the bone shaft can be sawed off from the medullary canal with an internal saw by "closed technique" without exposing the bone. The long bone is shortened after the morcellation and the displacement of the sawed-off cylindric piece by joining the proximal and distal portions of the bone. The shortening osteotomy is used more often than the lengthening osteotomy. The correction of the length is usually done only in the lower extremities. The correction of length is important because it avoids the nonphysiologic stresses to the skeletal system.

The shortening osteotomy is safer and more predictable than the lengthening procedure. The bone healing is also faster in the shortening osteotomy because no defects have to be bridged. In the shortening osteotomy, one also does not risk nerve or vessel damage by overstretching. The shortening osteotomy can usually be stabilized with a regular Küntscher nail. One must realize that the patient becomes shorter after a shortening osteotomy. The proportion of the trunk length to the extremity length is changed and becomes obvious if the shortening is greater than 3 cm. The trunk appears to be more massive and the arms longer. The soft tissue coverage in the shortening limb is increased and bulges. Because of this, femoral shortenings hinder the full extension or flexion of the knee joint. The decrease in muscle tone causes a relative instability of the ligamentous structures. This leads to an unstable knee. However, both the relative lengthening of the soft tissue coverage and its bulging, and the relative instability of the knee joint in femoral shortening osteotomies slowly correct themselves. The recovery period is proportional to the amount shortened. The shortening osteotomy of the tibia causes the identical changes in the soft tissue coverage, but affects both the talo-tibial and the talocalcaneal joint. The patient should be made aware of these changes before the operation. Shortening of the longer extremity is indicated when the limbs are of different lengths, regardless of the cause. Both legs can be shortened in cases in which the oversized stature leads to psychologic conflicts and changes. It is recommended that these psychologic effects be discussed with a psychiatrist before surgery. Any shortenings of great magnitude should be evenly distributed between the femur and tibia, not only for aesthetic reasons, but also because of the disproportionate diameters otherwise encountered while apposing the proximal and distal portions of the shortened bone. The latter effect would not allow for a solid intramedullary nailing. The necessity to distribute the shortening to both bones of the same extremity is also obvious in the preoperative roentgenograms. The exact amount of shortening is to be marked on the preoperative roentgenograms taken at a 1-m distance. The area of shortening is to be located in such a way that the diameters of the proximal and distal portions will sufficiently match, yielding satisfactory locking of the intramedullary nail in both fragments. The distance between the nail entry point and the distal osteotomy is measured in the preoperative roentgenogram and verified in situ by superimposing the Küntscher x-ray scale while fluoroscoping or by using the scale attached to the internal bone saw.

The skin incision and the reaming of the medullary canal with the flexible reamer guided by the ball-point guide pin are identical to the technique described for the intramedullary nailing of the corresponding bone. The medullary canal should be reamed open to the greatest extent possible in order to use the saw blade with the largest possible diameter. The appropriate eccentric disc is placed over the end of the internal saw's shaft. The largest possible saw blade is inserted into the medullary canal, using a handchuck fixed to the shaft. Then the saw's shaft, with the disc and the measuring device attached, is inserted, and the saw blade is guided to the distal osteotomy site under fluoroscopy. A notch is made at the distal osteotomy site by the saw. The measuring device rests firmly on the bone at the entry portal, while the shaft and the blade of the internal saw are withdrawn to the planned distance of shortening. The amount of shortening can be read directly from the measuring device. Once the measuring device is firmly attached to the shaft of the internal saw, the proximal osteotomy site is notched. The saw blade is then advanced back to the distal notch and the amount of shortening is again verified with the measuring device.

The bone is then completely separated at the distal osteotomy site. To avoid any jumping of the saw blade, the revolutions of the saw blade are slowly increased. Any remaining cortical spikes are cut by the use of the oscillating gear. The saw is then withdrawn to the proximal osteotomy site, where it circumferentially cuts the bone in such a way that the cylinder is not completely separated from the remaining bone. The saw blade is exchanged for an internal ball reamer. An eccentric disc is placed over the end of the saw's shaft when ball reaming. The wall of the cylinder to be resected is thinned by the internal ball reamer. Thereafter, the proximal osteotomy is completed by the internal saw armed with a saw blade. The internal saw is removed and a guide pin is inserted under image intensification into the distal fragment. An osteotomy hook is then inserted through the nail's entry portal into the interspace created by the osteotomy, so that the hook catches the remaining bone cylinder. Hammer the osteotomy hook retrograde with the slotted driver, thereby longitudinally splitting the cylinder to be removed. This action is repeated several times until at least two to three bony shells are created. The shells are then pushed aside with the same hook. The distal portion of the bone is pushed onto the proximal portion; the guide pin forms an "inner splint." The leg is removed from the traction apparatus for this procedure. The selected nail is driven over the nail driving guide under image intensification. While driving the nail through the osteotomy site, one must pay special attention to the correct rotational position and the retention of the longitudinal compression of the distal bone portion onto the proximal portion. The shells, the remnants of the resected bone cylinder, arrange themselves around the osteotomy site like shavings. The remaining operative technique is identical with that for closed intramedullary nailing of the femur.

The interlocking nail must be used if rotational stability cannot be maintained by the regular Küntscher nail.

In shortenings of 2 cm or less, the cylinder to be resected is mulched by the internal ball reamer after the completion of both osteotomies. The operative technique from there on is identical to that just described.

An especially intensive exercise program is necessary after all shortening osteotomies. If the ligamentous stability of the knee joint is insufficient, the knee joint must be splinted for the time being. After bilateral shortening osteotomies, training in ambulation must be stressed specifically.

Osteotomy as an Aid to Reduction

The osteotomy for the mobilization of a fresh fracture or a reducible pseudarthrosis can be performed closed by means of an internal bone saw. In fresh fractures, fragments and bone spikes, which render the reduction of a fracture impossible, may also be sawed off closed by the internal saw.

In pseudarthroses, the ligamentous structures can be divided and bone spikes can be cut off by the internal saw. If the mobilization of the pseudarthrosis by a distractor is impossible because of extensive scar formation, the osteotomy either proximal or distal to the pseudarthrosis can provide the correct alignment. The following closed intramedullary nailing of the fresh fracture or the pseudarthrosis can be done without any difficulty (figs. 388 through 392).

Particulars

Most of the closed osteotomies using the internal bone saw are done in the femur. The femoral osteotomy is easiest because only one bone must be severed. The medullary canal can be reamed to a large diameter and the osteotomy site is covered by a thick soft tissue envelope. The entry portal for the internal saw is identical to the nail's entry portal at the trochanter tip. Most of the closed osteotomies are performed by the foregoing method. The internal saw, however, can also be inserted into the femoral medullary canal from the entry portal in the medial femoral condyle, as described for the closed trochanter nailing. This approach may prove useful for the correction of a malaligned arthrodesis of the hip joint.

The correction of tibial malalignment always requires osteotomy of the fibula in addition to tibial osteotomy. The fibula can be fractured either manually or by an oblique osteotomy through a stab incision. The open fibula osteotomy should never be done at the same level as the tibial osteotomy. The tibial osteotomy must be cautiously performed because of the very thin anterior soft tissue cover. Injuries to the soft tissue can be avoided by using the oscillating internal saw rather than the rotational saw for the tibial osteotomy. The shortening of the tibia should never exceed 3 cm. The cylinder of the tibia that is to be resected is mulched by an internal ball reamer, in order to prevent soft tissue damage by avoiding the piercing of the fragments through the skin. The two fibular portions overlap one another during the longitudinal compression of the tibia. A resection of the fibula is unnecessary.

In the osteotomy of the humerus, it is important to avoid the section where the radial nerve crosses the humerus, i.e., at the transition of the middle and lower third.

Because of their narrow medullary canals, the bones in the forearm can only be osteotomized by an internal saw with very small saw blades. In these cases, the internal saw is used without its shaft.

Because the internal saw is rotating as fast as 8,000 rpm, parts of the saw blade, or the entire saw blade, or even the saw blade with its attached shaft can break off. These metallic pieces can be removed with long-handled forceps, which are introduced into the medullary canal under fluoroscopy. If a broken saw blade remains in the saw track, the blade must be maneuvered into the medullary canal by a hook or a guide pin, so that it can be retrieved by the longhandled pliers (figs. 371 and 372). To avoid this type of complication, one should always use new saw blades for each osteotomy.

The high rate of revolutions of the saw blade causes frictional heat at the osteotomy site and in the shaft of the internal saw. One should stagger the sawing in order to avoid possible heat necrosis of the bone.

Common Mistakes in Closed Osteotomies

The closed osteotomy is always terminated by a closed intramedullary nailing; therefore, the same mistakes can occur as in the Küntscher nailing of the corresponding bone.

The saw blade may be bent if it is inserted without caution and delicacy; consequently, the blade may break off entirely during the osteotomy. For this reason, the diameter of the saw blade selected should be 1 mm smaller than the last reamer used. If the internal saw separates only a small segment of the bone tube, either the eccentric disc was not attached to the saw shaft or the rotating drive was not exchanged for the oscillating gear after separating part of the bone tube.

It is difficult, in shortening osteotomies, to advance the internal saw distally into the medullary canal if the proximal osteotomy is mistakenly done first. Strong traction must be applied to align the axis of the bone being cut. The saw blade must then be partially withdrawn until it contacts the disc. The entire internal saw is then advanced in this configuration into the distal medullary canal. One must realise the added traction after this maneuver so that no error is made in measuring the shortening. If, for some reason, it is not possible to bring the internal saw to the selected distal osteotomy site, or the bone cannot be sawed through entirely, the internal saw must be inserted into the medullary canal from the medial femoral condyle. These complications do not occur during the tibial shortening osteotomy, because the bony cylinder to be resected is entirely mulched by the internal ball reamer.

If the osteotomy hook is advanced too far into the soft tissue while cleaving the bone cylinder, nerves and vessels can be damaged.

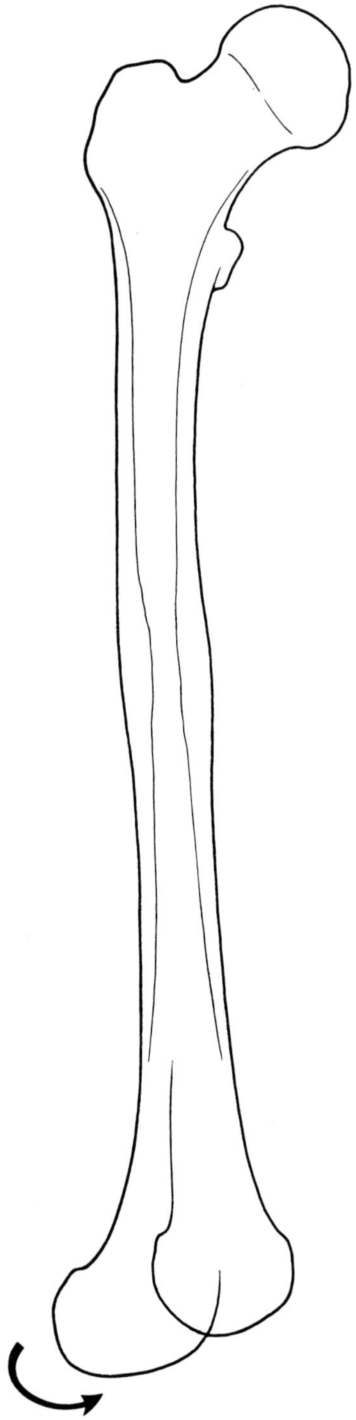

Figure 320 Healed fracture of the femur with rotational deformity.

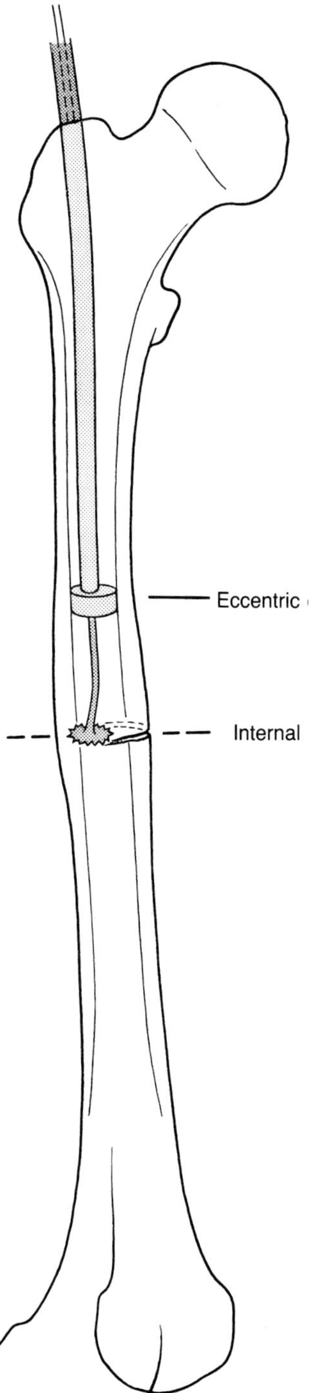

Figure 321 Osteotomy by internal saw after reaming.

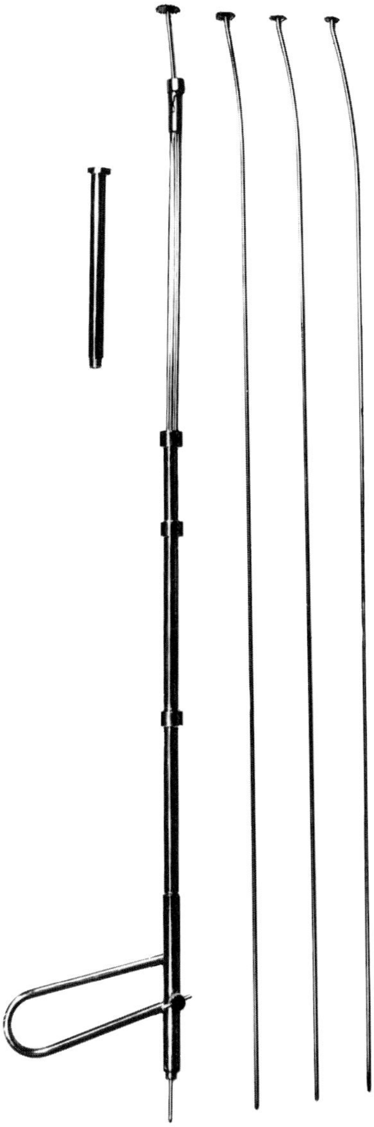

Figure 322 Internal saw with measuring device and extension.

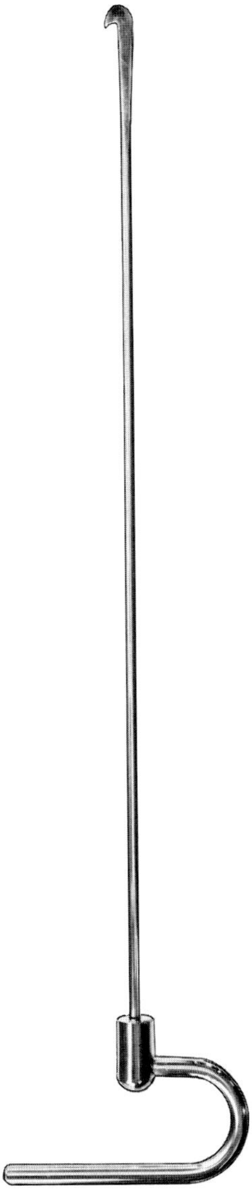

Figure 323 Internal osteotomy hook.

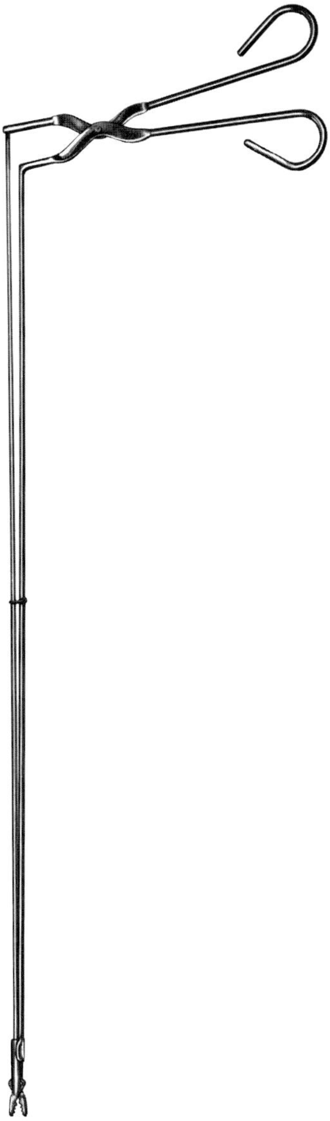

Figure 324 Long-handled forceps.

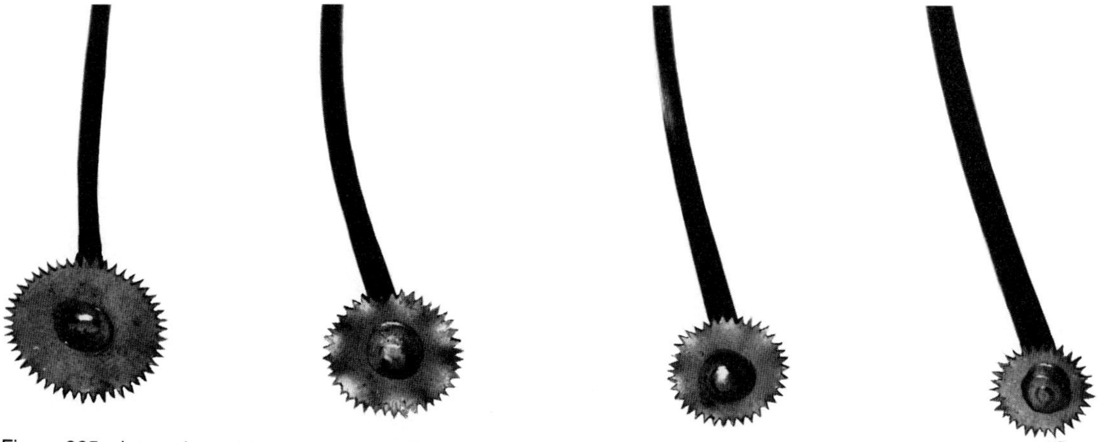

Figure 325 Internal saw blades in various diameters.

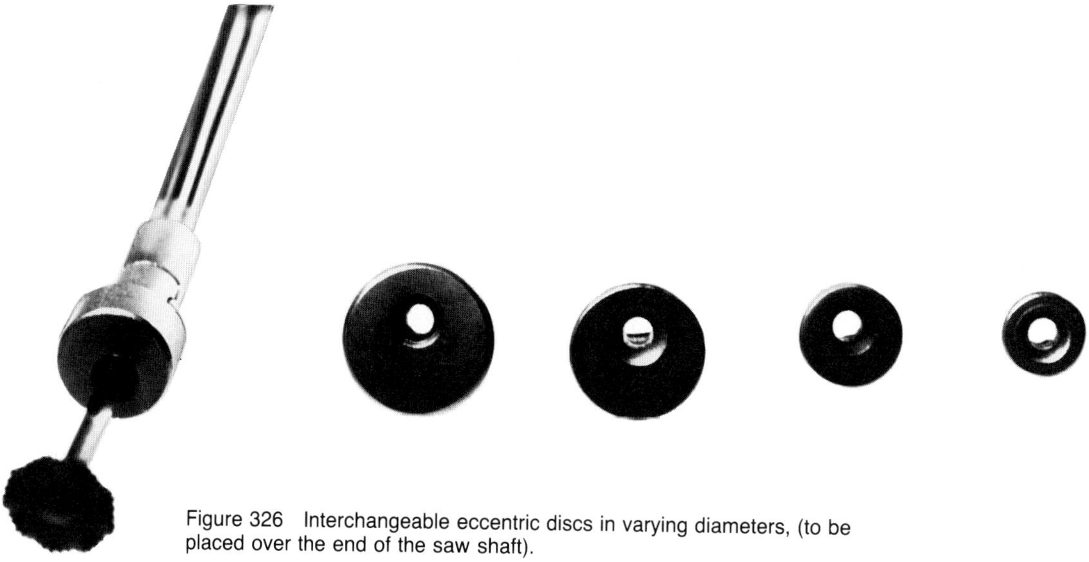

Figure 326 Interchangeable eccentric discs in varying diameters, (to be placed over the end of the saw shaft).

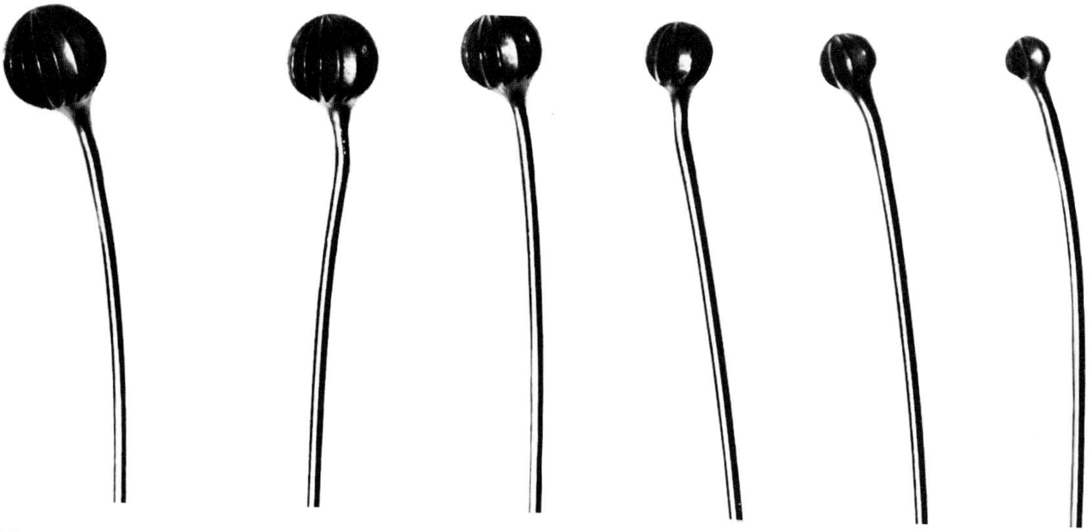

Figure 327 Internal ball reamers in varying diameters.

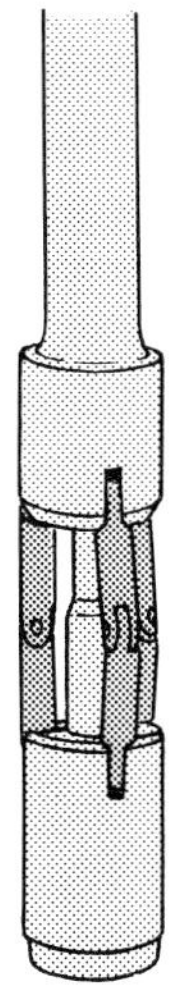

Figure 329

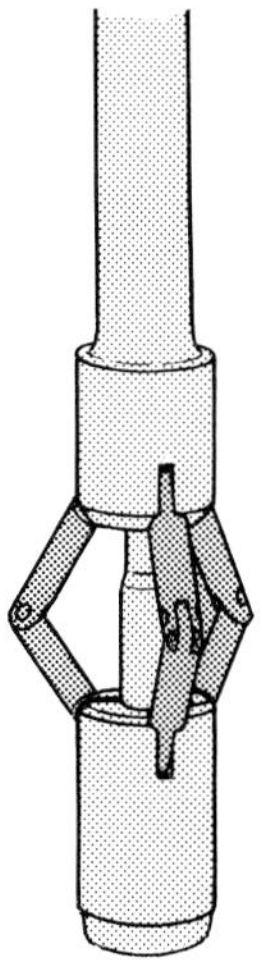

Figure 330

Figure 329 The closed spreader.

Figure 330 The open spreader.

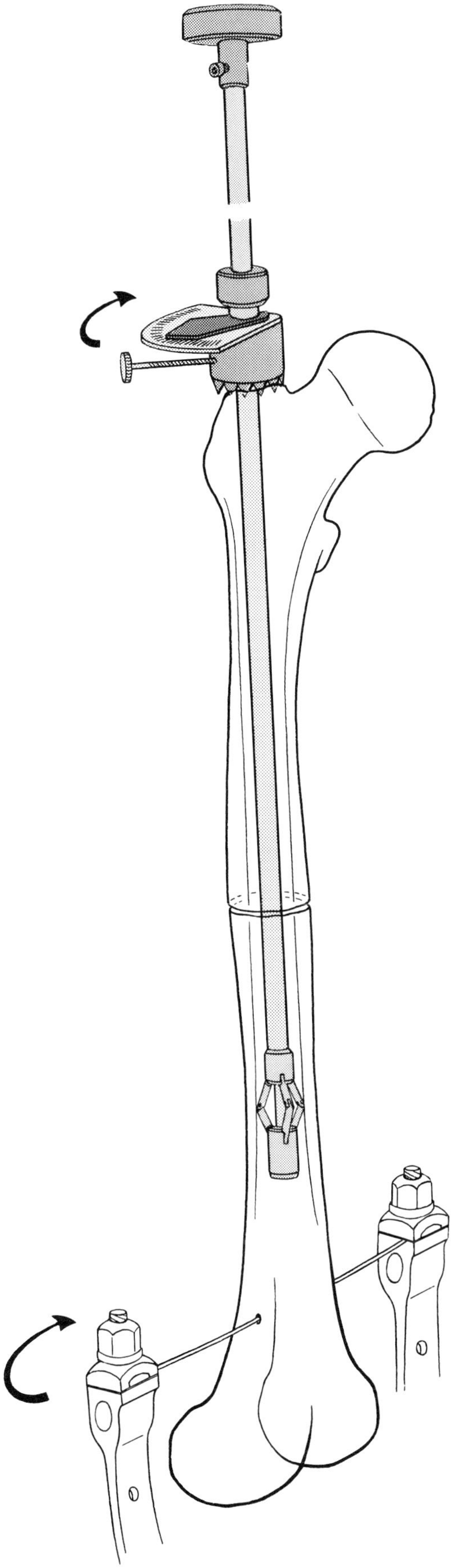

Figure 328 The protractor device inserted into the distal medullary canal and fixated by opening the spreader. When the Kirschner wire tractor is turned, the protractor indicates the corrected angle.

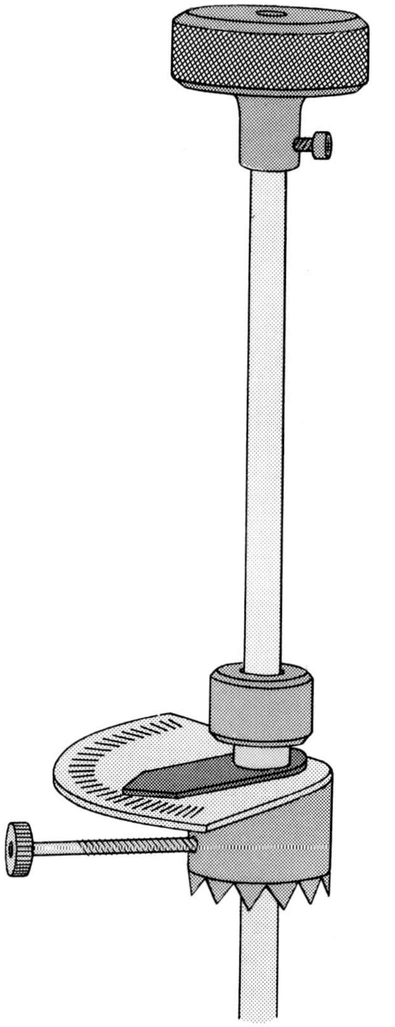

Figure 331 Top portion of the protractor device with scale and pointer.

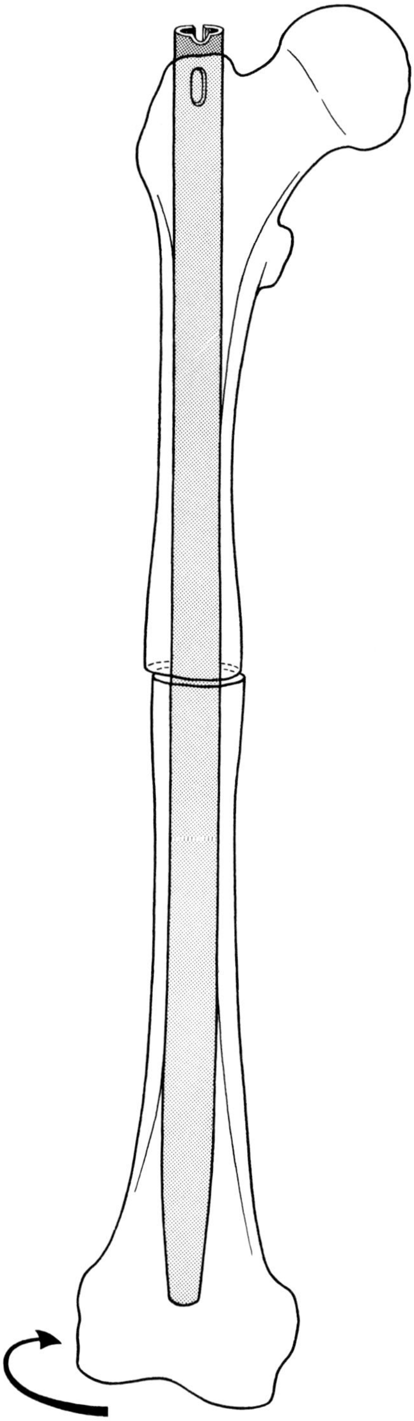

Figure 332 Completed intramedullary nailing after correction of the rotational deformity.

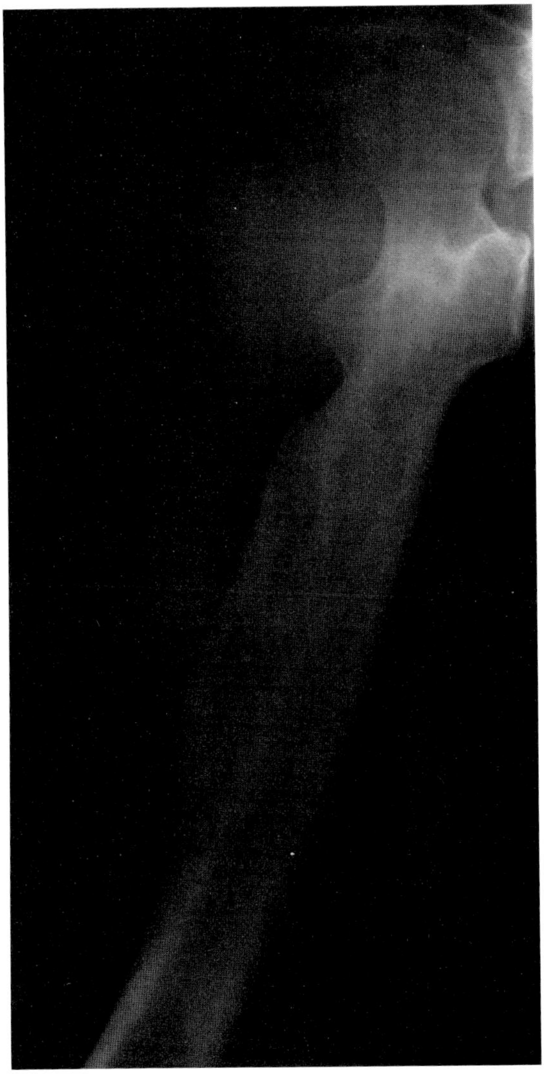

Figure 333 Healed femoral fracture with rotational deformity, lateral view.

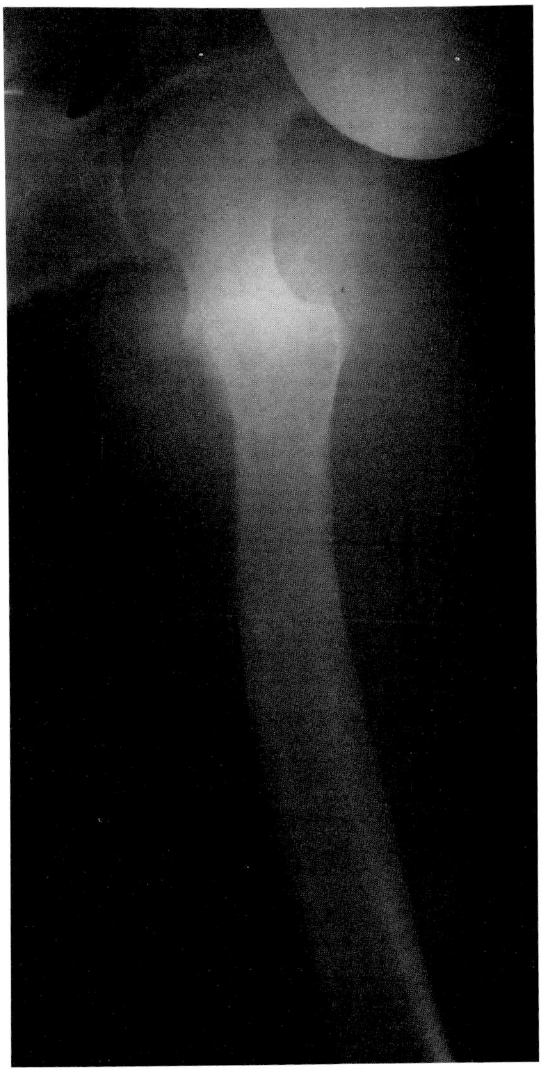

Figure 334 Comparison, lateral view of normal femur.

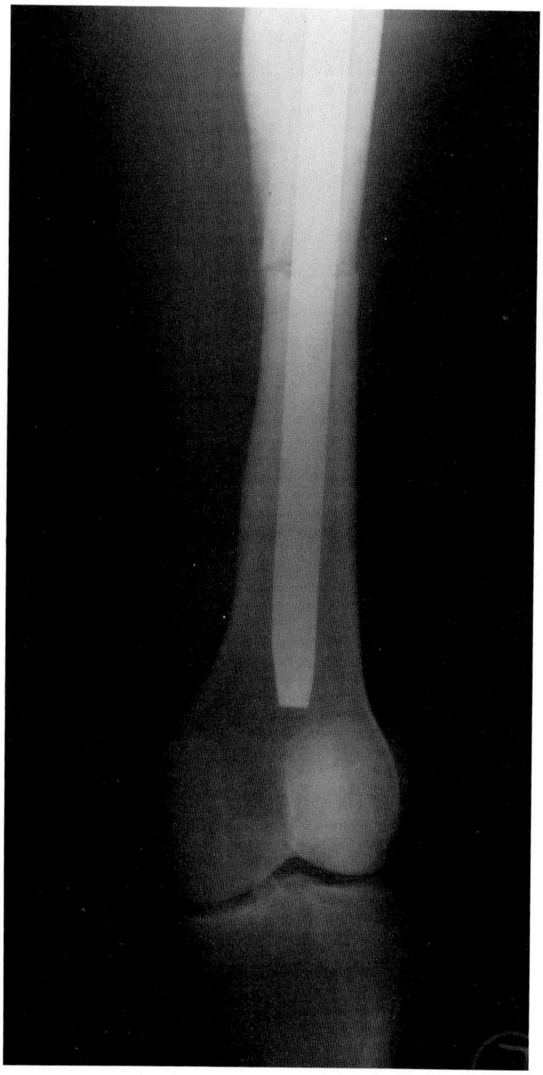

Figure 335 Completed intramedullary nailing after femoral osteotomy with an internal saw and correction of the rotational deformity, AP view.

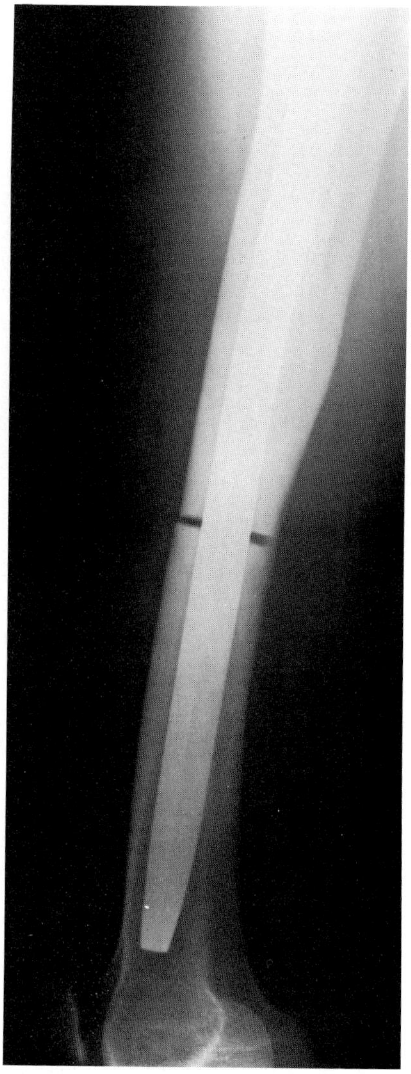

Figure 336 The same case, lateral view.

Figure 337 The same case after a completely healed osteotomy, ten months later, AP view. ►

Figure 338 The same case, lateral view. ►

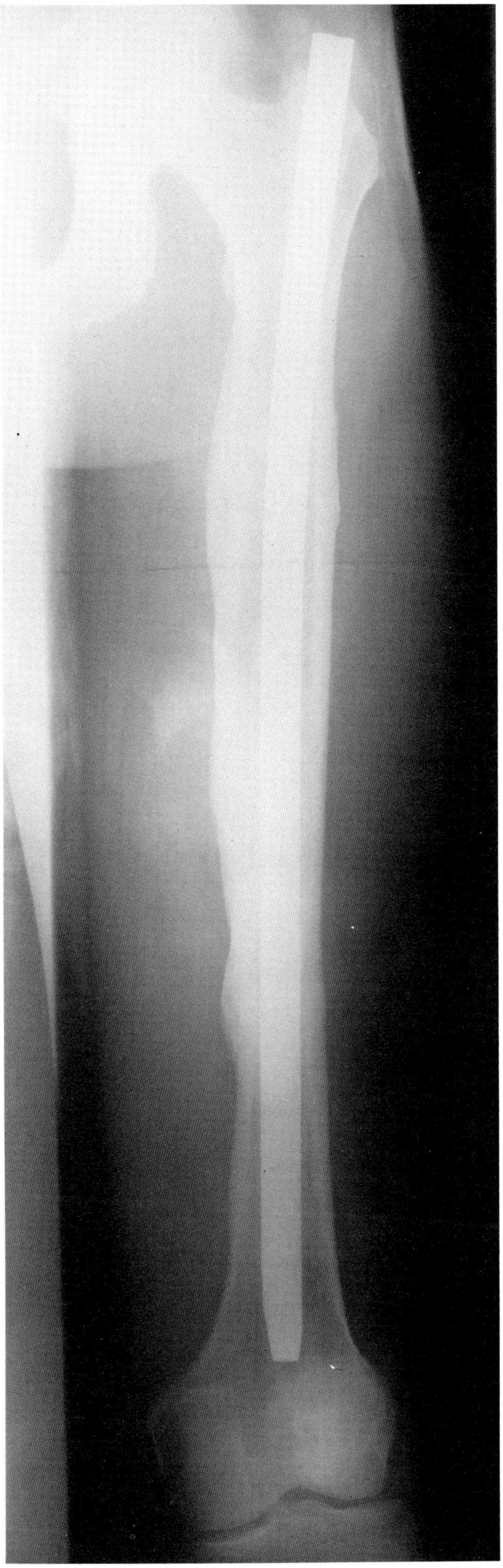

Figure 337

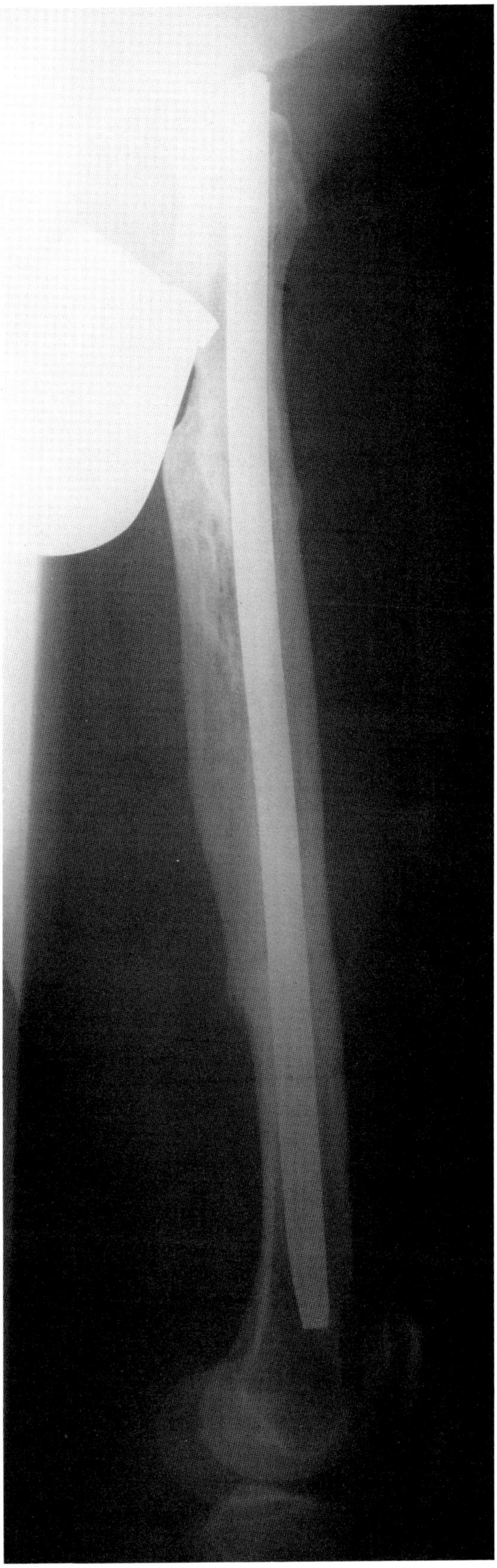

Figure 338

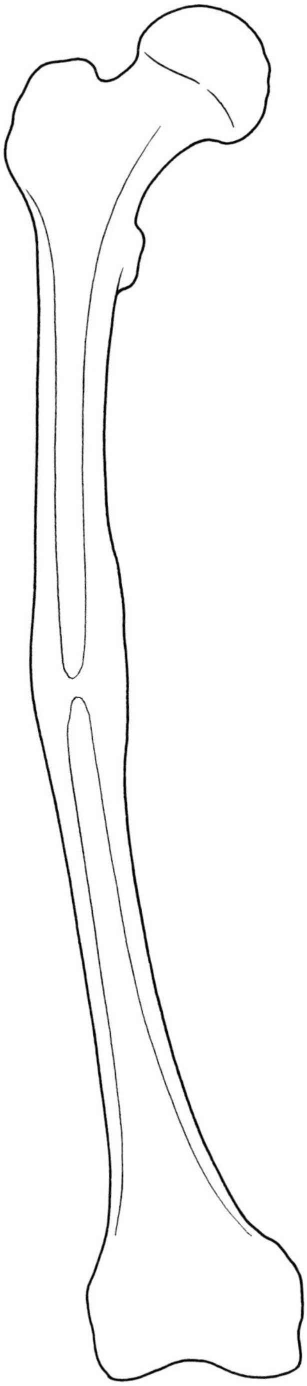

Figure 339 Healed femoral fracture with angulation deformity. The medullary canal is closed at the old fracture site.

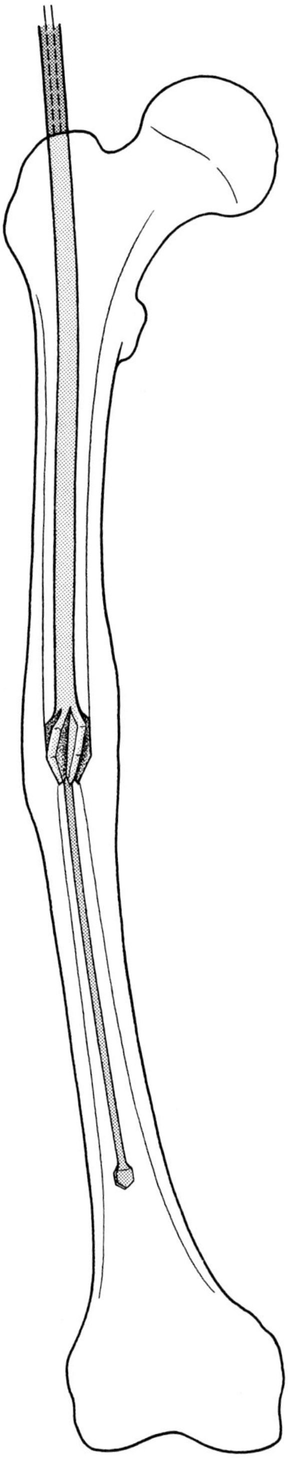

Figure 340 Reaming of the proximal medullary canal until reaching the old fracture site over a drill point guide pin, which was advanced into the distal medullary canal.

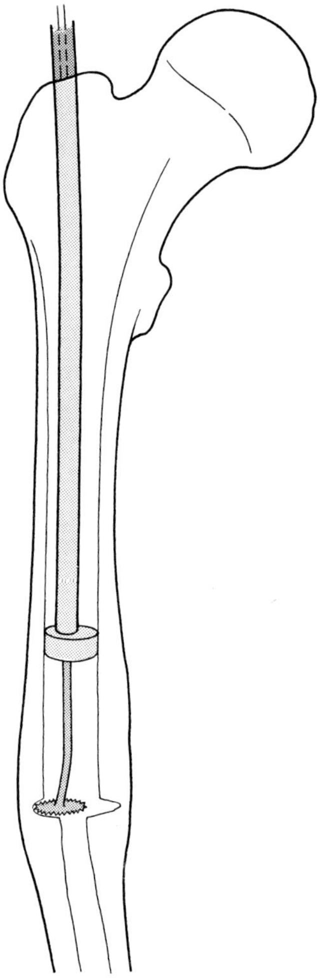

Figure 341 Osteotomy with an internal saw at the level of the old fracture site.

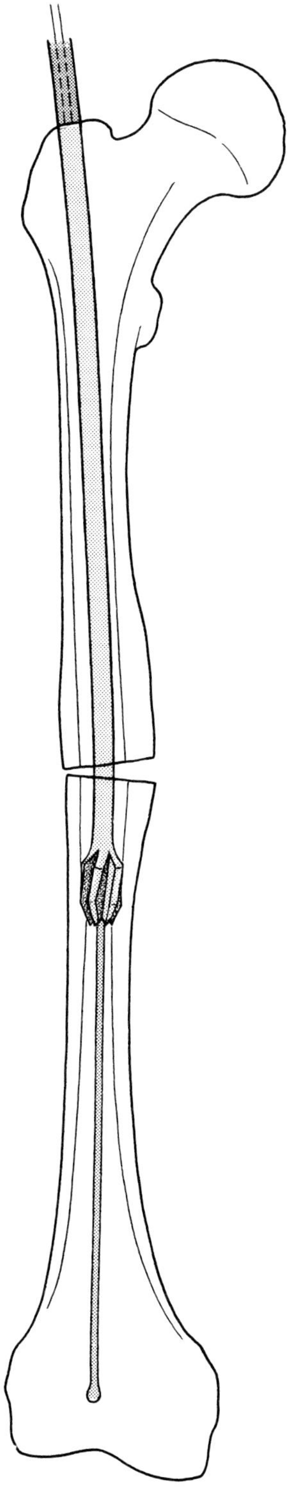

Figure 342 Reaming of the distal medullary canal over the guide pin after completing the osteotomy and correcting the angular deformity.

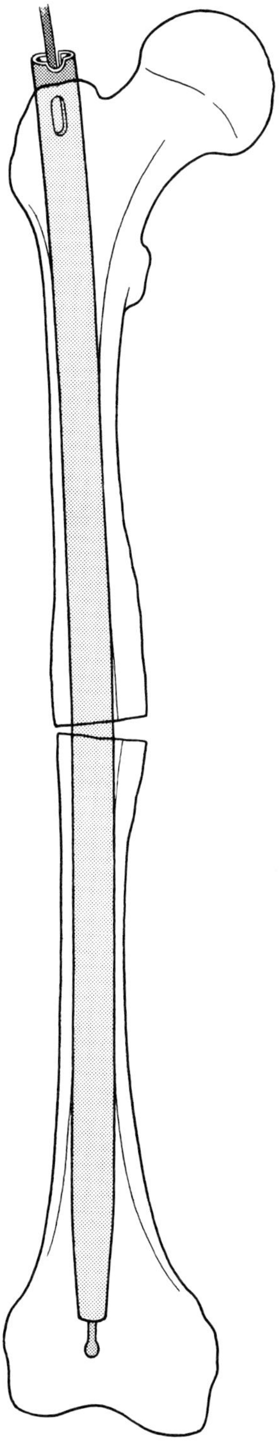

Figure 343 Completed femoral nailing after correction of the deformity.

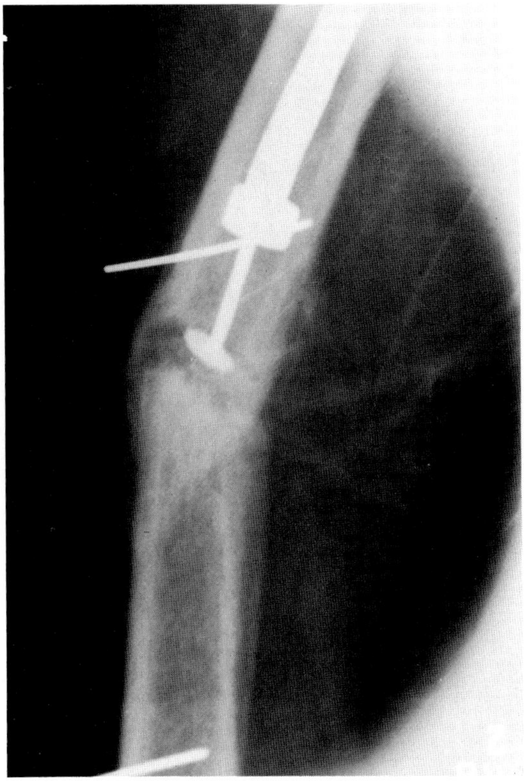

Figure 344 Correction of angular deformity of the femur with an internal saw. Instrument in the medullary canal.

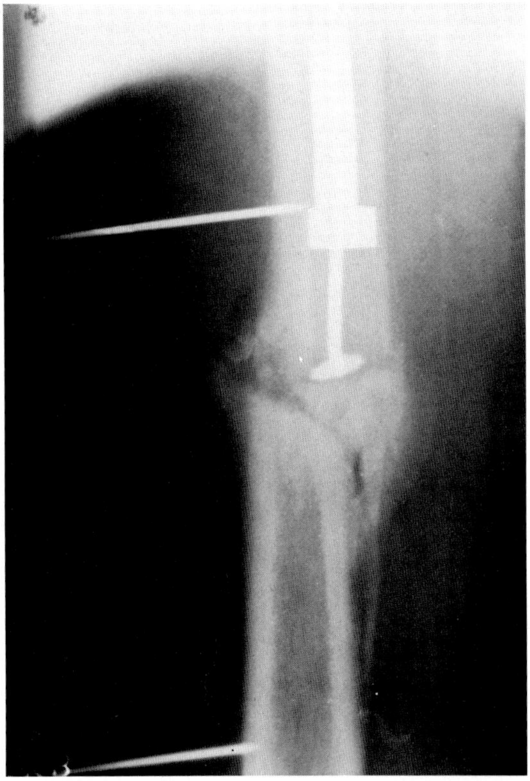

Figure 345 Sawing completed, malalignment corrected.

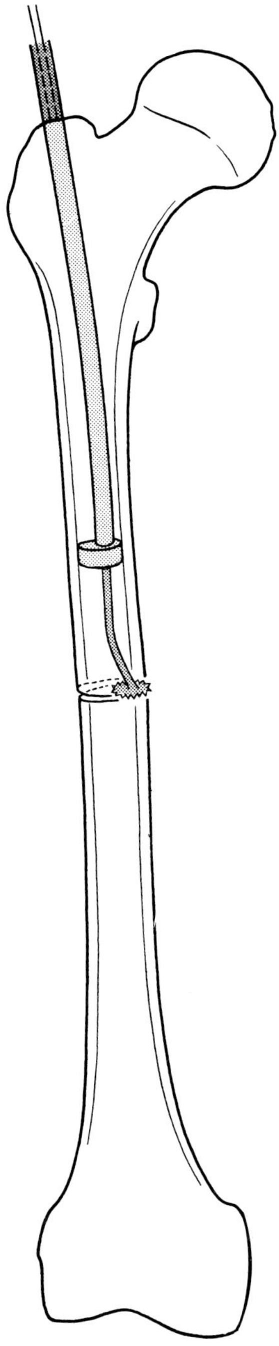

Figure 346 After reaming the medullary canal, osteotomy performed with an internal saw for the lengthening procedure.

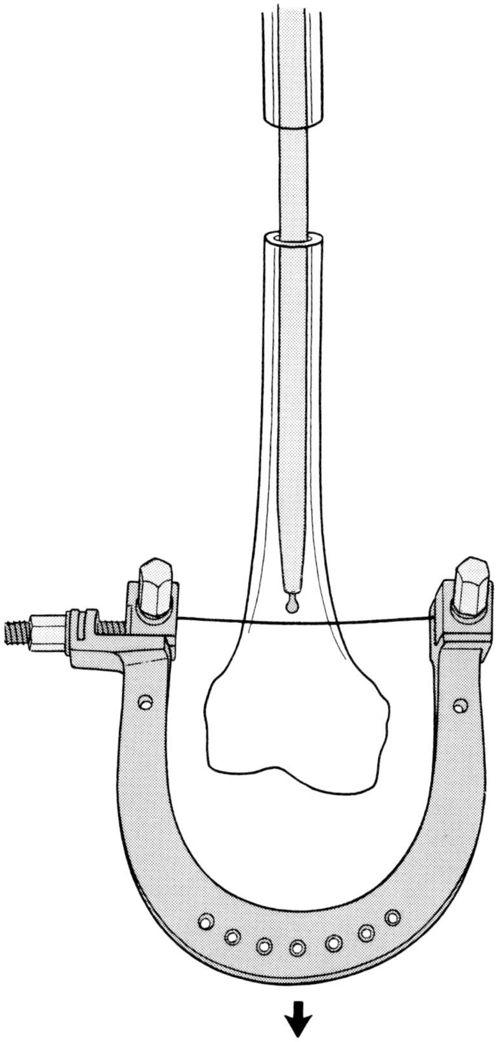

Figure 347 Lengthening of the extremity by use of the Kirschner wire tractor with a small intramedullary nail in situ.

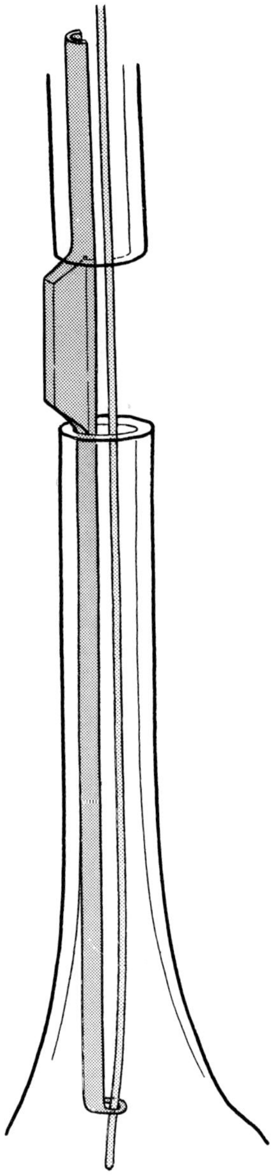

Figure 348 The spacer-nail with its spacer is inserted between the two fragments to maintain the lengthening. The axial alignment of the spacer-nail is maintained by the special thin guide pin through the spacer-nail's eyelet.

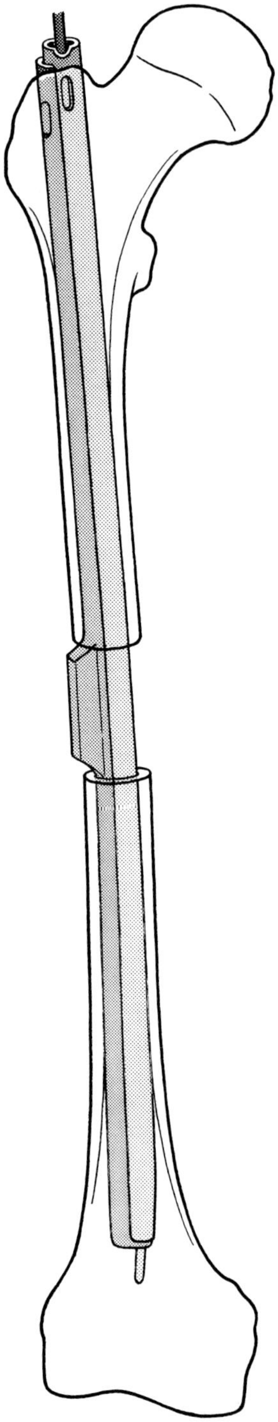

Figure 349 The spacer-nail with spacer is securely locked into place by adding the regular Küntscher nail.

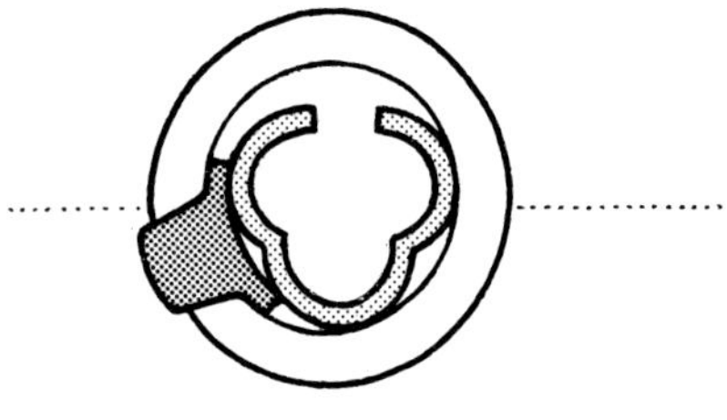

Figure 350 Cross section of the bone with the spacer-nail and regular Küntscher nail.

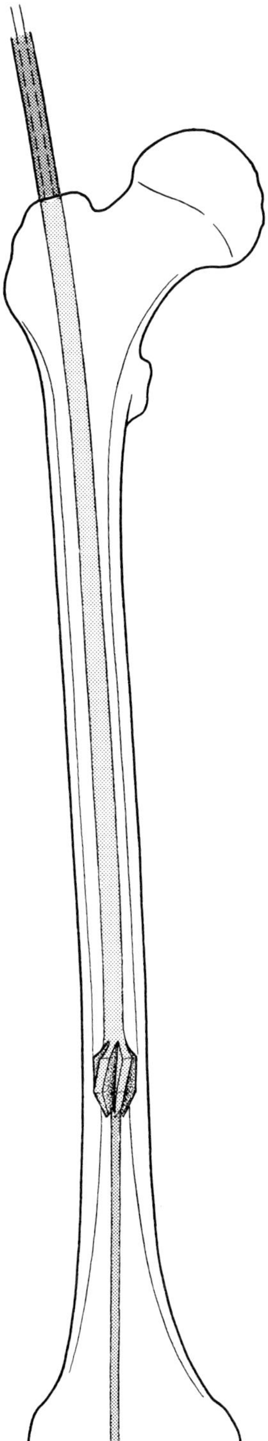

Figure 351 Reaming of the femoral medullary canal before inserting the internal saw.

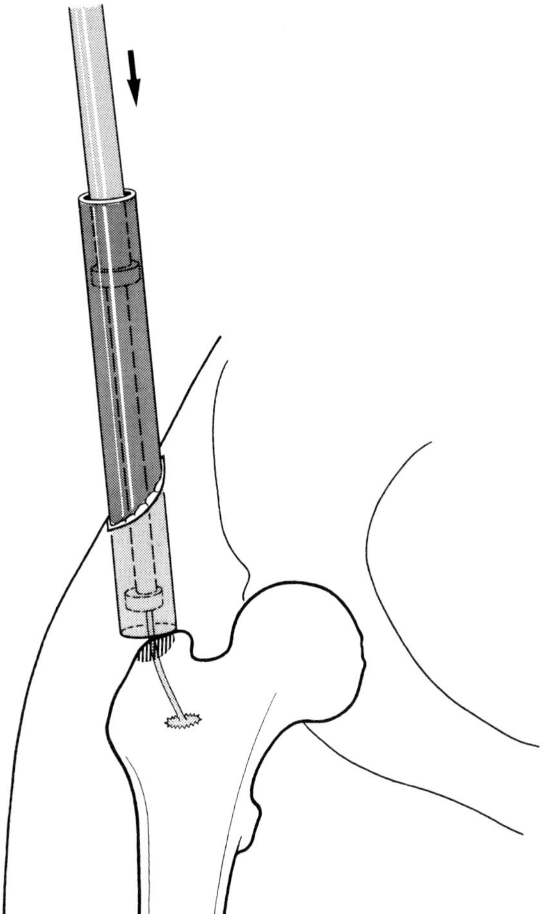

Figure 352 Insertion of the internal saw into the femoral medullary canal through the tubular soft tissue protector.

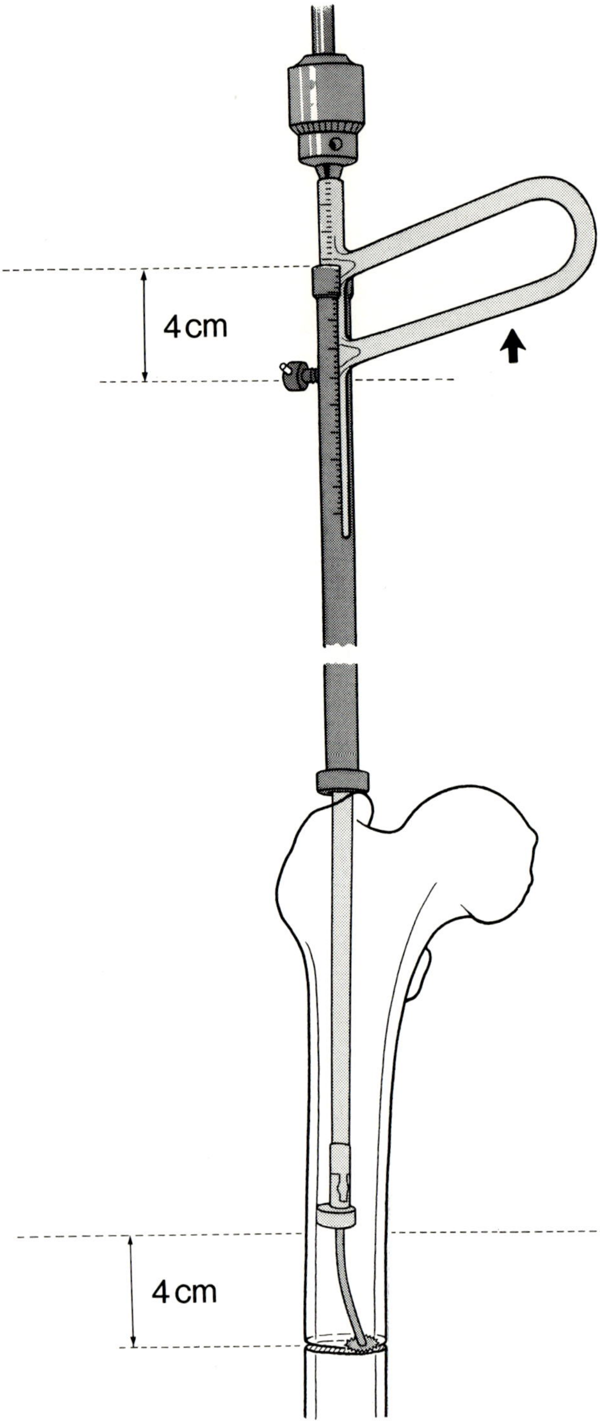

Figure 353 Internal saw with measuring device in place, distal osteotomy completed.

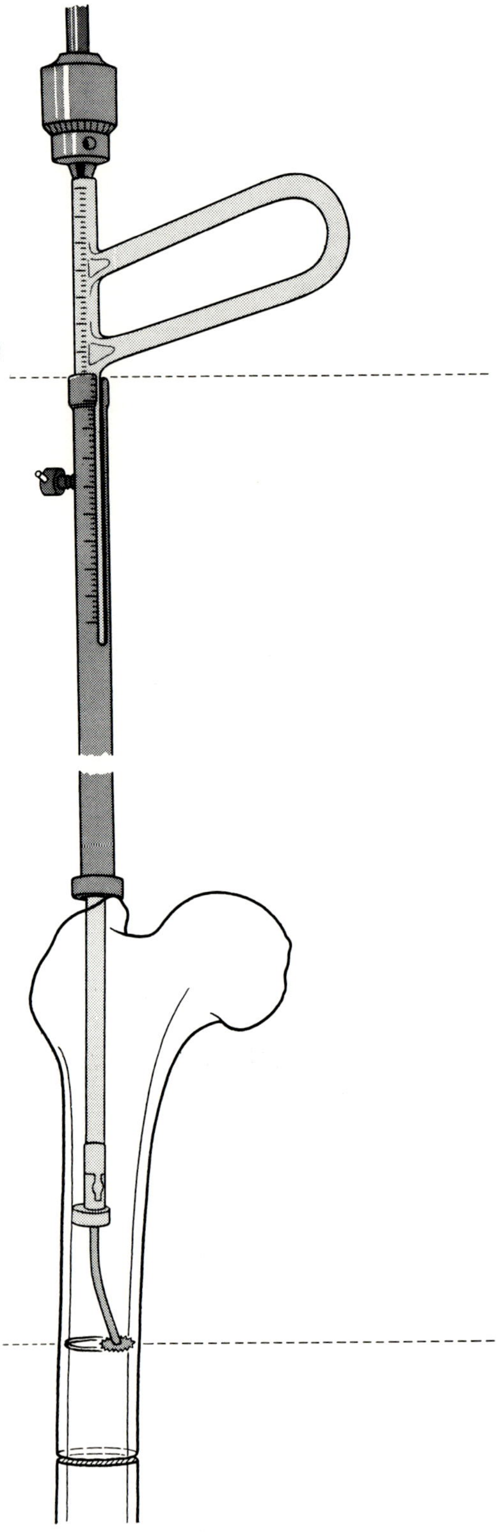

Figure 354 The site of the second saw cut as determined by withdrawing the internal saw the desired distance indicated on the measuring device.

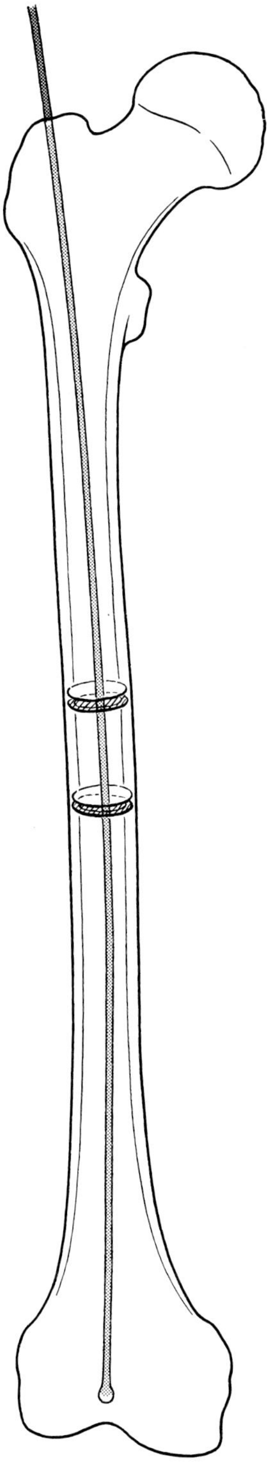

Figure 355 Both osteotomies completed.

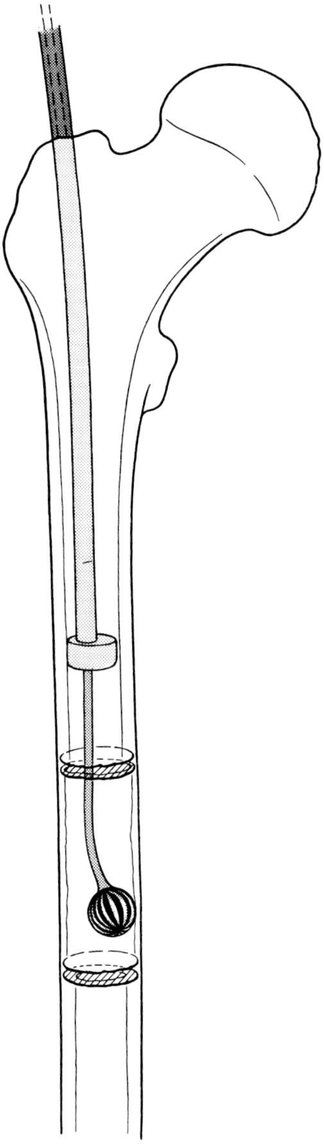

Figure 356 Thinning by the internal ball reamer of the cortex of the cylinder to be resected.

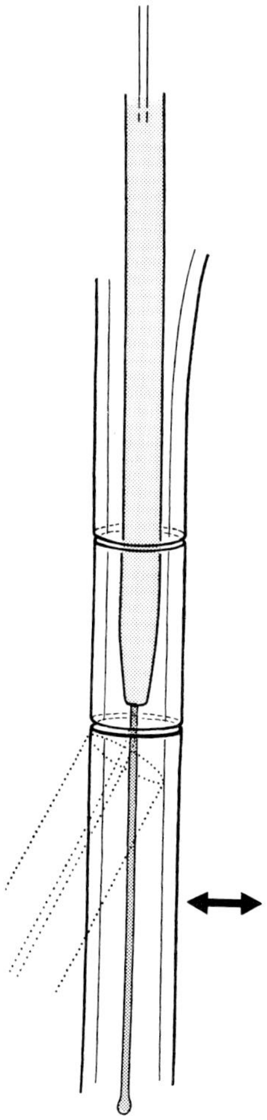

Figure 357 Splinting of the proximal osteotomy by intramedullary nail for complete separation of the distal osteotomy. Insertion of the guide pin avoids the displacement of the distal fragment.

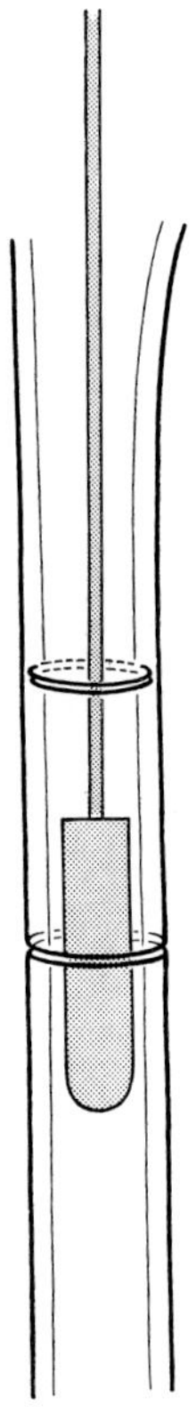

Figure 358 Auxiliary device aiding in the complete separation of the proximal osteotomy.

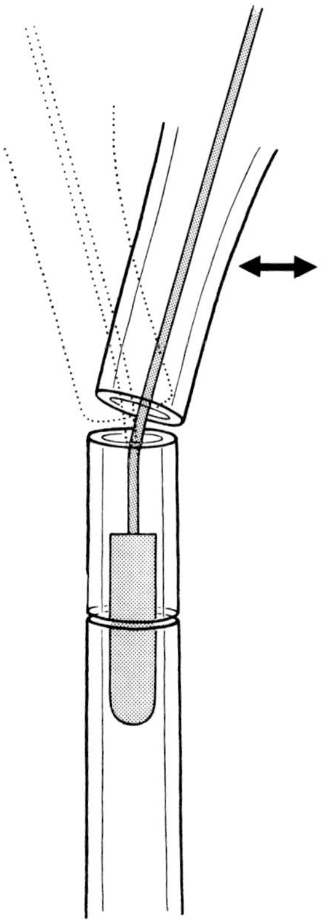

Figure 359 The proximal osteotomy is separated. The distal osteotomy was splinted by the auxiliary device.

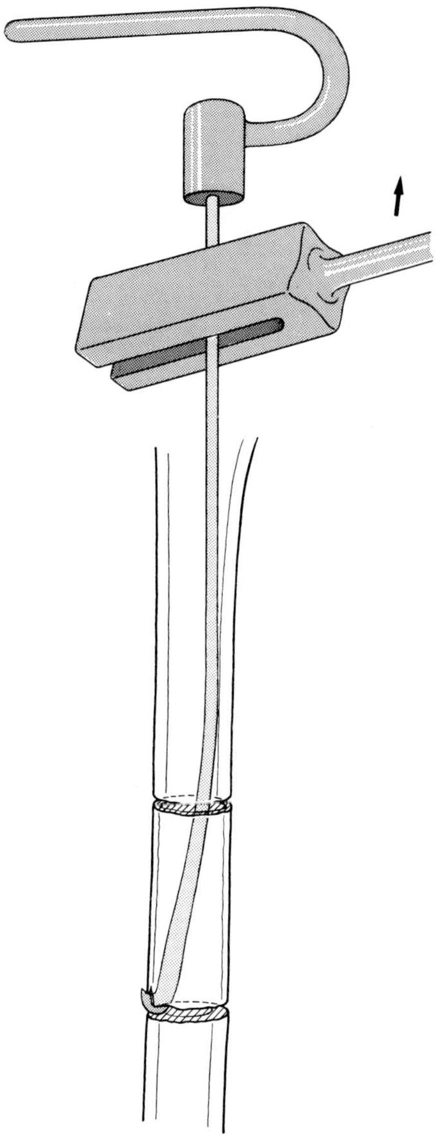

Figure 360 Cleavage by the internal chisel of the cylinder to be resected (the guide pin was deleted in the picture for clarification).

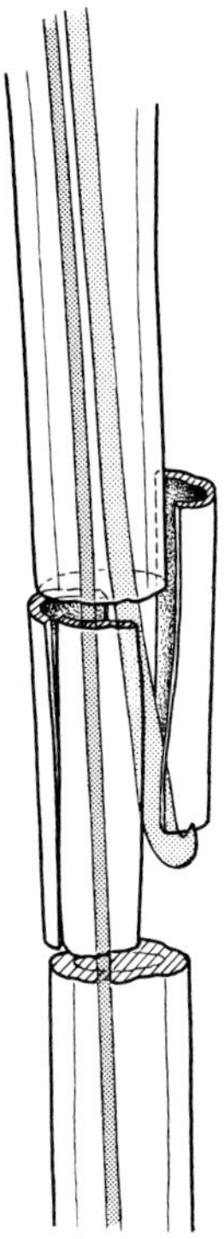

Figure 361 Removal of the bone shells by the internal chisel hook. The guide pin is in the medullary canal to secure the alignment.

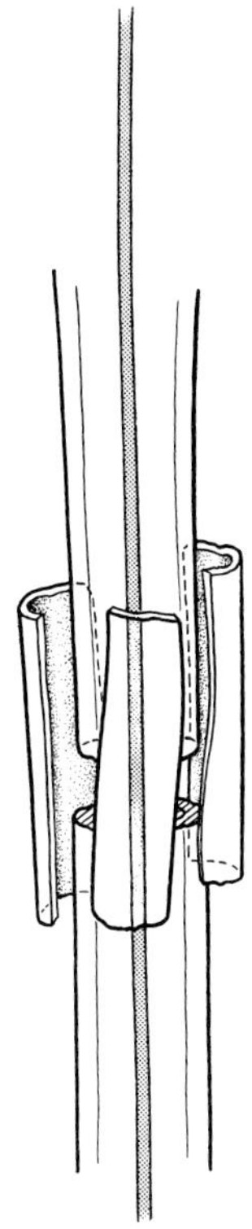

Figure 362 Shortening of the rim by pushing the distal portion onto the proximal portion, splinted internally by the guide pin.

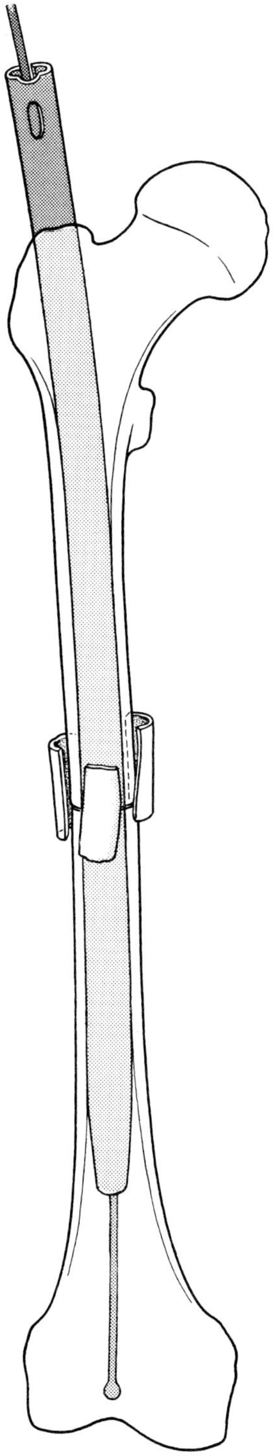

Figure 363 The intramedullary nailing of the femur after the shortening procedure. The bone shells position themselves around the osteotomy site.

Figure 364

Figure 365

Figure 364 The internal saw in the medullary canal during the distal osteotomy in the shortening procedure. Two staples are projected over the bone. The proximal osteotomy site is marked.

Figure 365 The proximal osteotomy is completed. The bone is already completely separated at the distal osteotomy site.

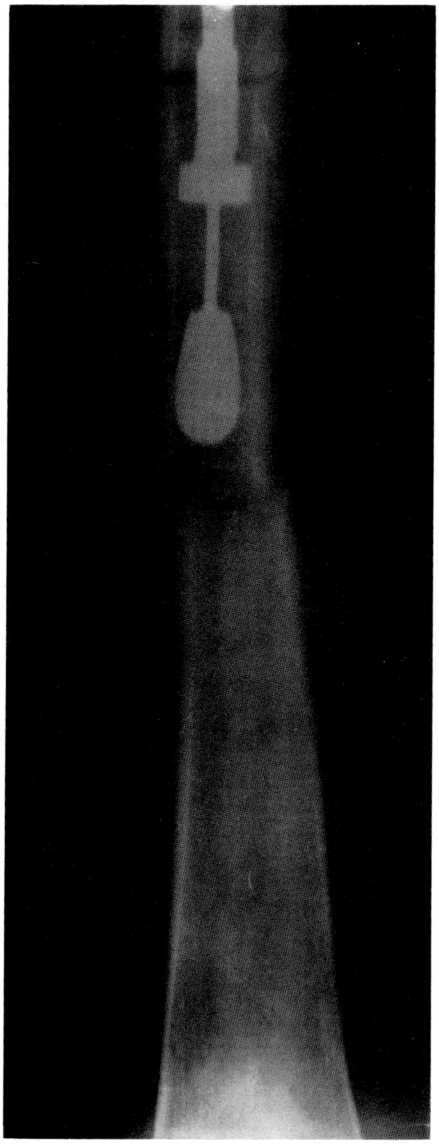

Figure 366

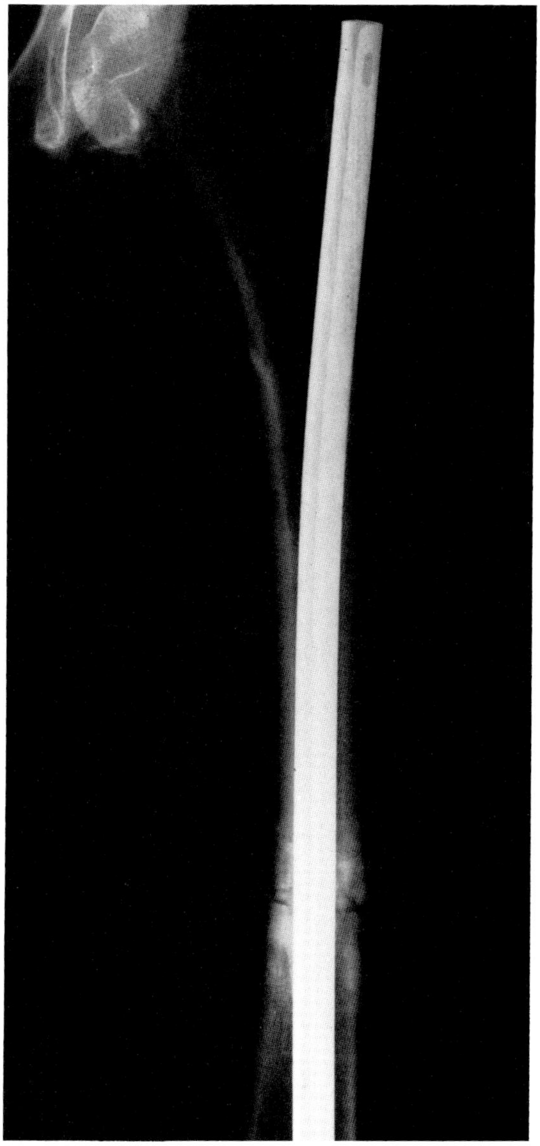

Figure 367

Figure 366 The cortex of the resected cylinder is thinned by an internal ball reamer.

Figure 367 The resected cylinder was split longitudinally by the internal chisel, the shells pushed aside, and the distal fragment pushed onto the proximal fragment. The intramedullary nailing is completed, AP view.

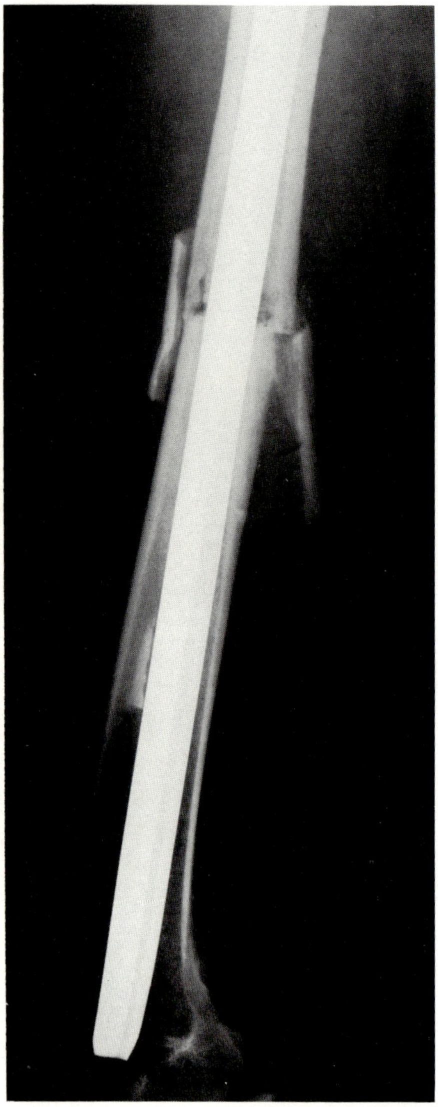

Figure 368 The same case as in figure 364 in lateral view. A displaced cortical fragment is visible anterior to the nail in the distal medullary canal.

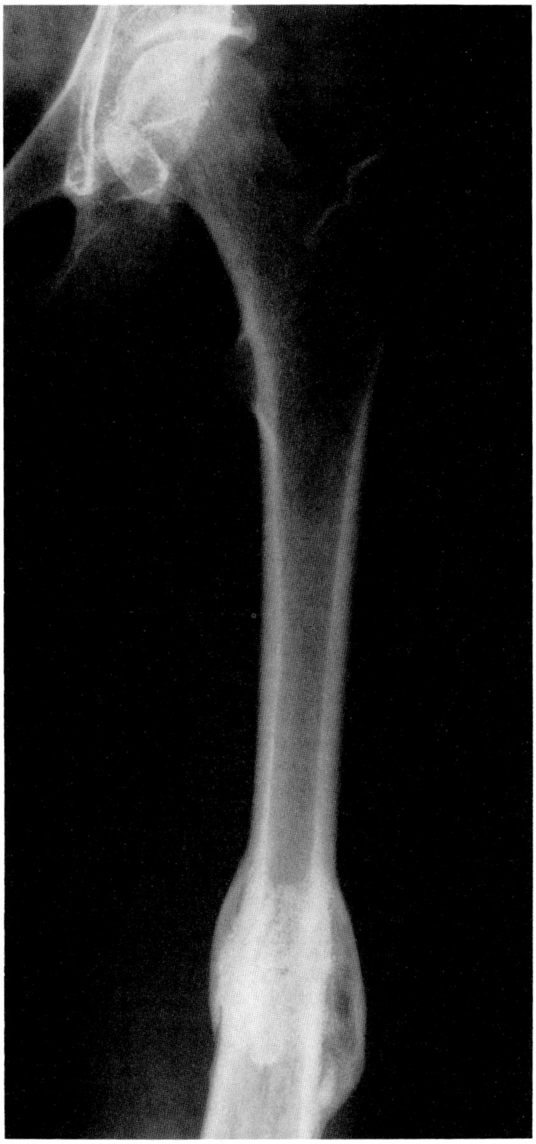

Figure 369 The same case eight months later, after complete bone healing and nail removal. The resected cylinder is partially resorbed, partially fused with the femur, like an autogenous graft, AP. view.

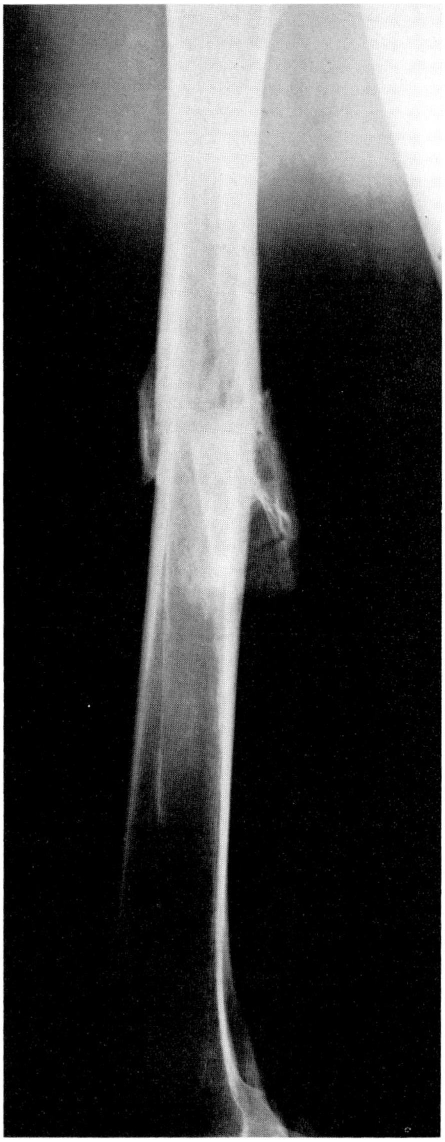

Figure 370 The same case in lateral view. The displaced cortical fragment in the distal medullary canal is nearly completely resorbed.

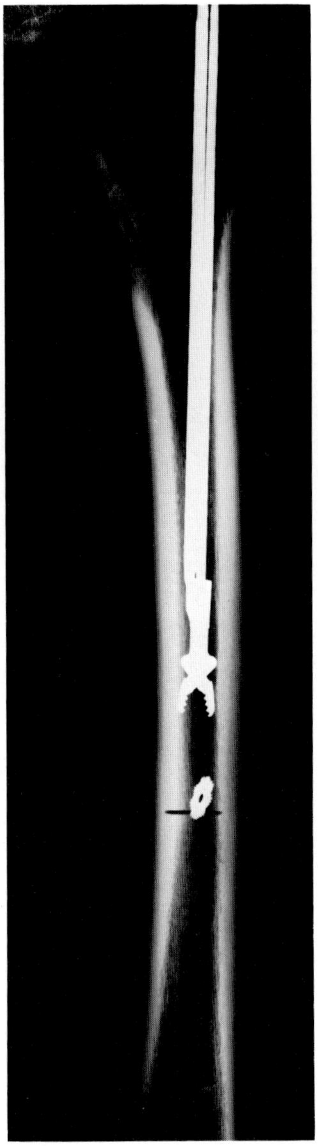

Figure 371

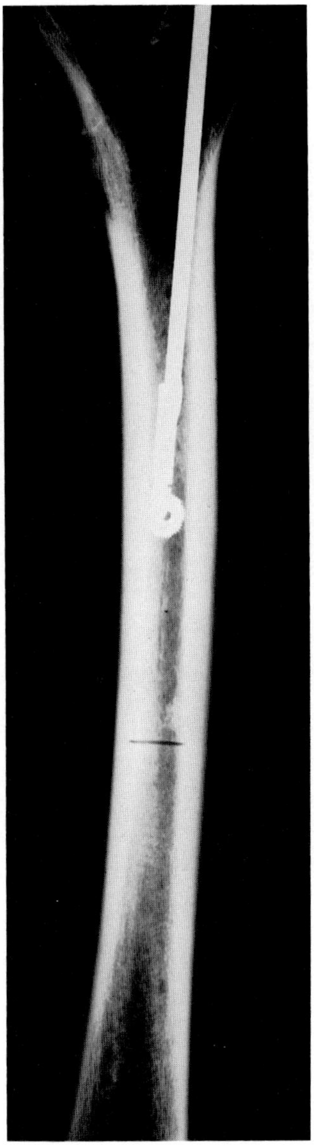

Figure 372

Figure 371 Detached saw blade in the medullary canal. A long-handled forceps is introduced into the medullary canal.

Figure 372 The detached saw blade is being removed from the medullary canal by the long-handled forceps in the medullary canal.

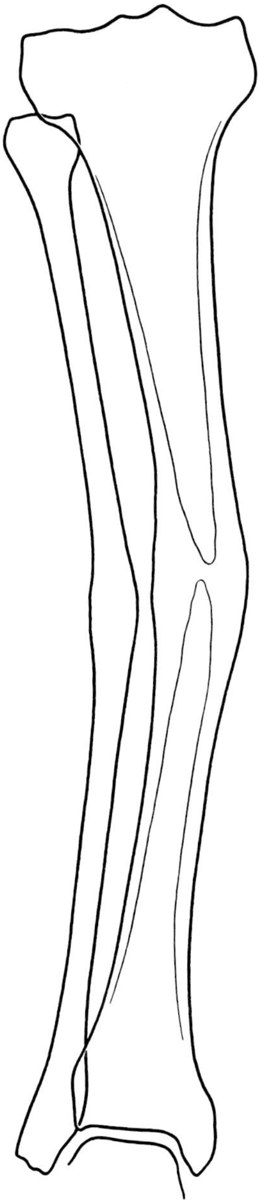

Figure 373 Healed fracture of the lower leg with angular deformity and closed medullary canal at the fracture site.

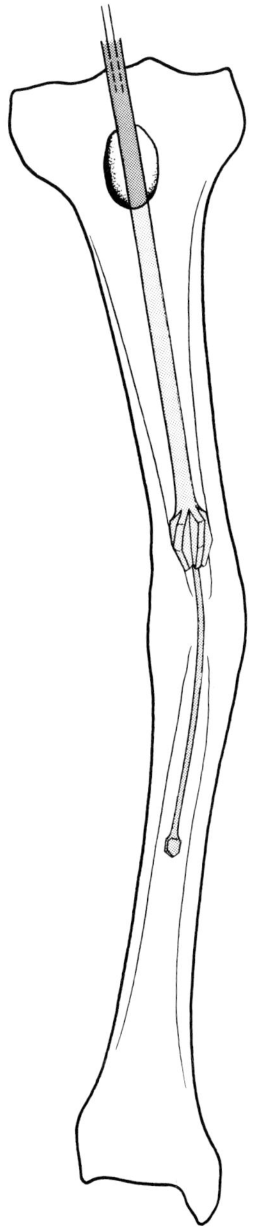

Figure 374 After a drill point guide pin perforates the closed portion of the medullary canal, the proximal medullary canal is reamed until the reamer reaches the previous fracture site.

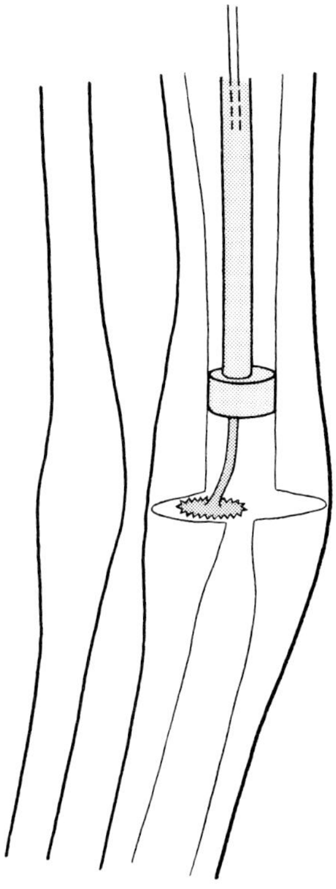

Figure 375 Osteotomy of the previous fracture site with an internal saw.

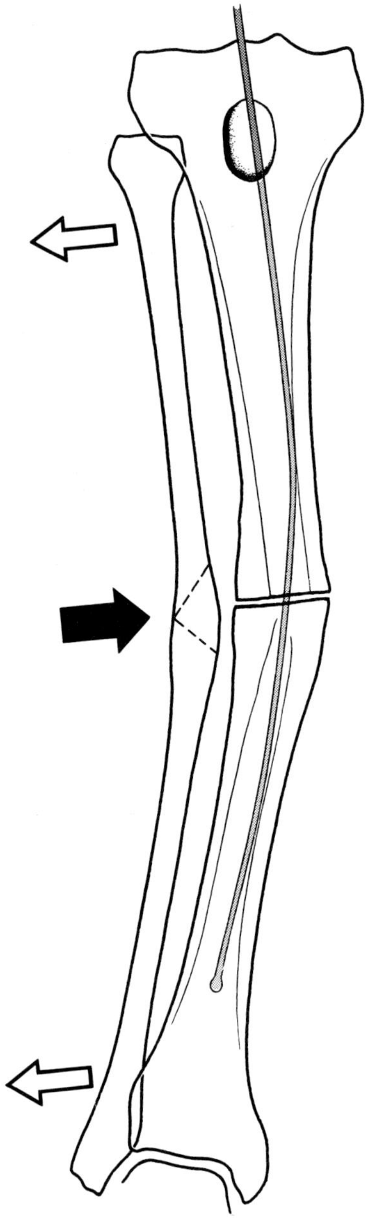

Figure 376 Manual fracture of the fibula. Protection of the soft tissue by a guide pin inserted into the tibia.

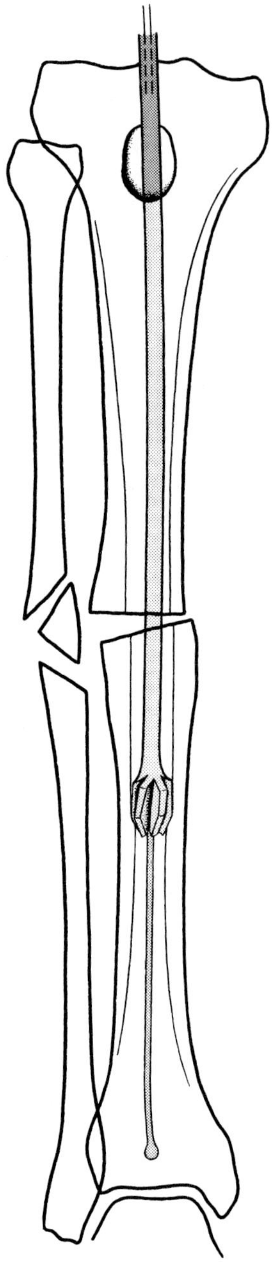

Figure 377 After correction of the deformity, reaming of the distal medullary canal of the tibia over the guide pin.

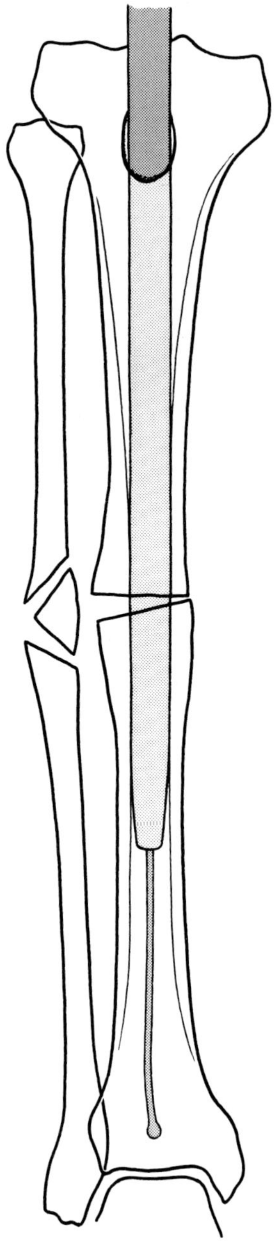

Figure 378 Intramedullary nailing of the tibia after the correction of the deformity.

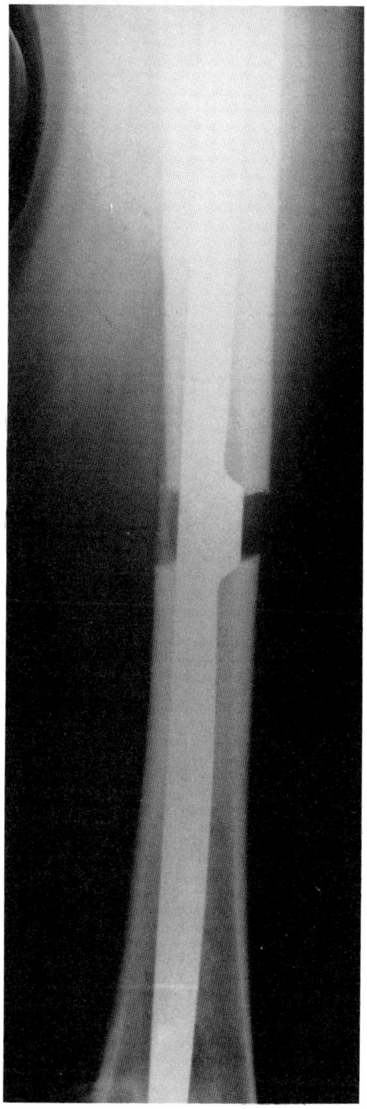

Figure 379

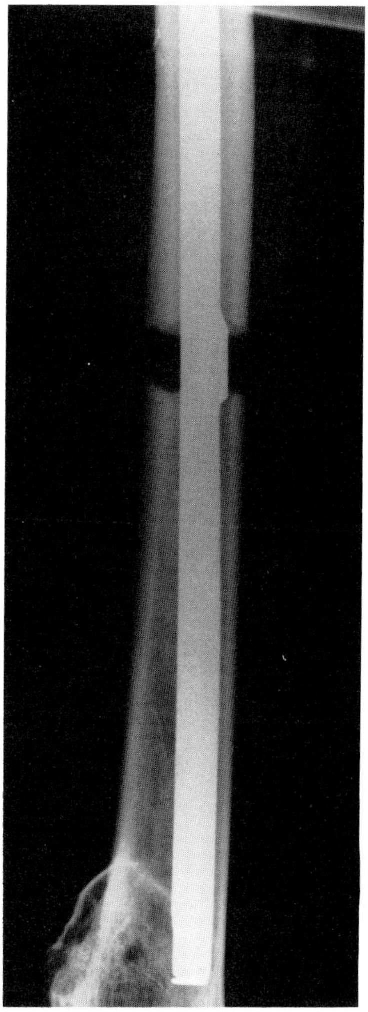

Figure 380

Figure 379 Completed osteotomy for lengthening of the femur. Nailing with a spacer-nail and a regular Küntscher nail. Saw dust of the osteotomy with the internal saw is visible in the interspace between the distal and proximal portions (no callus!). Oblique view to demonstrate the spacer of the spacer-nail.

Figure 380 The same lengthening osteotomy after nailing with a spacer-nail and a regular Küntscher nail, lateral view.

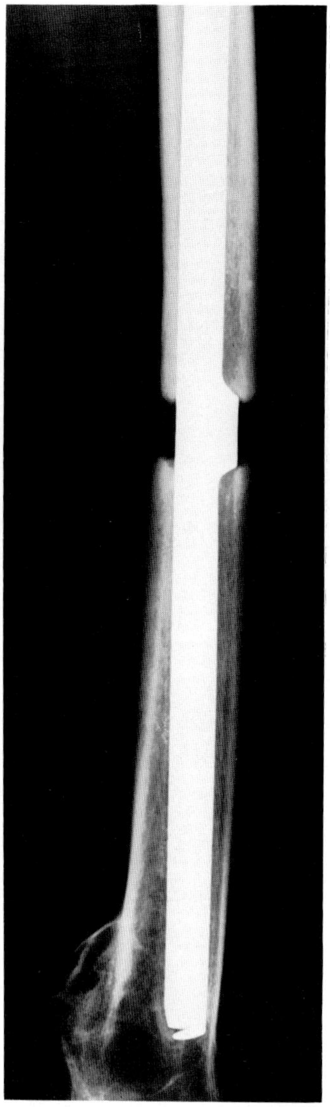

Figure 381

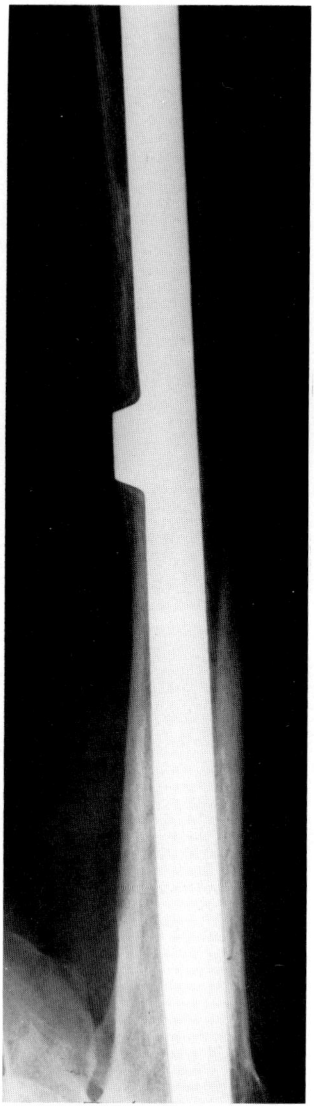

Figure 382

Figure 381 Seven months after lengthening osteotomy, the interspace is one-third covered by bone.

Figure 382 After 24 months, the interspace is completely bridged by bone.

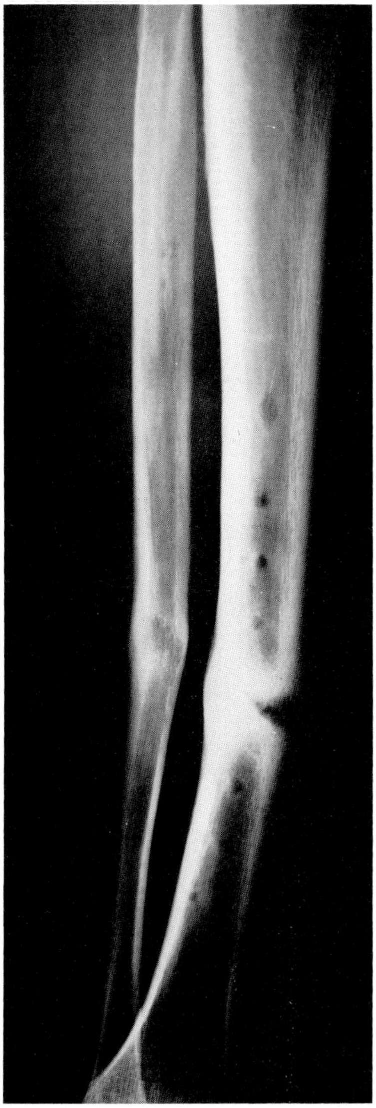

Figure 383

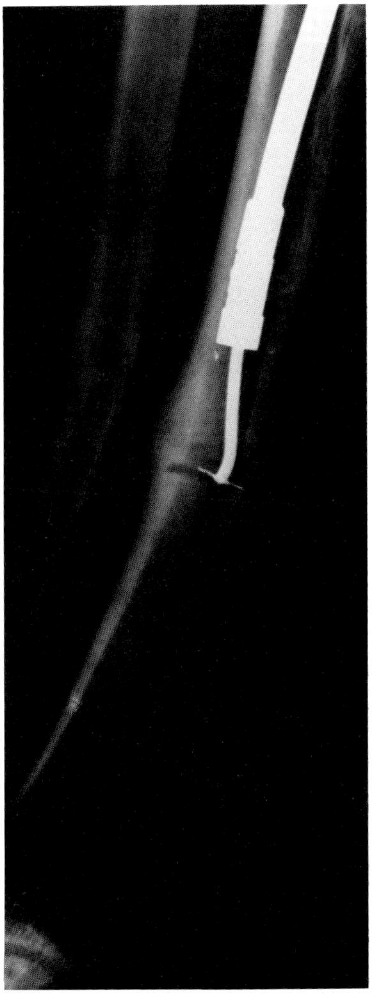

Figure 384

Figure 383 Healed fracture of the lower leg with angular deformity (antecurvation). Condition after compression plating.

Figure 384 The same situation, after reaming the medullary canal and osteotomy with an internal saw. Saw in action.

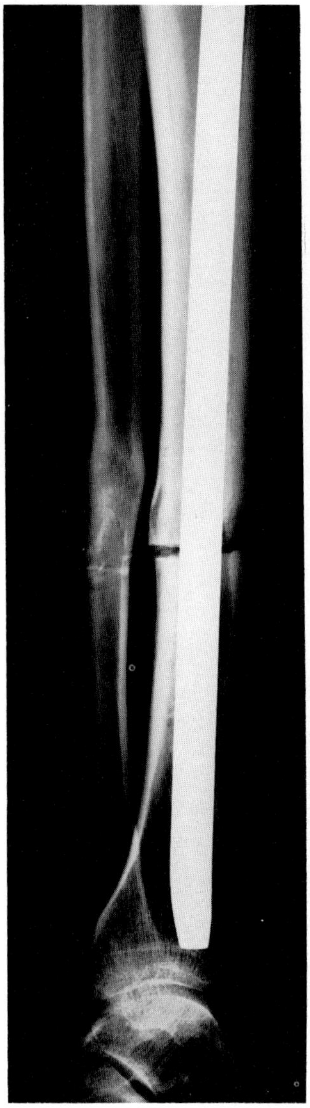

Figure 385

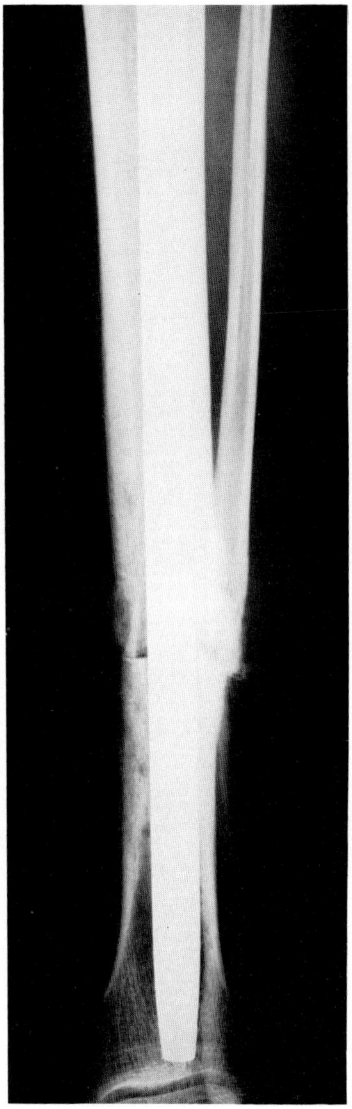

Figure 386

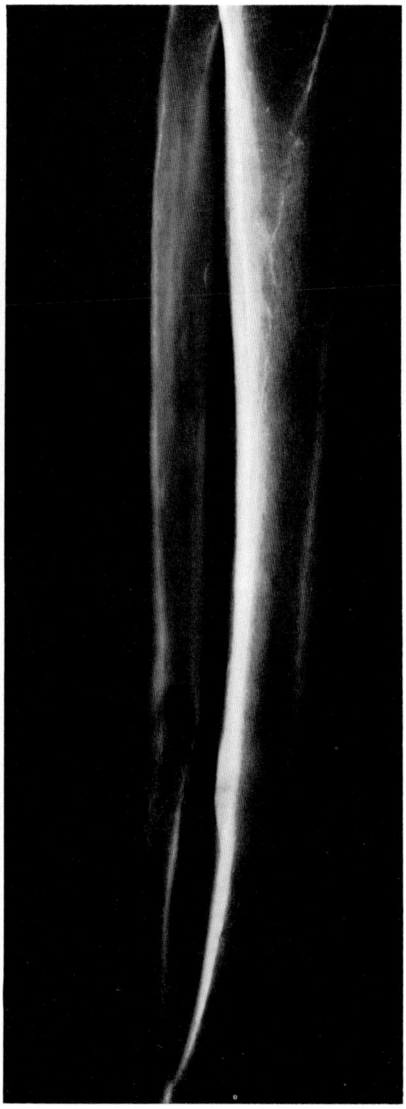

Figure 387

Figure 385 After reaming the distal medullary canal and after the osteotomy of the fibula with a sharp chisel, correction of the deformity and tibia nailing, lateral view.

Figure 386 AP view after complete tibia nailing.

Figure 387 The same case, 15 months later, after bone healing and nail removal, lateral view.

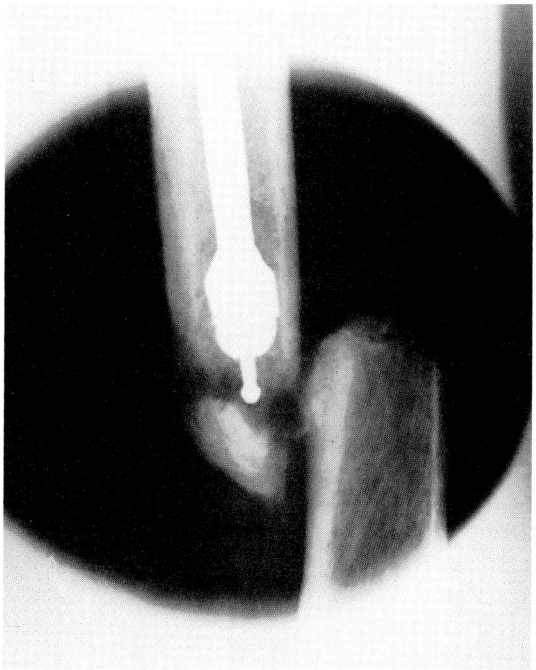

Figure 389 The internal saw is used as an auxiliary device for the reduction. Osteotomy of the proximal portion of the pseudarthrosis is performed at the level of the juxtapositioned end of the distal fragment in order to facilitate lateral alignment.

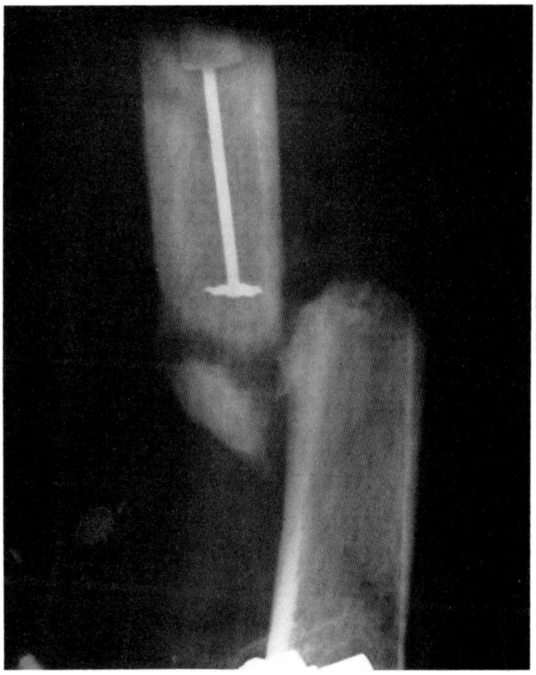

Figure 389 The internal saw is used as an auxiliary device for the reduction. Osteotomy of the proximal portion of the pseudarthrosis is performed at the level of the juxtapositioned end of the distal fragment in order to facilitate lateral alignment.

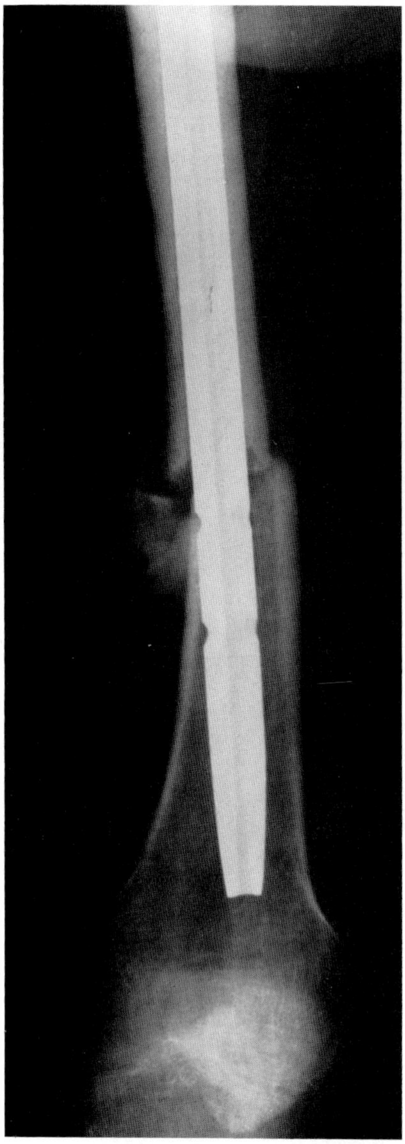

Figure 390 Condition after osteotomy—correction of the lateral malalignment and nailing of the pseudarthrosis. The sawed-off bone fragment is near the distal femoral portion.

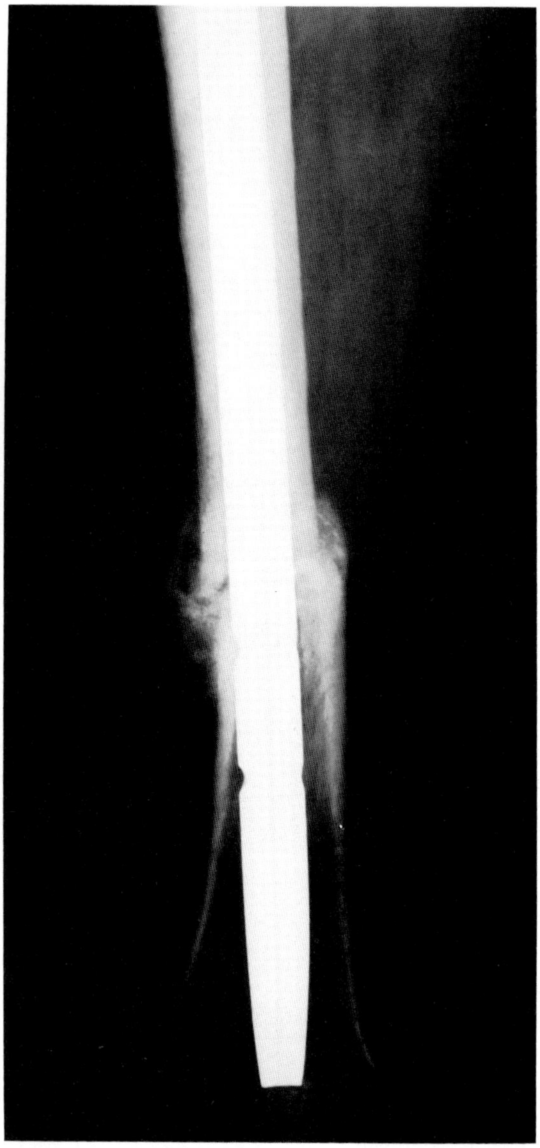

Figure 391 The same case three months later with good progress of bony healing of the pseudarthrosis. Partial resorption of the sawed-off bone fragment and partial fusion with the femur.

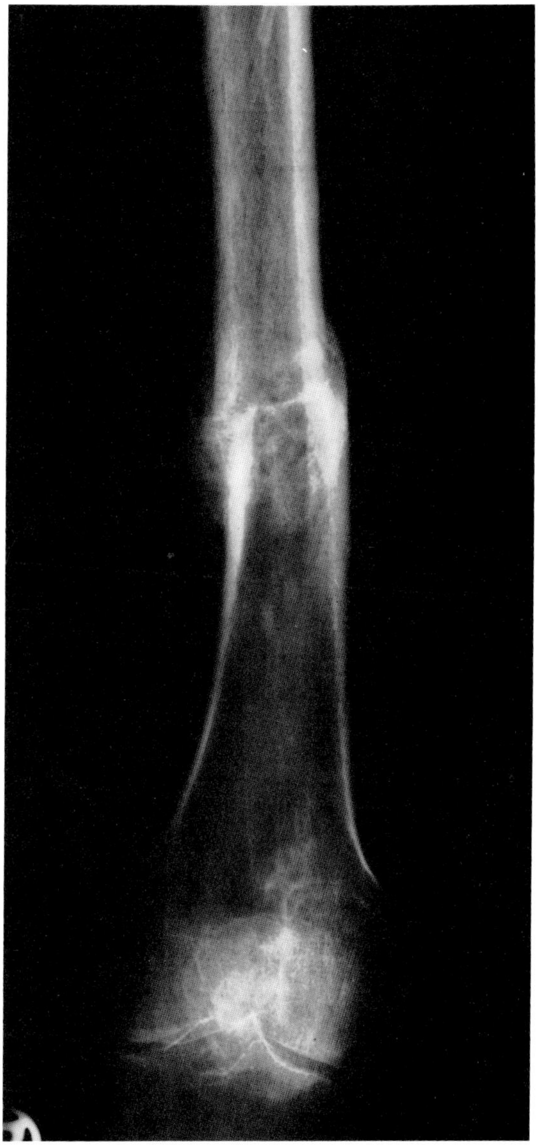

Figure 392 The same case after bone healing and nail removal. The bone fragment is barely visible.

Pathologic Fractures

Intramedullary nailing can usually be done in pathologic fractures of the metaphysis in long bones. This also pertains to pathologic fractures in systemic disease and in localized bone disease, for instance bone cysts and benign tumors. Pathologic fractures within the metaphysis of long bones caused by metastases should always be nailed if the patient can tolerate general anesthesia or nerve block. The intramedullary nailing can also enhance the bony healing of patients in the more advanced metastatic stages while they are being treated by radiation. The patient is spared part of his pain. The nursing of a bedridden patient is also greatly facilitated.

The intramedullary nailing of pathologic fractures caused by a primary malignant tumor is rarely indicated. It is done only to facilitate nursing in cases in which no other procedure can or should be done. The operative technique is identical to that described for closed intramedullary nailing of the corresponding bone. If the regular Küntscher nail does not provide satisfactory locking, an interlocking nail or compression nail must be used.

The reaming of the medullary canal in pathologic fractures caused by systemic bone disease should be performed cautiously to avoid splitting the bone. Bones that are highly fragile are best nailed with a special nail that does not demand maximal reaming.

Intramedullary nailing of pathologic fractures caused by metastasis of a radiation-sensitive tumor is done by reaming the medullary canal. The metastasis and the pertaining lymphs drainage area(s) must be irradiated as soon as possible after the operation. The radiation therapy reduces the risk of spreading tumor cells by the reaming and nailing and enhances the bone healing if the patient survives long enough. The risk of spreading the tumor by reaming is relatively insignificant in comparison to the usually poor prognosis of a tumor disease with known metastases. A biopsy of the pathologic fracture is taken under fluoroscopy with intramedullary gripping pliers or a sharp curette before the actual nailing of the bone. This is to be done even when the histology of the primary tumor is known.

Postoperative exercises can be started immediately if solid osteosynthesis has been obtained by the nailing. Pathologic fractures in the lower extremities are capable of weight-bearing postoperatively if sufficient cortical support exists at the fracture site and the nail is firmly locked.

The Küntscher nail is not removed after the nailing of any pathologic fracture caused by a malignant tumor. The bone healing is delayed in the nailing of pathologic fractures caused by systemic bone disease or by a local benign tumor. This must be taken into consideration when planning the nail removal.

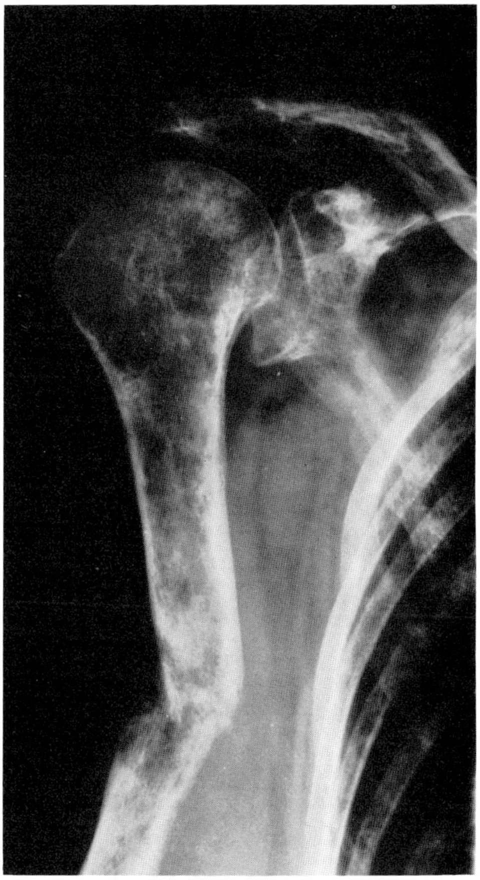

Figure 393 Pathologic fracture of the humerus with multiple metastases of breast cancer, AP view in 75-year-old female.

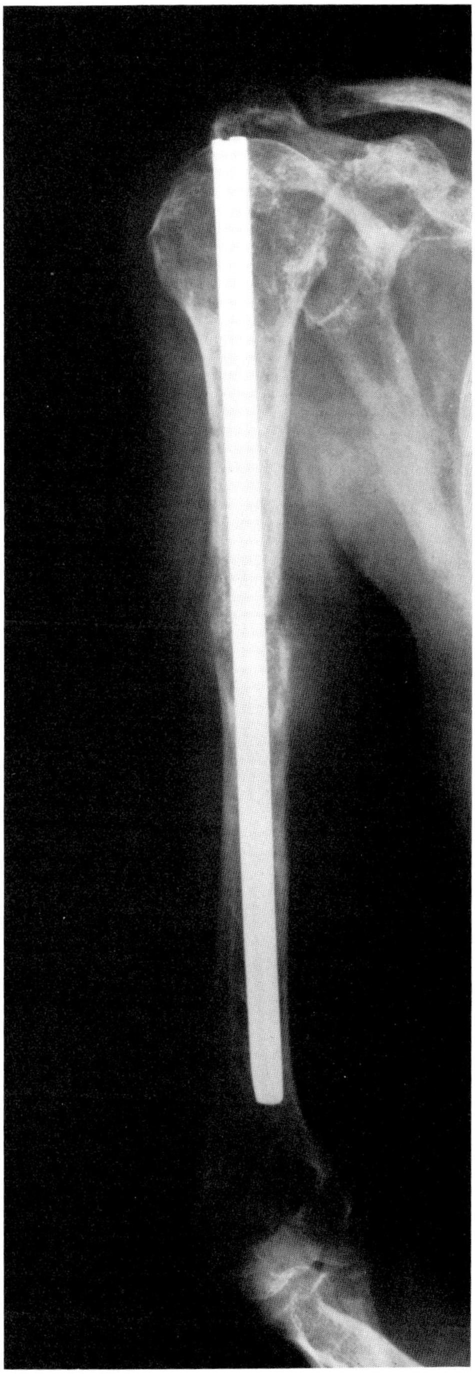

Figure 394 Because of severe pains, nailing of the humerus with a buried straight Küntscher nail, AP view. ▶

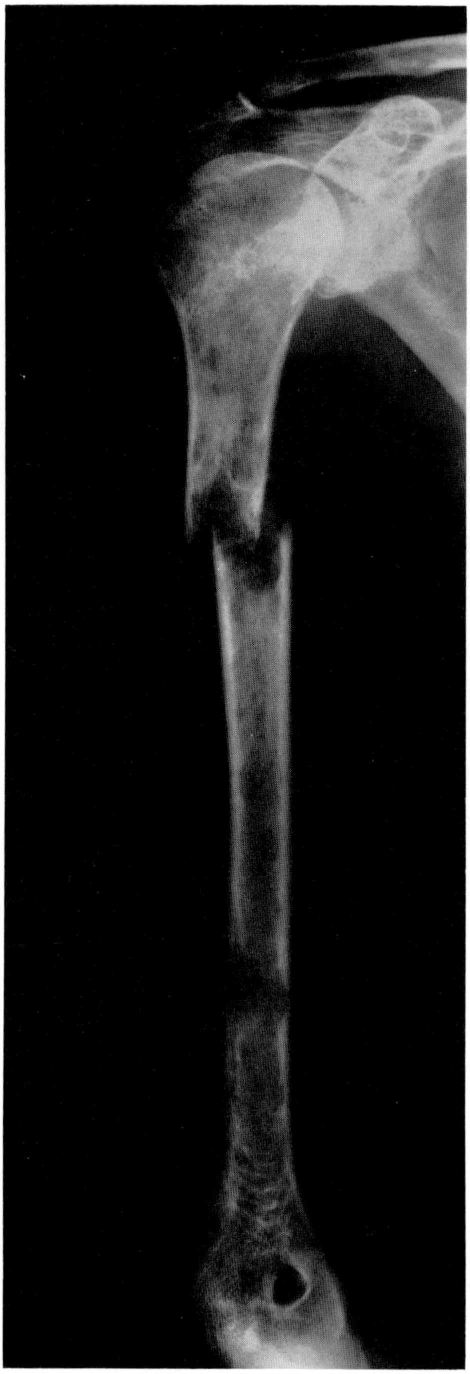

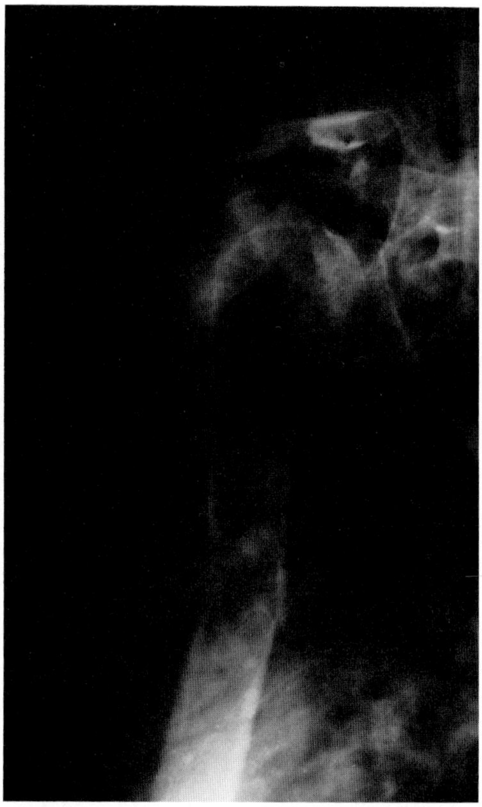

Figure 396 The same pathologic fracture in a lateral view, taken through the chest.

◀ Figure 365 Pathologic fractures of the humerus at the site of a larger metastasis of bone cancer with multiple bone metastases, AP view.

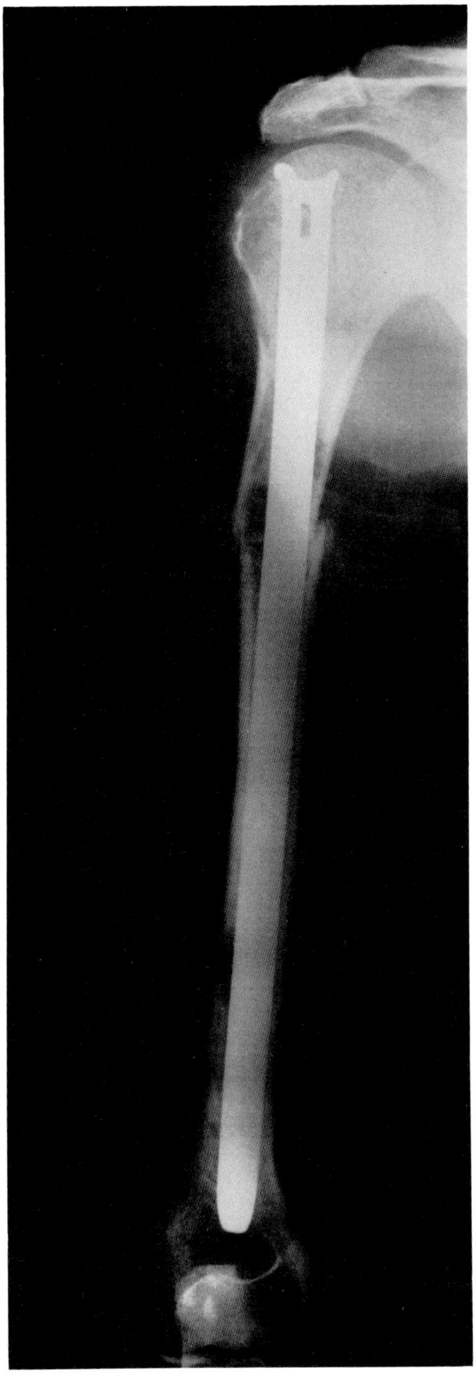

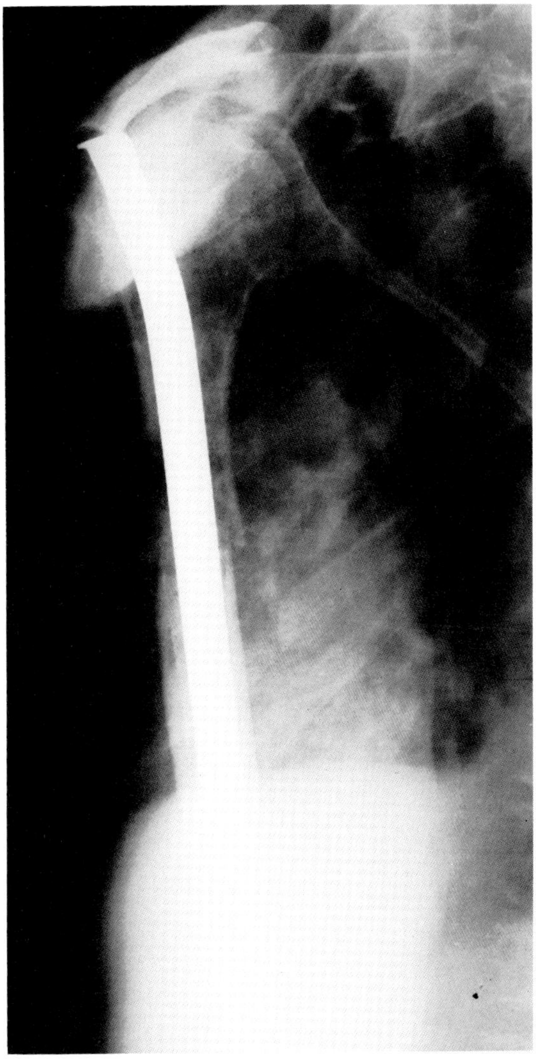

Figure 398 Lateral view taken through the chest after completed nailing.

◀ Figure 387 Condition after nailing of the pathologic fracture of the humerus with a bent cloverleaf nail. The fracture is compressed, AP view.

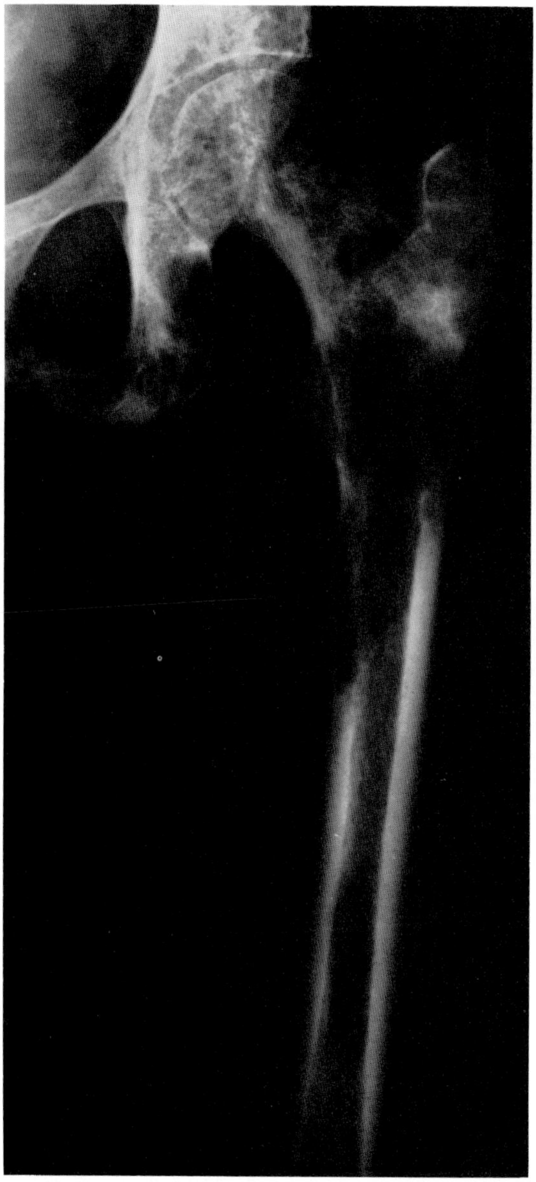

Figure 399 Multiple skeletal metastases of breast carcinoma. A huge metastasis in the subtrochanteric area of the femur.

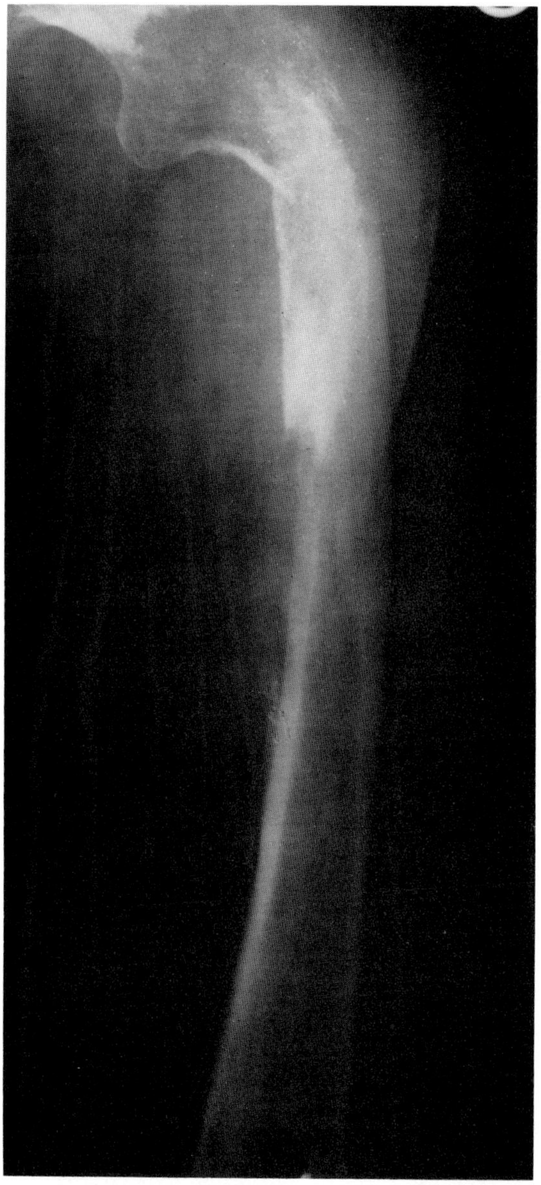

Figure 400 The same case four months later. Pathologic fracture in the area of the subtrochanteric metastasis.

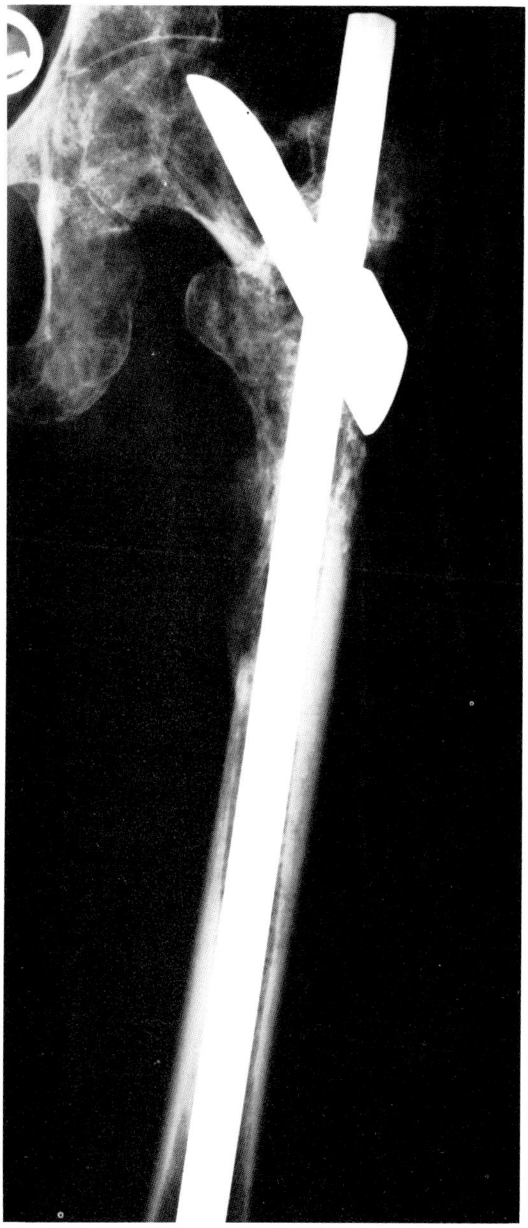

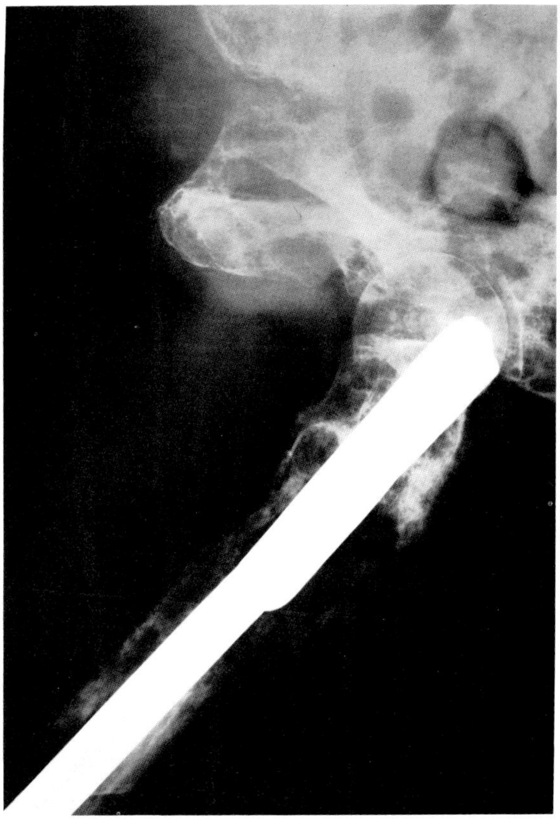

Figure 402 The same case after Y-nailing, lateral view.

◄ Figure 401 The same case after nailing of the pathologic fracture with a custom-made Y-nail, 14 mm in diameter, AP view.

Closed Shortening of the Femur

Utilizing a new type of intramedullary saw

Supplement by Robert A. Winquist, M.D.

History

As in nearly all practices of intramedullary nailing, the credit for intramedullary osteotomies certainly belongs to the unique, original mind of Gerhard Küntscher. This is an attempt to advance his work. In 1973, following the use of Küntscher's intramedullary saw, it was felt that some improvements could be made. Therefore, with the assistance of Raymond E. Pearson and the Boeing Company, several prototype models were designed. The premise for construction was to design a saw that made complete cuts, was simple in design, and had an accurate method of measurement. After many designs were tried, the final production, which was improved by the OEC Company, is now available and has been used for 153 cases of intramedullary osteotomies. The saw has a cam which offsets the blade, thus allowing advancement within the canal. The measuring device controls the depth of the saw as well as accurate measurement for femoral shortenings. The locking nut holds the measuring device in place and helps in controlling length measurements. The indexing plate is numbered from 0 to 40, and the indexing plunger moves in and out of the indexing plate. The T-drivehandle is used both to advance the blade and to turn the saw. The saw may be totally disassembled for cleaning. Blades and bushings vary in size, including 12-, 13-, 14-, 15-, 16-, and 17-mm diameters. They are actually undersized by 0.5 mm to allow easy insertion into a canal that is reamed to the appropriate size. Therefore, a 12-mm saw actually only measures 11.5 and is inserted into a canal reamed to 12 mm. In addition, there are three internal chisels for splitting of the fragment. One each for 12 to 13 mm; 14 to 15 mm; and 16 to 17 mm. A long metal x-ray scale must also be included in the set for accurate measurements.

Preoperative Evaluation

Patients with limb length inequality require a thorough evaluation of their spines, hips, knees, and feet to look for contractures as well as pre-existing deformity, which should be corrected. Limb length can be measured by a variety of methods. Variable height blocks to level the pelvis offer the most efficient clinical method of measurement. Scanograms or orthodiagrams are used to determine the degree of discrepancy in the pelvis, femur, tibia, and foot. An AP standing roentgenogram of the spine and pelvis, with the correct lift under the foot, offers the most accurate method of measuring the discrepancy. This may have to be supervised to be certain that the knees are straight and the patient is standing properly. An AP and lateral roentgenogram of the operative femur is examined to observe the amount of anterior bow and, particularly, the thickness of the linea aspera. The patient's hip rotation is inspected in the prone position, measuring internal and external rotation; these measurements are carefully recorded and used postoperatively to obtain appropriate rotary alignment. In addition, the patient is evaluated on the Cybex II for quadriceps power, and quadriceps rehabilitation is instituted six weeks prior to surgery. Prophylactic antibiotics are used, and the patient's blood is typed and cross-matched for two units of whole blood.

Table Position

The patient is placed in the lateral position on the fracture table, and the image intensifier is positioned to be certain that the trochanter can be visualized in two perpendicular planes. The rotation is carefully checked on the table and the position locked and remembered, so that correct rotation can be achieved at the conclusion of the case. The entire thigh is prepped, from the trochanter to the knee.

Surgical Starting Point

This is the most important step in the operation. An incision is made just proximal to the trochanter and carried down through the fascia. The trochanter is palpated and a sharp femoral awl inserted just inside the tip of the trochanter. The position is checked under AP and lateral image intensifier before making the hole, to be certain that it lines up centrally with the canal on both views. This ensures concentric reaming and easy passage of the saw down the canal.

Reaming

A ball-point guide pin is passed down to the subchondral bone of the distal femur. The length is measured and a correct nail length selected, allowing for the amount of femur to be shortened as well as subtracting an additional 2 cm. Reaming is started with an 8-mm end cutting reamer. The canal is reamed 1 to 2 mm larger than one would normally ream for a fracture. This allows insertion of a slightly larger saw, therefore making it easier to cut through the cortices. In females, generally a 13- to 14-mm saw is required; in males, a 14- or 15-mm saw. Again, the saw ranges are 12 to 17 mm. The proximal 3 cm of the femur is overreamed 0.5 mm to allow easier insertion of the saw. Since the proximal canal is not over-reamed, a tighter fit with the intramedullary nail and better control of rotation are obtained. Therefore, if the canal is reamed to 14 mm, the proximal trochanteric area is reamed to 14.5 mm, and a 14-mm saw is used as well as a 14-mm nail. If one uses the AO reaming system, the shaft of the reamer does not allow clearance of the canal, and therefore the reaming chips accumulate at the bottom of the bone. This makes it difficult to later drive the nail, and distraction is common at the osteotomy site. It is therefore important to use the 12.5 extra long end cutting reamer to clear the canal distally down to subchondral bone.

First Saw Cut

The ossimeter, a plastic scale, is used on the preoperative roentgenograms to determine the level of both cuts. The cuts should be made in approximately mid isthmus. The saw is then set using the long metal scale to measure the depth from the saw blade to the measuring device which rests on the trochanter. The locking nut is then tightened. The saw is inserted into the canal with a slight rotary motion, using pronation and supination of the wrist and passing the saw down to the appropriate level. It is extremely important that the assistant hold the measuring device firmly against the trochanter to establish the depth and maintain it during the early part of the saw cut. To advance the saw, one holds the indexing device with the left hand. The hypothenar eminence of the surgeon's hand is rested on the T-drive-handle. The indexing plunger is pulled out, and the hypothenar eminence pushes on the T-handle to advance it one hole. It is then locked and the saw turned in a circular fashion two to three times at each index. The saw will cut first through the anterior cortex, since it is the thinnest cortex. Occasionally the saw will become tight when it first cuts through and should be backed off 1 to 2 indexes and not forced in the cutting. It can then again be advanced. The saw is slowly advanced to the number 20, which brings it to its maximum cutting diameter. It is angulated slightly toward the posterior linea to facilitate cutting this thicker portion. The saw blade is then turned to the neutral zero position. In this closed position the saw is pulled back slightly. The saw is then let loose and left in the proximal canal. It is not used to manipulate the leg, since the saw and shaft can be bent with this abuse.

Leg Manipulation

The leg must now be manipulated. The posterior linea is broken through without difficulty. However, complete displacement of the shaft to tear the linea and periosteum has been known to greatly facilitate later displacement of the segmental fragments. The periosteum and linea are extremely strong and require fairly vigorous manipulation. The foot is removed from the foot plate and the femur angulated approximately 60 to 70 degrees in all directions to tear the periosteum. The shaft should be displaced 100 percent. Once this is completed, the leg is placed back in traction and again rotation checked.

Second Saw Cut:

The measuring device handle is advanced distally while the locking nut is carefully held in position. The handle advance from the locking nut is equal to the desired shortening. After the appropriate length is verified by the x-ray scale, the locking nut is secured to the handle. At this time the assistant must again push firmly against the measuring device to assume that it is well seated on the trochanter while the second cut is started. The saw is then advanced one hole at a time and the cut completed without difficulty. The saw is then removed. Only occasionally is the posterior cortex so thick that a percutaneous osteotome is inserted through a stab wound to complete the cut. This is more common in malunions or derotations through old callus than it is through an otherwise normal femur.

Splitting of the Fragment:

A special fragmenter was designed to expand inside the bone and split the fragment. Although successful, it was found to be an unnecessary piece of equipment, adding an extra step, and has therefore been eliminated from the procedure. Instead, the internal chisel is used and passed down to the distal cut. The segment of bone is hooked, and a slotted hammer is used to pound the hook proximally, using it as a splitting chisel. Generally one should make two cuts; one medially and one laterally. The hook is then rotated to move the fragments out of the way.

Displacement and Shortening:

This is the most difficult part of the entire procedure. It requires both an experienced scrubbed surgeon and an unscrubbed surgeon to manipulate the leg. Traction is completely released from the leg and the leg is shortened. The distal femoral shaft is used to push against the fragments and displace them out of the way. The scrubbed surgeon continues to use the internal chisel to displace the fragments as well. This manipulation can be difficult, requiring coordination between the two surgeons. Once it has been completed, the nail driving guide is inserted, again requiring accurate reduction in two planes with appropriate passage of the guide wire. The unscrubbed surgeon is by far the most important member of the team for this step. At this point, one must examine the fragments; any fragment that has turned on end generally can be flattened into place by external manipulation with either a leader glove or a mallet. If there is a problem with the fragment, the fracture is again distracted and the pieces worked out of the way.

Nail Driving:

At this point, the unscrubbed surgeon again plays a major role in maintaining correct rotation of the leg, and as the nail is being driven forward he must push firmly on the knee to prevent distraction. If distraction occurs, the nail can be overdriven slightly and then pulled back with the extractor to impact the fracture. The patient feels much more stable with it impacted and, therefore, this is preferably done under anesthesia. The wound is then closed. The patient is turned off the operating table into the supine position. Rotation is checked. If there is any question, the patient is turned prone to permit a more accurate check of rotation and to compare it to the preoperative measurements. The patient is then placed immediately in an antirotation boot to control rotation in the early postoperative phase.

Postoperative Care

Quadriceps exercises are begun the morning following surgery. As soon as patients are able to do a good quad set, they begin ambulation with weight-bearing as tolerated. In major discrepancies, use a knee splint for quadriceps insufficiency, and for shortening of more than 5 cm, use a single hip walking spica for approximately four weeks. For discrepancies less than 5 cm, the patient wears an antirotation boot at night for three weeks and takes it off during ambulation. No rotational problems have been known to occur after three weeks. The patient is discharged to his home when he is safe on crutches and is seen weekly in the office to be certain that rotation is correct. The patient continues on vigorous quadriceps rehabilitation, with careful supervision and monthly testing on the Cybex machine. The nail is removed approximately one year after the operation or when healing is solid.

Derotations and Malunions

The intramedullary saw can also be used for derotational osteotomies and malunions. These are done in a similar fashion as has already been described.

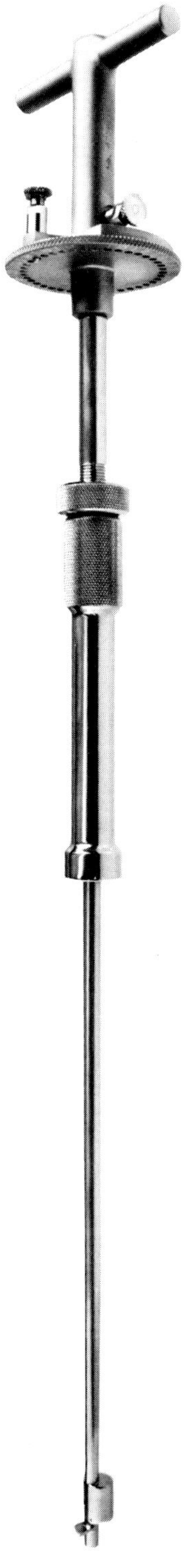

Figure 403. The O.E.C. Intramedullary Bone Saw.

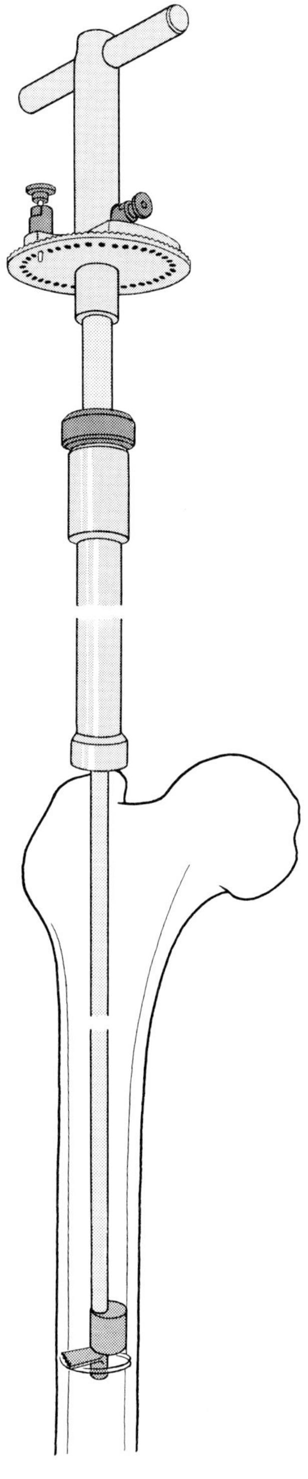

Figure 404 Saw positioned inside the shaft of the femur for first cut of intramedullary osteotomy.

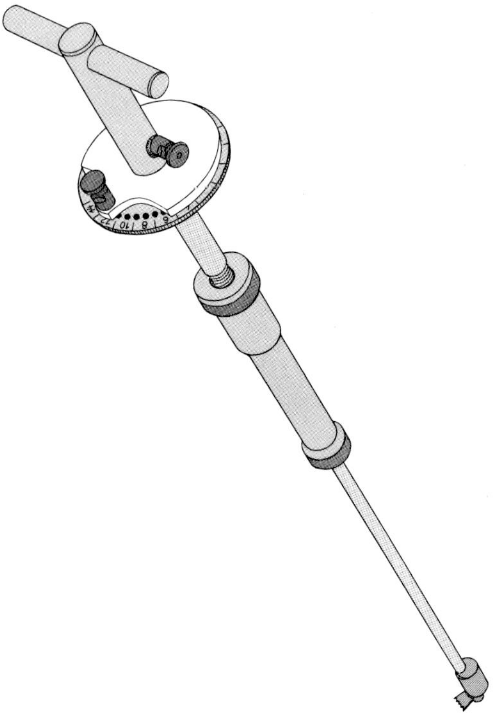

Figure 406 Indexing device controlling the saw blade extension relative to the cam.

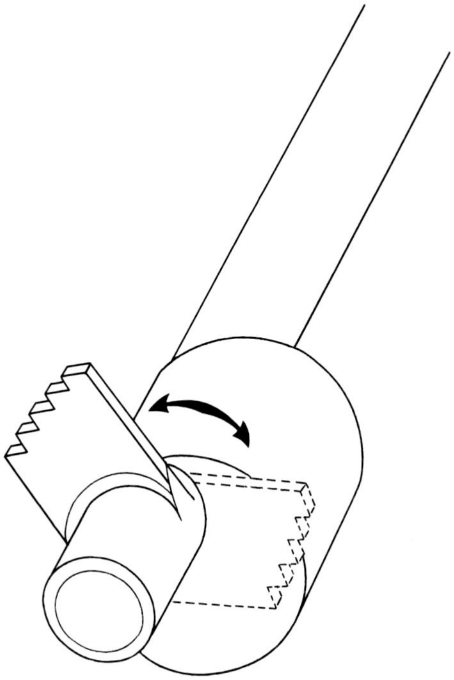

Figure 407 Saw blade and cam in various positions to each other.

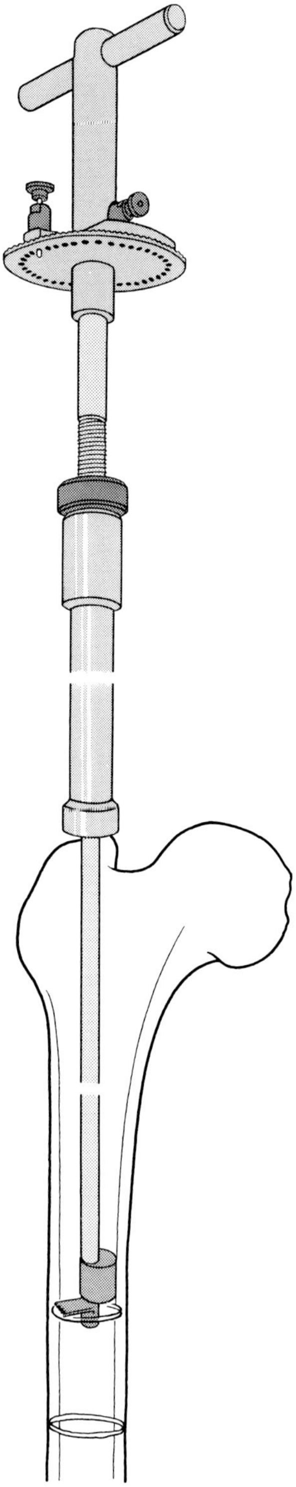

Figure 405 Second saw cut proximal of the first cut. The handle advance from the locking nut is equal to the desired shortening.

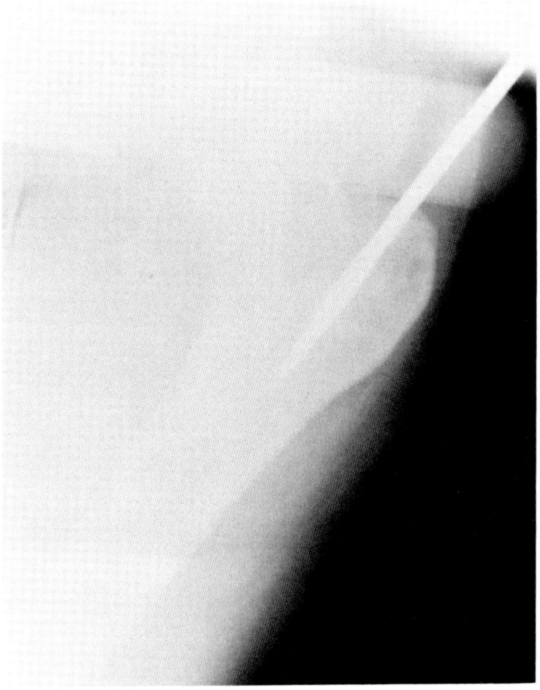

Figure 408 The correct surgical starting point is essential. It is checked with image intensifier.

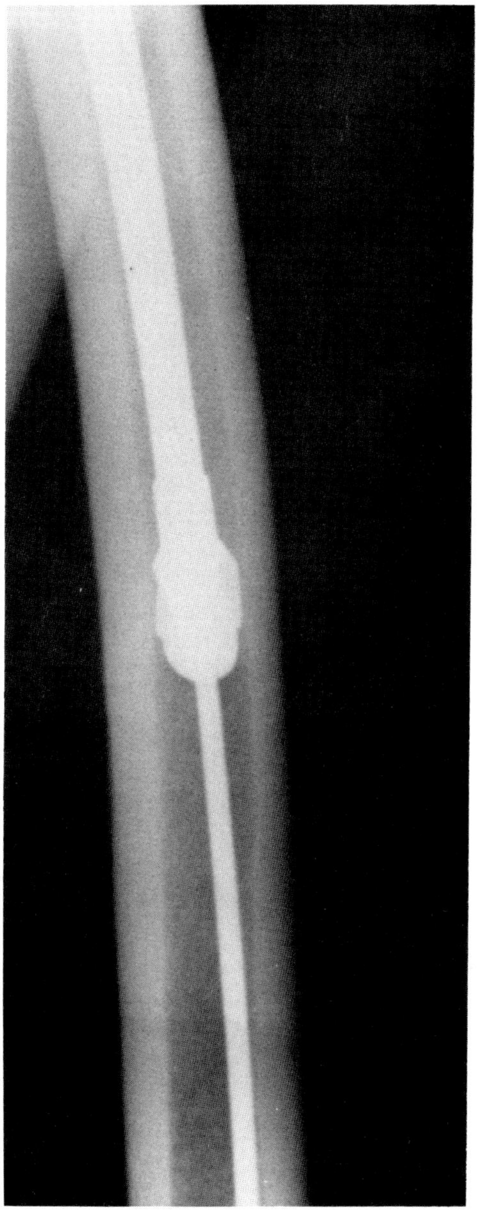

Figure 409 The canal is reamed to an appropriate size to accept the saw.

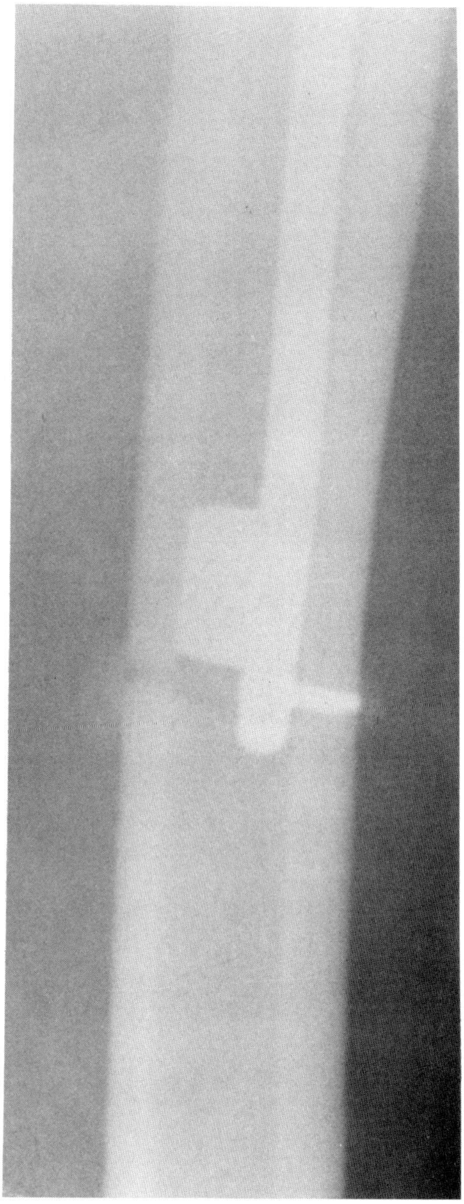

Figure 410 The distal saw cut is made first. The saw is in maximal expansion.

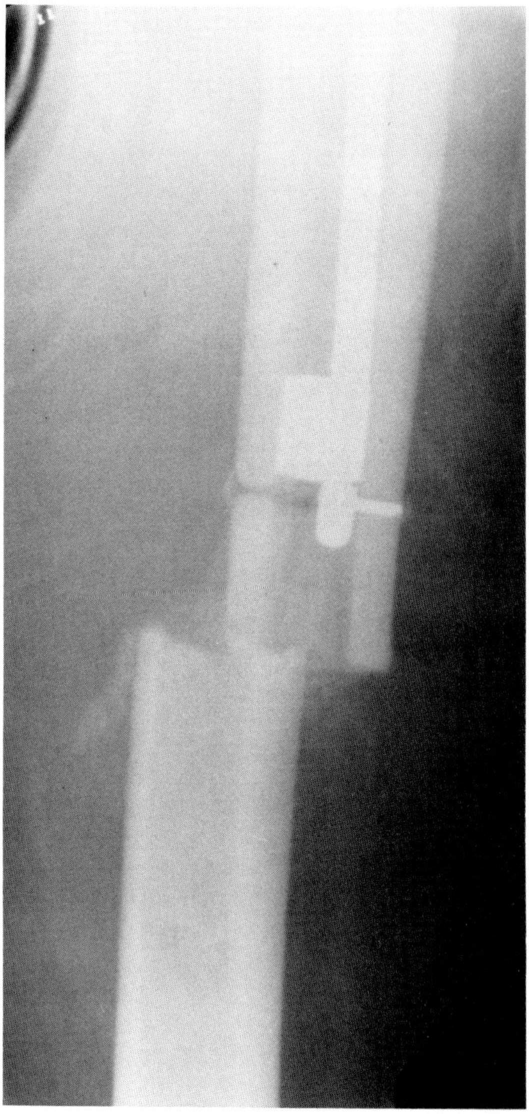

Figure 411 The distal saw cut is manipulated to both complete the break as well as tear the periosteum to ease later displacement of the fragments. The second saw cut is being completed.

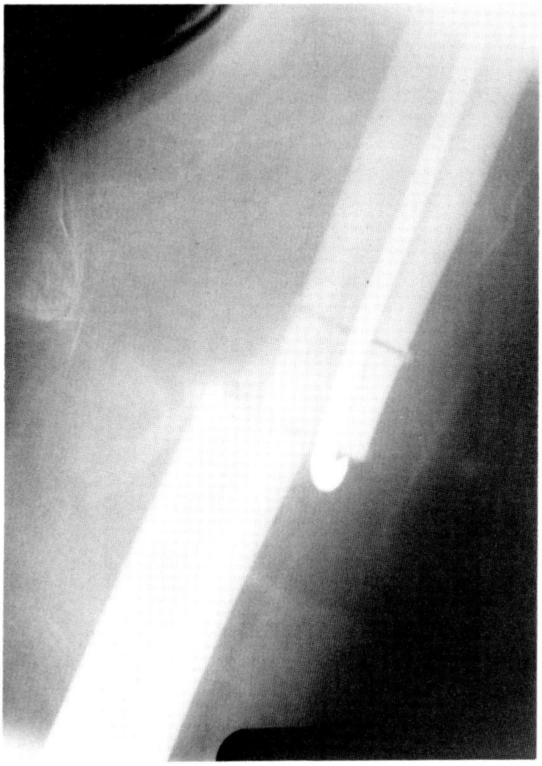

Figure 412 The internal chisel then splits the fragment. It may split in two like a piece of wood or may need to be split on two sides.

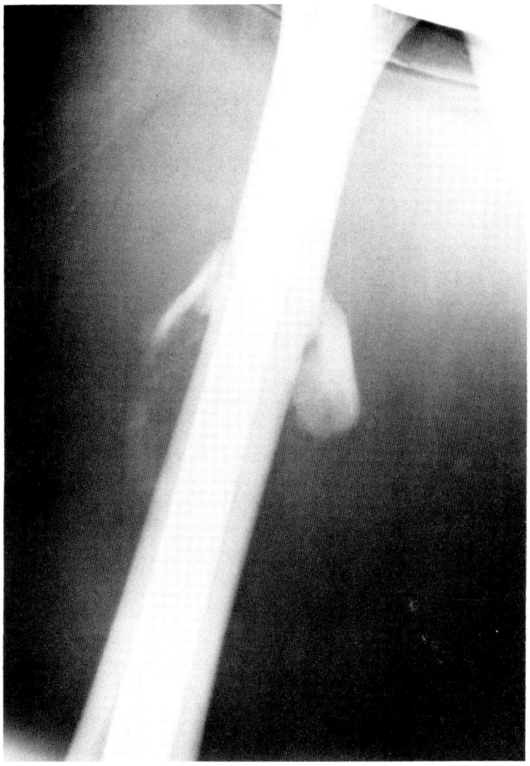

Figure 413 The fragments are displaced and the nail is inserted.

Bibliography

Fischer, S.: Über das Aufweiten der Markhöhle bei der Marknagelung. Chir. 12, 556 (1960)

Fischer, S.: Moderne Knochenbruchbehandlung. Hambg. Ärzteblatt 12, 470 (1960)

Fischer, S.: Methodik und Ergebnisse der Marknagelung der Unterschenkelbrüche. Kepner-Druck-Eppingen (1963)

Fischer, S.: Die Marknagelung. Chir. 36, 558 (1965)

Fischer, S.: Distraktor und Innensäge, wertvolle Hilfsmittel bei der Marknagelung der Pseudarthrose. H. f. Unfallheilkunde 94, 71 (1968)

Fischer, S.: Die Behandlung der spontanen per- und subtrochanteren Frakturen mit dem Y-Nagel mit G. Breitkreuz. Ztrlbl. f. Chir., 50, 1729 (1968)

Fischer, S.: Bisherige Ergebnisse der Anwendung der Knocheninnensäge. Chir. 5, 224 (1969)

Fischer, S.: Erfahrungen mit der Y-Nagelung nach Küntscher. H. f. Unfallheilkunde 106, 54 (1969)

Fischer, S.: Die geschlossene Beinlängenausgleichs-Osteotomie zur Vermeidung von Gelenkbeschwerden. Rehabilitation 3, 147 (1969)

Fischer, S.: Die Behandlung der Oberschenkeltrümmerfrakturen mit Distanznagel. Mschr. f. Unfallheilkunde 12, 509 (1969)

Fischer, S.: Hitzenekrosen bei Verwendung der Innensäge. Schriftreihe: Unfallmedizinische Tagungen der Landesverbände der gewerblichen Berufsgenossenschaften 11, 127 (1970)

Fischer, S.: Operative Beinverkürzung und Beinverlängerung nach dem Verfahren von Küntscher. Orthopäde 1, 50 (1972)

Fischer, S.: Röntgenstrahlenbelastung bei geschlossener Oberschenkelverkürzungs-Osteotomie. Chir. 44, 171 (1973)

Fischer, S.: Die Marknagelung von in Fehlstellung verheilten Frakturen und Pseudarthrosen. Chir. 44, 548 (1973)

Fischer, S.: Y-Nagel. Ztrbl. f. Chirurgie 100, 1020 (1975)

Götz, J., Klemm, K. und Schellmann, W. D.: Osteosynthese infizierter Femurpseudarthrosen mit dem Verriegelungsnagel. Arch. orthop. Unfall-Chir. 90, 275–284 (1977)

Hempel, D.: Gefahren und Schäden im Operationssaal aus der Sicht des Chirurgen. Chir. 40, 385–388 (1969)

Hempel, D.: Grundsätzliche Indikationsfehler bei operativer Therapie. (Hauptreferat 87. Tagung Dt. Ges. f. Chirurgie 1970) Lagenbecks Archiv 327, 821 (1970)

Hempel, D.: Die Marknagelung der frischen Fraktur. Chir. 44 (1973)

Hempel, D. und Zimmermann, H.-G.: Indikation zur Trochanternagelung als sofort belastbarer Osteosynthese bei Frakturen im Trochanterbereich.
114. Tagung Vereinigung Nordwestdt. Chir. 7. 12. 1974, Hamburg. Ztrlbl. Chir. (1975)

Hempel- D.: Trochanternagelung nach Küntscher; *Film:* Erstaufführung Deutscher Chirurgenkongreß München 1977. Ref. Langenbecks Arch. Kongreßband 1977/Film C1255 des IWF Göttingen

Hempel, D.: Trochanternagelung nach Küntscher. Publikationen zu Wissenschaftlichen Filmen, Sekt. Med., Ser. 4, Nr. 5/C 1255 (1977) 11 s

Hempel, D.: Beseitigung von Torsions- und Winkelfehlstellungen nach Femurfrakturen mit einer modifizierten Küntscher'schen Innensäge.
120. Tagung Vereinigung Nordwestdt. Chir. 3. 12. 1977 Hamburg Ztrlbl. Chir.

Hempel, D.: Verbesserte geschlossene Osteotomie durch aufsetzbares Meßgerät und oscillierenden Sägeantrieb. Chir. 49, 525 (1978)

Kaeßmann, H.-J.: Stabile Osteosynthese durch den Kompressionsnagel. Innere Schienung kombiniert mit einem dosier- und ablesbaren axialen Druck. Chir. 37, 272 (1966)

Kaeßmann, H.-J. und Weber, H.-G.: Der Kompressionsnagel, eine Modifikation des Marknagels nach Küntscher. Bruns'Beitr. 217, 325–320 (1969)

Kaeßmann, H.-J. und Weber, H.-G.: Die Technik der Kompressionsnagelung. Ztrlbl. Chir. 15, 496 (1969)

Kempf, I, Große, A. und Lafforgue, D: L'apport du verrouillage dans l'enclouage centro-médullaire des os longs. Revue de Chirurgie orthopédique 64, 635–651 (1978)

Klemm, K. und Schellmann, W. D.: Dynamische und statische Verriegelung des Marknagels. Mschr. Unfallheilk. 75, 568–575 (1972)

Klemm, K.: Die Stabilisierung infizierter Pseudarthrosen mit Verriegelungsnagel. Langenbecks Arch. Chir. 334 (Kongreßbericht 1973)

Küntscher, G.: Praxis der Marknagelung. Schattauer Verlag, Stuttgart (1962)

Küntscher, G.: Die geschlossene Osteotomie der langen Röhrenknochen. Chir. 33, 273 (1962)

Küntscher, G.: Die geschlossene Verkürzungsosteotomie. Z. Orthop. 98, 123 (1964)

Küntscher, G.: Die Innensäge (intramedulläres Osteotom). Chir. 35, 413 (1964)

Küntscher, G.: Erfahrungen mit der geschlossenen Osteotomie. Chir. 36, 69 (1965)

Küntscher, G.: Zur Frage der Implantatentfernung. Chir. 2, 85 (1971)

Küntscher, G.: Die Technik der geschlossenen Osteotomie. Mschr. Unfallheilkunde 75, 505 (1972)

Willenegger, H. und Roth, W.: Die antibakterielle Spüldrainage als Behandlungsprinzip bei chirurgischen Infektionen. DMW 87, 1485 (1962)

INDEX